FINAL YEAR DIPLOMA IN PHARMACY

Pharmaceutical Chemistry II

Theory and Practical

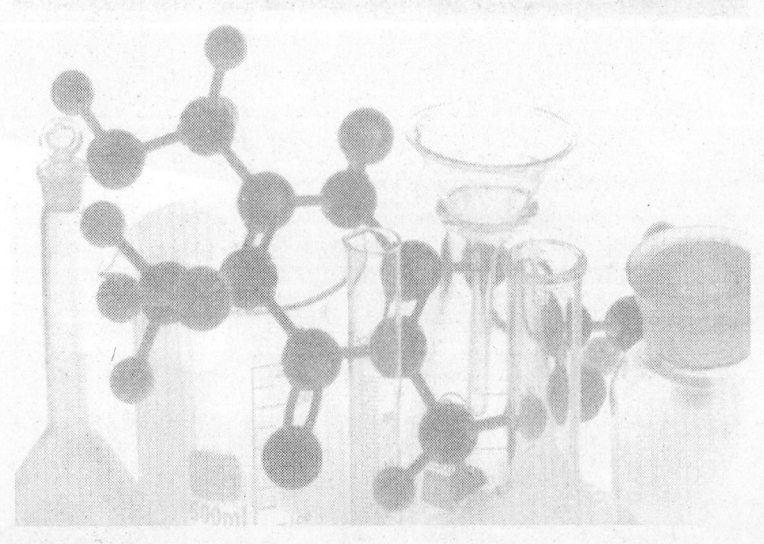

FINAL YEAR DIPLOMA IN PHARMACY

Pharmaceutical Chemistry II

Theory and Practical

Prof VN Rajasekaran

Formerly
Joint Director of Medical Education (Pharmacy)
Tamil Nadu
and
Professor of Pharmaceutical Chemistry
Madras Medical College, Chennai
and
Madurai Medical College, Madurai

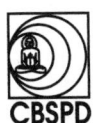

CBSPD

CBS Publishers & Distributors Pvt Ltd

New Delhi • Bengaluru • Chennai • Kochi • Kolkata • Lucknow • Mumbai
Hyderabad • Jharkhand • Nagpur • Patna • Pune • Uttarakhand

FINAL YEAR DIPLOMA IN PHARMACY

Pharmaceutical Chemistry II

Theory and Practical

ISBN: 978-81-239-2938-5

Copyright © Author and Publisher

CBS Edition: 2016

Reprint: 2017, 2018, 2019, 2020, 2021, 2023

Published by Satish Kumar Jain and Produced by Varun Jain for

CBS Publishers & Distributors Pvt Ltd

4819/XI Prahlad Street, 24 Ansari Road, Daryaganj, New Delhi 110 002, India.
Ph: 011-23289259, 23266861, 23266867 Fax: 011-23243014   Website: www.cbspd.com

e-mail: delhi@cbspd.com; cbspubs@airtelmail.in.
Corporate Office: 204 FIE, Industrial Area, Patparganj, Delhi 110 092
Ph: 011-4934 4934   Fax: 011-4934 4935   e-mail: publishing@cbspd.com; publicity@cbspd.com

Branches

- **Bengaluru:** Seema House 2975, 17th Cross, KR Road, Banasankari 2nd Stage, Bengaluru 560 070, Karnataka, India
  Ph: +91-80-26771678/79   Fax: +91-80-26771680   e-mail: bangalore@cbspd.com
- **Chennai:** 7, Subbaraya Street, Shenoy Nagar, Chennai 600 030, Tamil Nadu, India
  Ph: +91-44-26680620, 26681266   Fax: +91-44-42032115   e-mail: chennai@cbspd.com
- **Kochi:** 42/1325, 1326, Power House Road, Opp KSEB, Power House, Ernakulam 682 018, Kerala, India
  Ph: +91-484-4059061-65/67   Fax: +91-484-4059065   e-mail: kochi@cbspd.com
- **Kolkata:** 147, Hind Ceramics Compound, 1st Floor, Nilgunj Road, Belghoria, Kolkata 700 056, West Bengal, India
  Ph: +033-25633055, 033-25633056   e-mail: kolkata@cbspd.com
- **Lucknow:** Basement, Khushnuma Complex, 7-Meerabai Marg (Behind Jawahar Bhawan), Lucknow 226 001, UP, India
  Ph: 0522-4000032   e-mail: tiwari.lucknow@cbspd.com
- **Mumbai:** PWD Shed. Gala no. 25/26, Ramchandra Bhatt Marg, Next to JJ Hospital Gate no. 2, Opp. Union Bank of India, Noorbaug, Mumbai 400 009, Maharashtra, India
  Ph: 022-66661880/89   Mob: 0-8424005858   e-mail: mumbai@cbspd.com

Representatives

- **Hyderabad** 0-9885175004 • **Jharkhand** 0-9811541605 • **Nagpur** 0-9421945513
- **Patna** 0-9334159340 • **Pune** 0-9623451994 • **Uttarakhand** 0-9716462459

Printed at SRK Graphics, Delhi, India

PREFACE

Persistent requests from the students and staff of the Diploma in Pharmacy institutions in Tamilnadu motivated me to write this book. This book follows faithfully the E.R.'91 syllabus and should be found useful by those for whom it is intended. The coverage is limited to only the drugs in the syllabus.

Introduction to structure and chemical nomenclature is confined and limited to drugs marked with an asterisk in the syllabus and additionally those with simple structure only in order to present a book to the student which follows the syllabus faithfully in this respect. Otherwise classification of drugs under each topic, their physical and chemical properties, stability and storage, uses, official pharmaceutical preparations and brand names are fully covered for all the drugs mentioned in the syllabus.

The list of drugs and pharmaceutical preparations given under 'official' are from the latest Indian Pharmacopoeia and the British Pharmacopoeia, that is, I.P. '96 and B.P. '93. Where any drug is official in an earlier I.P. or B.P., it is specifically mentioned.

I hope and trust that this book will be found useful, instructive and of immense benefit by the staff and students of the Diploma in Pharmacy institutions.

A section on Practical is also included for the convenience of the students which, I hope, will go a long way towards meeting the complete needs of the students in practical, in that they will now have both theory and practical in one text book.

V.N.RAJASEKARAN

CONTENTS

SECTION B - PRACTICAL

SYLLABUS

THEORY

1. Introduction to the nomenclature of organic chemical systems with particular reference to heterocyclic system containing upto 3 rings.

2. The chemistry of the following pharmaceutical organic compounds, covering their nomenclature, chemical structure, uses and the important physical and chemical properties (chemical structure of only those compounds marked with asterisk *).

The stability and storge conditions and the different types of pharmaceutical formulations of these drugs and their popular brand names.

Antiseptics and Disinfectants-Proflavine*, Benzalkonium chloride, Cetrimide, Chlorocresol*, Chloroxylenol, Formaldehyde solution, Hexachlorophene, Liquefied phenol, Nitrofurantoin.

Sulfonamides-Sulfadiazine*, Sulfathiazole, Sulfadimethoxine, Sulfamethoxypyridazine, Sulfamethoxazole, Cotrimoxazole, Sulfacetamide*.

Antileprotic Drugs–Clofazimine, Thiambutosine, Dapsone*, Solapsone.

Anti-tubercular Drugs-Isoniazid*, PAS*, Streptomycin, Rifampicin, Ethambutol*, Thiacetazone, Ethionamide, Cycloserine Pyrazinamide*.

Antiamoebic and Anthelmintic Drugs-Emetine, Metronidazole*, Halogenated hydroxyquinolines, Diloxanide furoate, Paromomycin, Piperazine*, Mebendazole, D.E.C.*.

Antibiotics-Benzyl Penicillin*, Phenoxymethyl Penicillin*, Benzathine Penicillin, Ampicillin*, Cloxacillin, Carbenicillin, Gentamycin, Neomycin, Erythromycin, Tetracycline, Cephalexin, Cephaloridine, Cephalothin, Griseofulvin, Chloramphenicol.

Antifungal agents–Undecylenic acid, Tolnaftate, Nystatin, Amphoterecin, Hamycin.

Antimalarial Drugs–Chloroquine*, Amodiaquine, Primaquine, Proguanil, Pyrimethamine*, Quinine, Trimethoprim.

Tranquillizers–Chloropromazine*, Prochlorperazine, Trifluoperazine, Thiothixene, Haloperidol*, Triperidol, Oxypertine, Chlordiazepoxide, Diazepam*, Lorazepam, Meprobamate.

Hypnotics–Phenobarbitone*, Butobarbitone, Cyclobarbitone, Nitrazepam, Glutethimide*, Methyprylon, Paraldehyde, Triclofos Sodium.

General Anaesthetics–Halothane*, Cyclopropane*, Diethylether*, Methohexital sodium, Thiopental sodium. Trichloroethylene.

Antidepressant Drugs–Amitriptyline, Nortryptyline, Imipramine*, Phenelzine, Tranylcypromine.

Analeptics-Theophylline, Caffeine*, Coramine*, Dextroamphetamine.

Adrenergic Drugs-Andrenaline Noradrenaline, Isoprenaline*, Phenylephrine, Salbutamol, Terbutaline, Ephedrine*, Pseudoephedrine.

Adrenergic Antagonists–Tolazoline, Propranolol*, Practolol.

Cholinergic Drugs–Neostigmine*, Pyridostigmine, Pralidoxime, Pilocarpine, Physostigmine*.

Cholinergic Antagonists–Atropine*, Hyoscine, Homatropine, Propantheline*, Benztropine, Tropicamide, Biperiden*.

Diuretic Drugs–Furosemide*, Chlorothiazide, Hydrochlorothiazide*, Benzthiazide, Urea*, Mannitol*, Ethacrynic acid.

Cardiovascular Drugs–Ethyl nitrite*, Glyceryl trinitrate, Alphamethyldopa, Guanethidine, Clofibrate, Quinidine.

Hypoglycaemic Agents - Insulin, Chlorpropamide*, Tolbutamide, Glibenclamide, Phenformin*, Metformin.

Coagulants and Anti-Coagulants–Heparin, Thrombin, Menadione, Bishydroxycoumarin, Warfarin sodium.

Local Anaesthetics–Lignocaine*, Procaine*, Benzocaine.

Histamine and Antihistaminic Agents–Histamine, Diphenhydramine*, Promethazine, Cyproheptadine, Mepyramine, Pheniramine, Chlorpheniramine*.

Analgesics and Anitpyretics–Morphine, Pethidine*, Codeine, Methadone, Aspirin*, Paracetamol*, Analgin, Dextro propoxyphene, Pentazocine.

Non-steroidal Anti-inflammatory Agents–Indomethacin*, Phenylbutazone*, Oxyphenbutazone, Ibuprofen.

Thyroxine and Antithyroids–Thyroxine*, Methimazole, Methylthiouracil, Propylthiouracil.

Diagnostic Agents–Iopanoic Acid, Propyliodone, Sulfobromophthalein sodium, Indigotindisulfonate sodium (Indigo carmine), Evans blue, Congo red, Fluorescein sodium.

Anticonvulsants, Cardiac glycosides, Antiarrhythmics, Antihypertensives and Vitamins.

Steroidal Drugs–Betamethasone, Cortisone, Hydrocortisone, Prednisolone, Progesterone, Testosterone, Oestradiol, Nandrolone.

Anti-neoplastic Drugs - Actinomycins, Azathioprine, Busulphan, Chlorambucil, Cisplatin, Cyclophosphamide, Daunorubicin hydrochloride, Fluorouracil, Mercaptopurine, Methotrexate, Mytomycin.

PRACTICAL

1. Systematic qualitative testing of organic drugs involving solubility determination, melting point and / or boiling point, detection of elements and functional groups (10 compounds).

2. Official identification tests for certain groups of drugs included in the I.P. like barbiturates, sulfonamides, phenothiazines, antibiotics etc. (8 compounds).

3. Preparation of three simple organic preparations.

SOLUBILITY DESCRIPTIONS

The solubility descriptions in this book denote the following ranges :-

Description	Approximate quantities of solvent by volume required to dissolve 1 part of solute by weight.
Very soluble	Less than 1 part
Freely soluble	From 1 to 10 parts
Soluble	From 10 to 30 parts
Sparingly soluble	From 30 to 100 parts
Slightly soluble	From 100 to 1,000 parts
Very slightly soluble	From 1,000 to 10,000 parts
Practically insoluble	More than 10,000 parts

SECTION A

THEORY

CHAPTER - 1

INTRODUCTION

Valency is the combining capacity of an element or a radical. Some may be monovalent, some divalent and some trivalent etc. A list of these is given below :

Monovalent (one valency)

–H	hydrogen	–Na	-	sodium
–OH	hydroxyl	–K	-	potassium
–Cl	chloride	–Hg	-	mercurous
–Br	bromide	–Ag	-	silver
–I	iodide			
$-NO_3$	nitrate	$-CH_3^-$	-	methyl (alkyl-symbol R)
$-HCO_3$	bicarbonate	$-C_6H_5^-$	-	phenyl (aryl)
$-NH_4$	ammonium	$-C_6H_5CH_2^-$	-	benzyl (aralkyl)

Divalent (two valencies)

SO_4 < sulphate		Hg = mercuric
CO_3 < carbonate		Ba = barium
O = oxygen		Zn = zinc
Mn = magnanese		Pb = lead
Mg = magnesium		Fe = ferrous
Ca = calcium		

Trivalent (three valencies)

N	(either 3 or 5)	nitrogen	Cr	chromic
Sb	”	antimony	Fe	ferric
As	”	arsenic	Al	aluminium
P	”	phosphorus		

1

Tetravalent (four valencies)

C. carbon

A monovalent element or radical, since its valency is one, will combine with only one equivalent of another monovalent element or radical.

Example : NaCl

Likewise a divalent element or radical, which has two valencies, will combine with one equivalent of another divalent element or radical.

Example :- $CaCO_3$. Like this for trivalent elements etc.

Two equivalents of a monovalent element or radical will combine with one equivalent of a divalent element or radical.

Eg :- Na_2CO_3

Similarly three equivalents of a monovalent element or radical will combine with one equivalent of a trivalent element of radical, eg: - $FeCl_3$ (ferric chloride). Likewise four equivalents of a monovalent element will combine with one equivalent of a tetravalent element.

Eg : - CH_4 (Methane).

Therefore to understand the structure of any substance a knowledge of the valencies of the components involved is necessary.

In the structure of organic compounds, the elements or radicals are linked by covalent bonds which is indicated by a line drawn between the components.

Eg : - CH_4.

Structural formula

$$\begin{array}{c} H \\ | \\ H-C-H \\ | \\ H \end{array}$$

In this structure, the four valencies of carbon are fully satisfied by four monovalent hydrogen atoms. However when the valencies are not fully satisfied like this, a double bond or a triple bond may form part of the structure

Eg : - Ethylene
$$\begin{array}{c} H-C=C-H \\ | \quad | \\ H \quad H \end{array}$$

Here two hydrogen atoms satisfy two valencies of each of the two carbon atoms. The other two valencies are satisfied by setting up another link between the carbon atoms themselves. Therefore a double bond comes into existence. In the same way acetylene $CH \equiv CH$ has one valency of each carbon satisfied by one hydrogen and the other three valencies by the carbon atoms between themselves by establishing a triple bond.

Benzene is a ring compound with the formula.

C_6H_6 or

There are three double bonds in the structure. Benzene has 6 carbon atoms to each of which is attached a single hydrogen atom. If each carbon atom is attached to two carbon atoms, one on either side, even then including the hydrogen atom only three valencies are satisfied. Therefore a double bond comes into being on one side of the carbon atom so that each carbon atom may have all the four valencies accounted for.

3

So benzene can also be depicted as below :

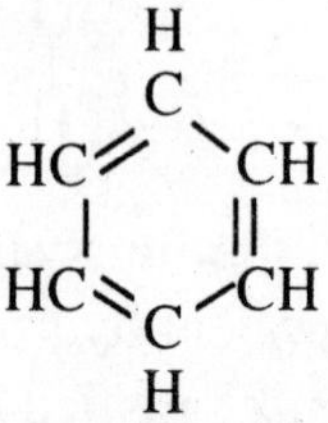

$$\begin{array}{ccc} & \overset{\displaystyle H}{\underset{\displaystyle C}{}} & \\ HC & & CH \\ | & & || \\ HC & \underset{\displaystyle C}{} & CH \\ & \overset{\displaystyle}{H} & \end{array}$$

Usually the hydrogen atoms are not indicated in the structures. Therefore it is better to calculate the number of other atoms or radicals and if any valencies are still left unsatisfied, it may be safely assumed that in the absence of a double or triple bond, the valencies are satisfied by the required number of hydrogen atoms. Even if there is a double bond, there is scope for the presence of hydrogen atoms also subject to the condition that the number of valencies satisfied does not exceed the valency number of the element.

Examples :

(1)   Cyclopropane 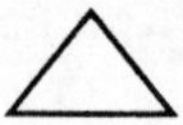   or

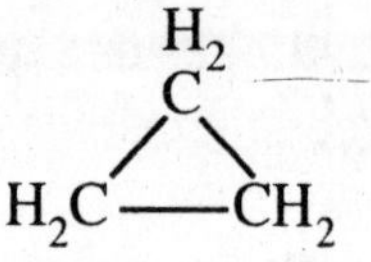

(2)   Cyclohexene 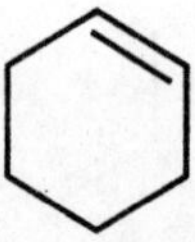   or

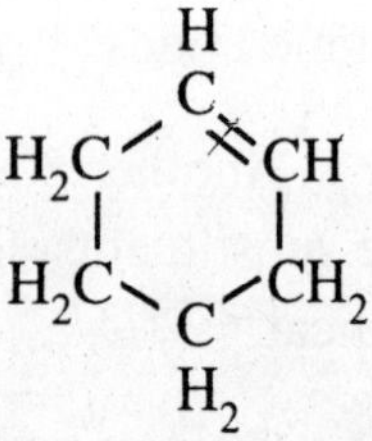

(3)   Pyridine 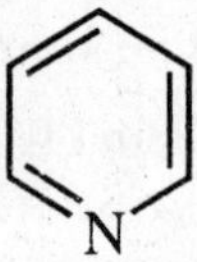   or

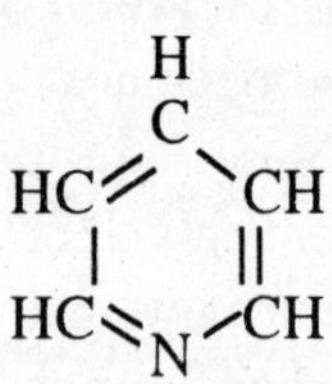

4

In this structure please note the trivalent nitrogen atom whose three valencies are satisfied by a single bond with one carbon atom on one side and by a double bond with another carbon atom on the other side.

(4)   Piperidine 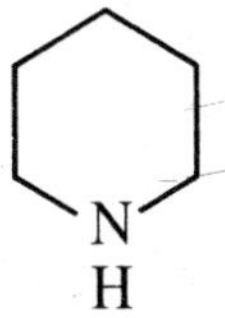   or

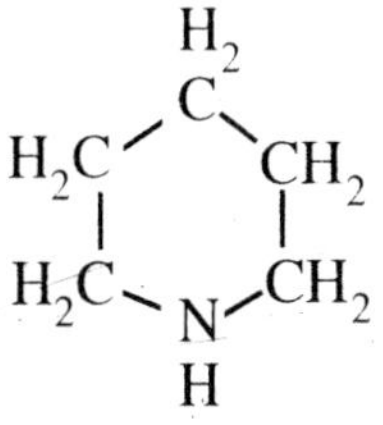

(5)   Thiophen 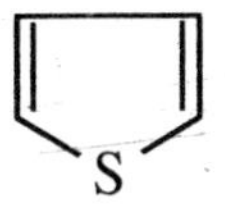   or

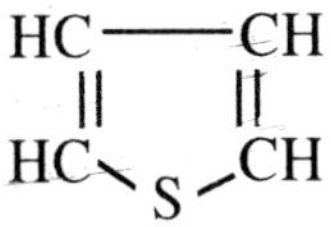

Piperidine is prepared by reduction of pyridine. Note that there are no double bonds now. The carbon atoms and the nitrogen atom have each acquired one hydrogne atom more. Since all the valencies are satisfied now, there is no need for double bonds.

Another point to be noted is that the atoms and radicals are substituents, that is they come in place of another atom or radical.

Consider the structure of phenol.

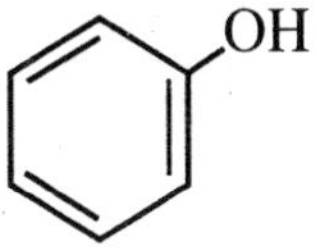

or

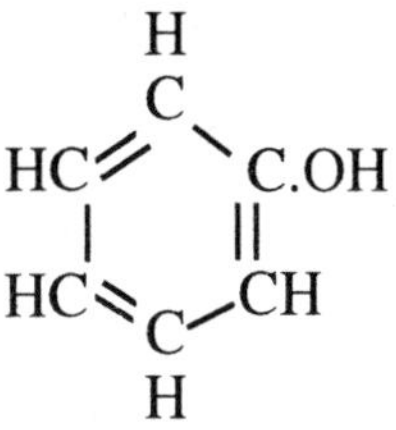

In this structure the -OH group has come in place of a hydrogen atom. It has replaced a hydrogen atom. The structural formula can also be written as C_6H_5OH. If another substituent such as a nitro group is introduced into the nucleus, it will take the place of a hydrogen atom at another position.

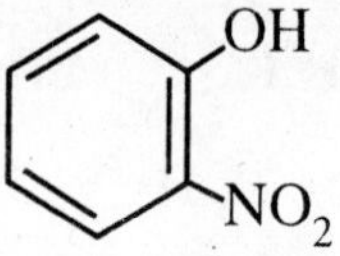

or 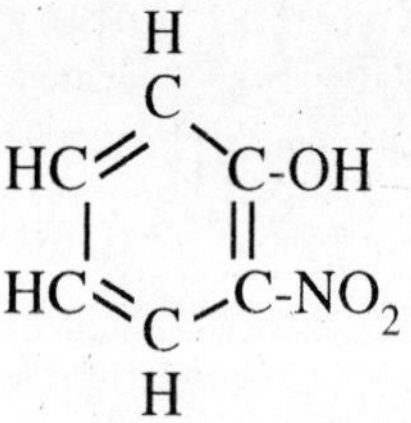   or $C_6H_4(OH)NO_2$

CHAPTER - 2

CARBOCYCLIC AND HETEROCYCLIC COMPOUNDS

Organic compounds may be classified as below :-

(1) Aliphatic Compounds : The molecules of these compounds are made up of open chains only.

(2) Carbocyclic or homocyclic compounds : The molecules of these compounds are made up of one or more closed chains or rings formed from carbon atoms only. They may be further divided into:-

(a) Alicyclic compounds : These compounds resemble the aliphatic compounds in many ways. However they possess a ring structure. The saturated alicyclic hydrocarbons have the general formula C_nH_{2n} and do not contain a double bond. Examples are cycloparaffins such as cyclopropane. They may be relatively simple compounds or may contain bridged or fused rings, eg : steroids.

(b) Aromatic compounds : Many organic compounds such as benzene, naphthalene, anthracene etc. are known as compounds of aromatic character. They differ from the aliphatic and alicyclic compounds in many ways. Simple aromatic compounds such as benzene contain at lease six carbon atoms in a ring containing three double bonds. Aromatic compounds are known also as benzenoid compounds. Naphthalene and anthracene are fused ring aromatic hydrocarbons in that two and three benzene rings have fused to form them.

(3) Heterocyclic compounds

In these compounds the rings are not entirely composed of carbon atoms only as in the case of carbocyclic compounds. They may contain one or more other atoms known as heteroatoms. The usual heteroatoms are nitrogen, oxygen and sulphur. The heterocyclic systems may be simple, fused or bridged. The bridging or fusing may be with carbocyclic systems. The heterocyclic compounds may be saturated, unsaturated or partly saturated. The most common heterocyclic systems present in drugs are those of five and six members.

Many drugs have heterocyclic structures. Examples are several antibiotics such as penicillin, alkaloids such as quinine and morphine, vitamins such as thiamine and nicotinamide, antitubercular compounds such as I.N.H. etc. Therefore it is essential that one should have a thorough knowledge of the structure of basic heterocyclic compounds to be able to understand fully the structures of various drugs.

CARBOCYCLIC COMPONDS

The common basic aromatic compounds with their conventional numberings are given below :-

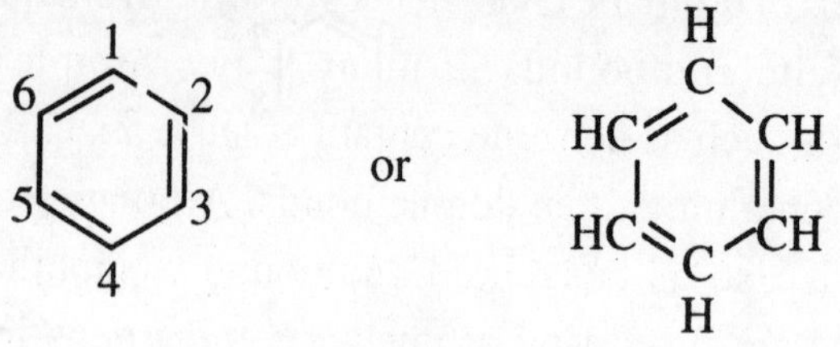

BENZENE

8

(Numbering may start anywhere on the nucleus and may proceed in a clockwise or anticlockwise direction)

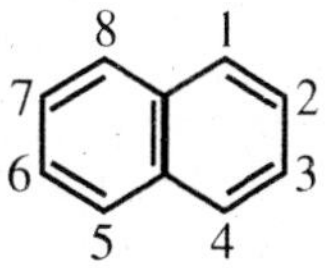

or

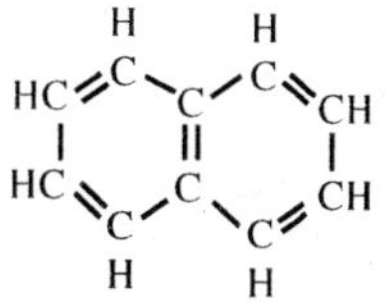

NAPHTHALENE

(1)

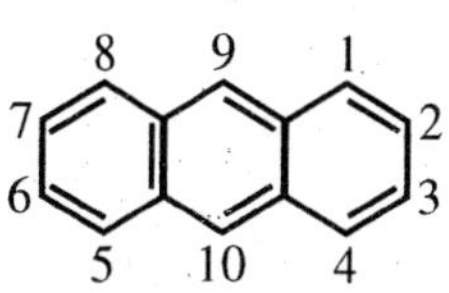

or

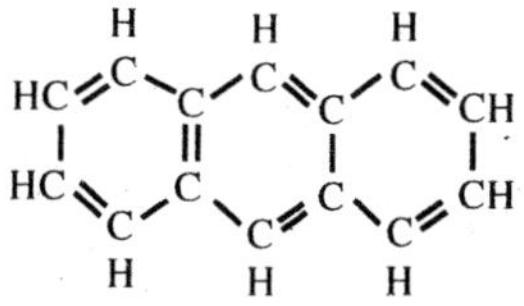

ANTHRACENE

(2)

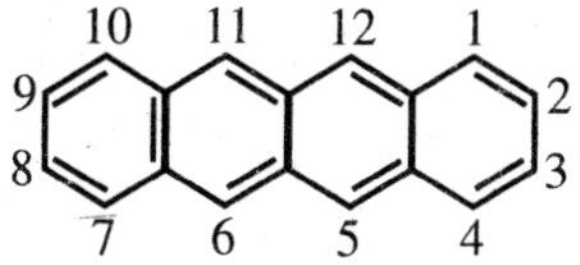

NAPHTHACENE

(3)

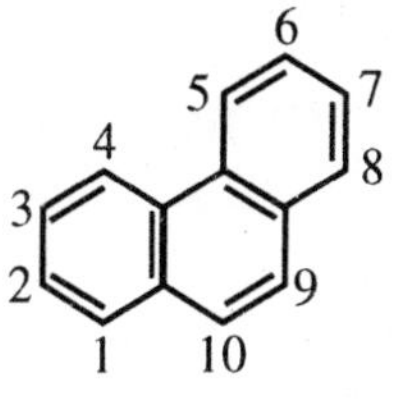

PHENANTHRENE

(4)

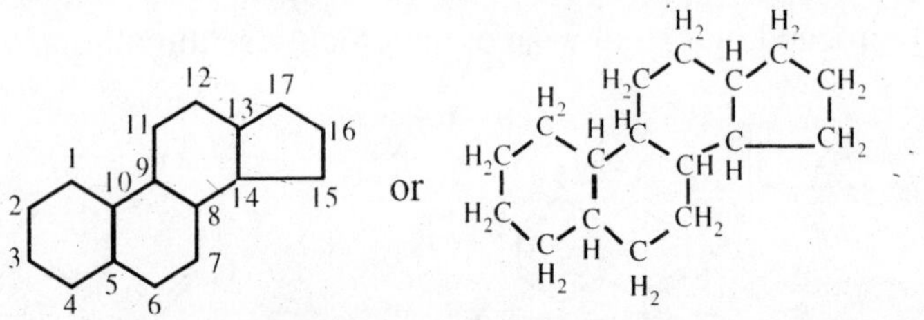

CYCLOPENTANOPERHYDROPHENANTHRENE

This is the steroid nucleus. Steroid hormones and cardiac glycosides have this basic structure. It is made up of one fully saturated phenanthrene nucleus (that is, upto 13 and 14 carbon atoms) fused with one cyclopentane ring (that is, from the 13th carbon atom to the 17th carbon atom.)

HETEROCYCLIC COMPOUNDS

The numbering of heterocyclic compounds is as follows. The heteroatom is usually numbered as 1. Nitrogen occurs as the most common heteroatom. If there is any other heteroatom present in the ring along with nitrogen, it is given the next higher position. Thus if sulphur is present along with nitrogen, sulphur gets the no.1 position. However if oxygen is present along with sulphur and nitrogen, it gets the no.1 position followed by sulphur and nitrogen in that order.

Basic Heterocyclic Compounds

(1)   Three-membered (with one hereatom)

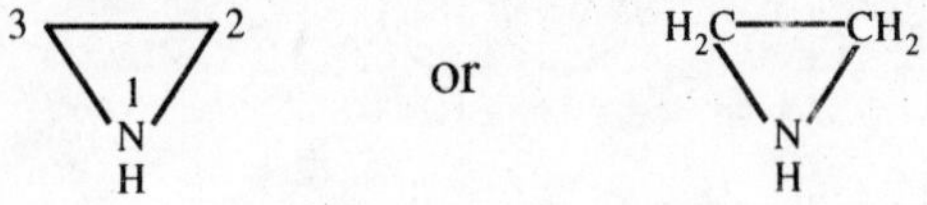

or

AZIRIDINE

10

(2) Five membered (with one heteroatom)

PYRROLE

PYRROLIDINE
(Saturated form of pyrrole)

FURAN

THIOPHEN

(3) Five-membered (with two heteroatoms)
a) With two nitrogen atoms

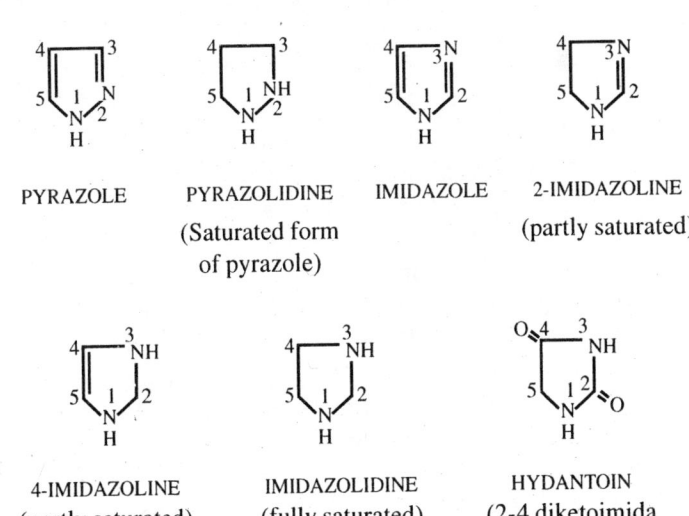

PYRAZOLE

PYRAZOLIDINE
(Saturated form
of pyrazole)

IMIDAZOLE

2-IMIDAZOLINE
(partly saturated)

4-IMIDAZOLINE
(partly saturated)

IMIDAZOLIDINE
(fully saturated)

HYDANTOIN
(2-4 diketoimida
zolidine)

b) With one nitrogen and one oxygen atoms

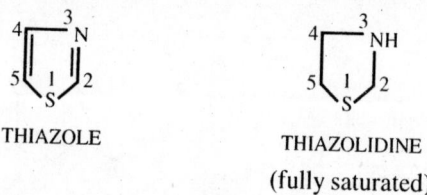

OXAZOLE

OXAZOLIDINE
(fully saturated)

c) With one nitrogen and one sulphur atoms

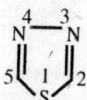

THIAZOLE

THIAZOLIDINE
(fully saturated)

d) With two nitrogen atoms and one sulphur atom

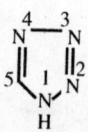

1,3,4 - THIADIAZOLE

e) With four nitrogen atoms

1,2,3,4, - TETRAZOLE

(4) Six-membered (with one heteroatom only)

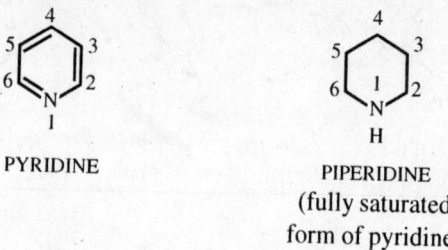

PYRIDINE

PIPERIDINE
(fully saturated
form of pyridine)

(5) Six-membered (with two heteroatoms)
a) With two nitrogen atoms

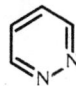
PYRIDAZINE

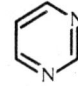
PYRIMIDINE

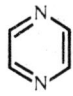
PYRAZINE

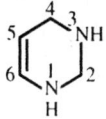

1,2,3,4-TETRAHYDRO
PYRIMIDINE
(partly saturated
pyrimidine)

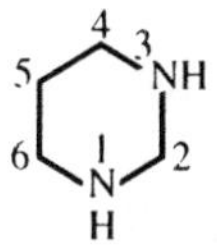

PERHDRO
PYRIMIDINE
(fully saturated
pyrimidine)

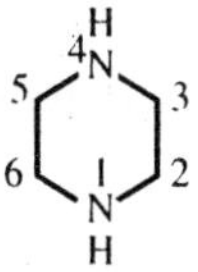

PIPERAZINE
(fully saturated
form of pyrazine)

b) With one nitrogen atom and one sulphur atom

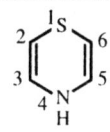

1,4-THIAZINE

c) With two nitrogen atoms

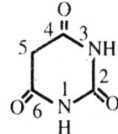

BARBITURIC ACID

(6) Fused rings
a) Heterocyclic rings fused to carbocyclic rings

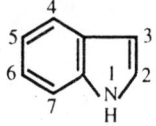

INDOLE
(pyrrole fused with
a benzene ring)

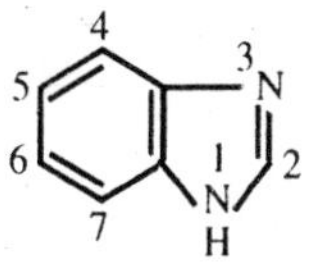

BENZIMIDAZOLE
(imidazole fused with
a benzene ring)

13

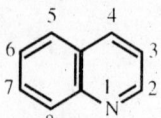

QUINOLINE
(pyridine fused with
a benzene ring)

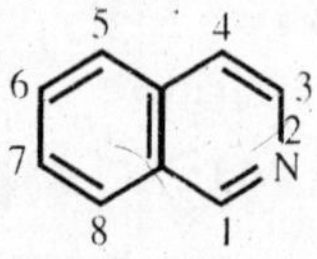

ISOQUINOLINE
(pyridine fused
with a benzene ring)

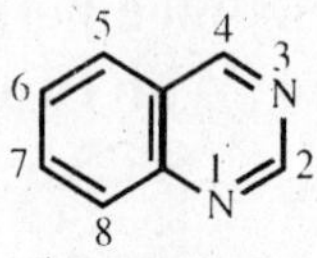

QUINAZOLINE
(pyrimidine fused
with a benzene ring)

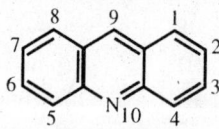

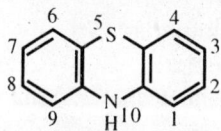

ACRIDINE
(pyridine fused with
two benzene rings)

PHENOTHIAZINE
(thiazine fused with
two benzene rings)

(b) Heterocyclic rings fused to heterocyclic rings

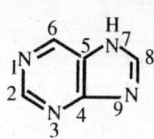

PURINE
(Pyrimidine fused
to imidazole)

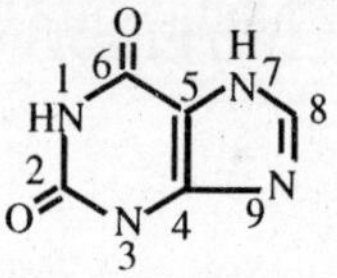

XANTHINE
(Tetrahydrodiketopyrimidine
fused to imidazole)

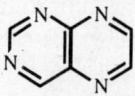

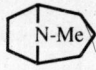

PTERIDINE
(Pyrimidine fused
to pyrazine)

TROPANE
(Pyrrolidine fused
to piperidine.
The common nitrogen
atom is methylated).

CHAPTER 3

NOMENCLATURE OF ORGANIC COMPOUNDS

Initially when the organic compounds were being discovered, they were given common or trivial names such as acetic acid etc. Later when it was realised that there were millions of organic compounds, naming them suitably became a problem. So the IUPAC system of nomenclature according to the structure of the organic compound was adopted in 1958.

As you should be already aware, the hydrocarbons, that is, compounds made of carbon and hydrogen only are divisible into saturated hydrocarbons or alkanes and unsaturated hydrocarbons such as alkenes (compounds containing double bonds) and alkynes (compounds containing triple bonds).

The alkanes upto the 10th carbon atom are given below :-

CH_4	-	Methane	C_6H_{14}	-	Hexane
C_2H_6	-	Ethane	C_7H_{16}	-	Heptane
C_3H_8	-	Propane	C_8H_{18}	-	Octane
C_4H_{10}	-	Butane	C_9H_{20}	-	Nonane
C_5H_{12}	-	Pentane	$C_{10}H_{22}$	-	Decane

From the above it is clear that the general formula of alkanes is C_nH_{2n+2}

In the same way the alkenes or olefines may also be classified starting from ethylene, $CH_2=CH_2$. Similarly the alkynes also may be classified starting from acetylene, $CH\equiv CH$. The members of these classes may also be called as homologous series and members belonging to a homologous series such as alkanes or alkenes or alkynes have similar chemical properties but differ in physical properties, that too in a graded manner. Derivatives of hydrocarbons such as alcohols, aldehydes, ketones, acids etc. also form homologous series.

Long chain straight or branched chain hydrocarbons are named according to certain rules. In the case of long chain straight saturated hydrocarbons there is no problem since the numbering can start from either end (that is, from the left or right) giving the same name. But in the case of branched chain compounds, the carbon atoms are not present in a linear fashion, that is, there may be one or more branches at intervals and the naming becomes difficult.

In this context, the alkyl groups are important. Alkyl groups are derived from alkanes by the removal of one hydrogen atom. For example methane (CH_4) becomes methyl (CH_3-). Similarly we get ethyl (C_2H_5-) from ethane (C_2H_6), propyl (C_3H_7-) from propane (C_3H_8), butyl (C_4H_9-) from butane (C_4H_{10}) and so on.

The rules that should be followed in the nomenclature of organic compounds are as below :-

1. The linear straight chain or the longest straight chain of carbon atoms in the compound is found out. In the example given below, the longest chain has eight carbon atoms.

$$CH_3 - CH - CH_2 - CH_2 - CH_2 - CH - CH_2 - CH_3$$
$$\qquad\quad | \qquad\qquad\qquad\qquad\qquad\quad |$$
$$\qquad\quad CH_3 \qquad\qquad\qquad\qquad CH_2 - CH_3$$

In this compound there are two branches, a methyl and an ethyl groups. The rule of nomenclature is that the substituted carbon atoms should have the lowest possible numbers. So the naming has to start from the left and move to the right. Since there are 8 carbon atoms in the straight chain, it can be called as octane or more correctly as a sub-stituted octane. The positions of the substituents should be correctly indicated by numbers.

2. If the alkyl groups present are not the same but different, they should be indicated in alphabetical order. So the compound in the above example may be named as

$$\overset{1}{C}H_3 - \overset{2}{C}H - \overset{3}{C}H_2 - \overset{4}{C}H_2 - \overset{5}{C}H_2 - \overset{6}{C}H - \overset{7}{C}H_2 - \overset{8}{C}H_3$$
$$\qquad\quad | \qquad\qquad\qquad\qquad\quad |$$
$$\qquad\quad CH_3 \qquad\qquad\qquad\quad CH_2\text{-}CH_3$$

6-ethyl-2-methyloctane

Please note the hyphens between the numbers and the alkyl groups.

3. If the same group is present at more than one place, they are indicated by numbers separated by commas. An example is given below :-

$$\overset{1}{C}H_3 - \overset{2}{C}H_2 - \overset{3}{C}H - \overset{4}{C}H - \overset{5}{C}H - \overset{6}{C}H_2 - \overset{7}{C}H_3$$
$$\qquad\qquad\qquad | \quad\; | \quad\; |$$
$$\qquad\qquad\quad CH_3 \; CH_3 \; CH_3$$

This compound may be named as *3,4,5-trimethylheptane*.

4. As far as the substituents present in cyclic compounds such as the cycloalkanes, the same rules are applied.

Example :

17

This compound may be named as *1,3-dimethyl-4-ethylcyclohexane*. Incidentally a cyclic compound is known by applying the prefix cyclo to its name. In the above example the 6-membered compound which is actually hexane is known as cyclohexane as it is cyclic compound.

Functional groups

The task of naming the organic compounds is made simpler by taking into account any functional group or groups present. A functional group consists of an atom or a group of atoms joined together in a characteristic manner and has specific and characteristic chemical properties.

For example, take the case of compounds having the alcoholic -OH group (alcohols). They all have similar chemical properties. For instance all the alcohols liberate hydrogen on reaction with metallic sodium. It is easy to classify the organic compounds based on the functional group(s) present into distinct homologous series. For this purpose the following rules are applied :-

1. Find out the functional group present and use this as the prefix or the suffix in the name of the compound. For example a compound containing the -OH group may be named as methanol (CH_3OH) since -OH group may be indicated by the words -ol suffixed to the name.

2. Then find out the number of carbon atoms comprising the longest chain containing the functional group. Using this, fix the name of the alkane corresponding to the carbon number.

3. Give the lowest number to the carbon carrying the functional group or is part of the functional group.

4. Name the compound using the above three rules.

Study the following example :-

$$\overset{1}{C}H_3-\overset{2}{C}H_2-\overset{3}{C}H_2-\overset{4}{C}H-\overset{5}{C}H_2-\overset{6}{C}H_2-\overset{7}{C}H_2-\overset{8}{C}H-\overset{9}{C}H_2-\overset{10}{C}H_3$$
$$\qquad\qquad\qquad\quad | \qquad\qquad\qquad\qquad\quad |$$
$$\qquad\qquad\qquad\quad OH \qquad\qquad\qquad\qquad\quad C_2H_5$$

Here the functional group is an alcoholic -OH. So it is given the prefix -ol (Rule 1). Secondly it is a 10-carbon chain corresponding to the saturated hydrocarbon decane. The -OH group is attached to the 4th carbon atom. So the compound may be named as *8-ethyl-4-decanol*.

Another example is given below :-

$$\overset{6}{C}H_3-\overset{5}{C}H_2-\overset{4}{C}H = \overset{3}{C}H-\overset{2}{C}H_2-\overset{1}{C}HO$$

There are two functional groups present here, that is, a double bond (alkene) and an aldehydic group (-CHO). Both can be combined together in the naming. Since the aldehydic group is indicated by the suffix -al, the compound can be named as *3-hexenal*. Please note that there are six carbon atoms in the chain. So the compound is derived from the alkane hexane. The double bond is between the 3rd and the 4th carbon atoms. So the suffix -ene is used to indicate that it is also an alkene in addition to being an aldehyde.

The important functional groups present in the organic compounds are given below :-

Compound	Functional Group	Suffix(s) (or) Prefix(p)	Example
Alkane	---	-ane(s)	$CH_3CH_2CH_3$ (Propane)
Alkene	$\diagdown C = C \diagup$	-ene(s)	$CH_3CH=CHCH_3$ (2-Butene)
Alkyne	$-C \equiv C-$	-yne(s)	$CH_3C \equiv CCH_3$ (2-Butyne)
Alcohol	$-OH$	-ol(s)	CH_3CHCH_3 $\quad$ OH (2-Propanol)
Aldehyde	$-C = O$ $\quad$ H	-al(s)	$CH_3CH_2CH\text{-}CH_3$ $\quad$ CHO (2-Butanal)
Ketone	$-C = O$	-one(s)	$CH_3 - C - CH_3$ $\quad$ ‖ $\quad$ O (2-Propanone or acetone)
Ether	$-C - O - C-$	--	$CH_3\text{-}O\text{-}CH_3$ (Methoxymethane or dimethyl ether)
Halide	$-X$ (X=F,Cl,Br or I)	-yl halide(s)	$CH_3CH_2CH_2Cl$ (n-propyl chloride)
Nitro compound	$-NO_2$	Nitro(p)	$CH_3CH_2CH_2NO_2$ (1-Nitropropane)

Compound	Functional Group	Suffix(s) (or) Prefix(p)	Example
Amino compound	$-NH_2$	Amino(p) or Amine(s)	$CH_3CH_2CH_2NH_2$ (1-Aminopropane or 1-Propaneamine)
Carboxylic acid	$-COOH$	-oic acid(s)	$CH_3CH_2CH_2CH_2COOH$ (1-Pentanoic acid)
Acid anhydride	$-\overset{\text{O}}{\underset{\text{}}{C}}-O-\overset{\text{O}}{\underset{\text{}}{C}}-$	-oic anhydride(s)	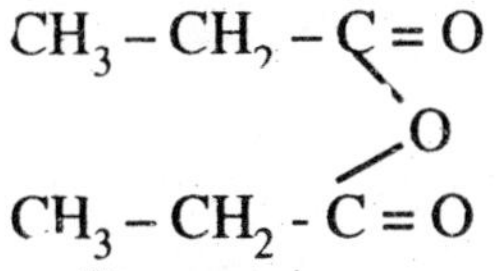 $CH_3-CH_2-C=O$ with O bridging to $CH_3-CH_2-C=O$ (Propanoic anhydride)
Amide	$-\overset{\text{}}{\underset{\text{O}}{C}}-O-NH_2$	-amide(s)	$CH_3CH_2CONH_2$ (Propionamide)
Acyl halide	$-\overset{\text{}}{\underset{\text{O}}{C}}-X$	-oyl halide(s)	CH_3CH_2COCl (Propionyl chloride)
Arene	--	--	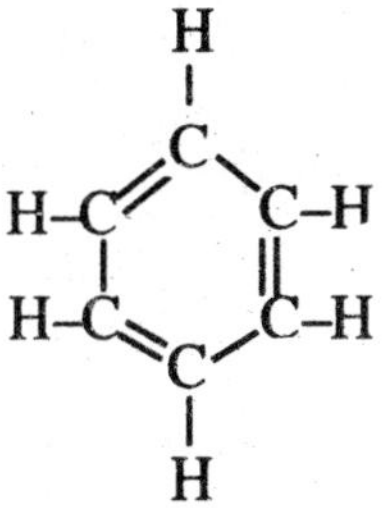 (Benzene)

(Benzene)

CHAPTER 4

TOPICAL ANTI-INFECTIVES
(Antiseptics and Disinfectants)

A disinfectant or a germicide is a chemical substance which destroys microorganisms. Spores of the microorganisms are not usually killed by disinfectants. Disinfectants may also be more specifically named as bactericides, fungicides, virucides, amoebicides etc., when they are used to kill bacteria, fungi, viruses, amoebae etc. respectively. They can be used for the external sterilization of instruments, articles, surfaces etc., and also for room sterilization. Sterilization is the total elimination of all kinds of microorganisms including their spores and the product thus obtained is said to be sterile. An antiseptic is a substance which destroys the microorganisms by inhibiting their growth. They can be safely applied to the skin or mucous membrane to prevent sepsis. The same substance can be used. as a disinfectant or an antiseptic and this is dependent upon the concentration in which it is used. A good example is phenol or carbolic acid.

Antiseptics and disinfectants exert their action through various mechanisms. Some of them oxidise the bacterial protoplasm, some tend to denature the bacterial proteins which include the bacterial enzymes also and some act like detergents thereby increasing the permeability of the bacterial cell membrane.

CLASSIFICATION

Antiseptics and disinfectants are also known as topical anti-infectives because they are always used locally or on specific surfaces to prevent infection and sepsis. They are classified as below :-

a) **Phenols**
   1. Liquefied phenol
   2. Chlorocresol
   3. Chloroxylenol
   4. Hexachlorophene

b) **Cationic Surface Active Agents**
   1. Benzalkonium chloride solution
   2. Cetrimide

c) **Dyes**
   Proflavine

d) **Miscellaneous**
   1. Formaldehyde solution
   2. Nitrofurantoin

1. PHENOL

Phenol is derived from benzene structurally and may be called as hydroxybenzene. Its structure is given below :

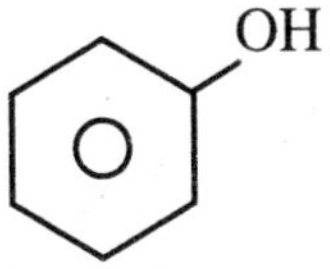

It is also known as carbolic acid. It is official as phenol and also as liquefied phenol. Liquefied phenol contains 80% w/w of phenol and water 20% w/w.

Physical Properties

Phenol consists of colourless or faintly pink, needle shaped crystalline masses. It has a characteristic, phenolic odour. The crystals turn pink on prolonged exposure to air and light due to oxidation. Phenol is deliquescent. It is soluble (1 in 15) in

23

water and freely soluble in alcohol, solvent ether, glycerol, chloroform, fixed oils and volatile oils. Phenol is very caustic when applied on the skin undiluted. The causticity is greatly reduced when phenol is dissolved in alcohol, glycerol or fixed oils. Phenol is stable and solutions of phenol may be sterilized by autoclaving.

Chemical Properties

Phenol answers the tests for phenolic -OH group :-

a) A violet colour is produced when ferric chloride test solution is added to a solution of phenol.

b) When bromine water is added to a solution of phenol, a white or yellowish white precipitate is produced. When more bromine water is added, the precipitate at first dissolves and then becomes permanent.

c) Though phenol has acidic properties, it is neutral to litmus. It does not react with metallic carbonates. However it dissolves easily in solutions of sodium or potassium hydroxide forming the phenoxides or phenates.

d) Phenol can be nitrated easily by heating with concentrated sulphuric and nitric acids. It is converted into yellow picric acid or 2 : 4 : 6-trinitrophenol.

Stability and Storage

As already stated, phenol turns pink on exposure to air and light. It is also deliquescent, that is it absorbs water from the atmosphere and dissolves in the water absorbed forming a solution. So phenol should be stored in a well closed container protected from light (amber glass containers) in a cool place, preferably at a temperature not exceeding 15°C.

Uses

Phenol can be used in the following ways :-

1. **Antiseptic and Disinfectant :** As an antiseptic and disinfectant, phenol is used against Gram positive and Gram negative bacteria. Aqueous solutions upto 1% are antiseptic and from 1-2% are disinfectant.

2. **Antimicrobial preservative.**

3. **Antipruritic :** A 0.5% solution of phenol is occasionally used to relieve itching.

4. **Analgesic :** Phenol is used as an analgesic in dentistry, mouth ulcers and tonsillitis as a solution in glycerol.

Official

Phenol, I.P., B.P.
Liquefied Phenol, B.P.
Phenol Glycerin, B.P.
Phenol and Glycerol Injection, B.P.
Oily Phenol Injection, B.P.

Brand Names

Carbolic acid, Phenylic acid.

LIQUIFIED PHENOL

Liquefied phenol contains 80% w/w of phenol and the rest is water. It is a colourless liquid which may become pink on keeping. It has a characteristic phenolic odour. All its other properties and uses are the same as that of phenol.

Storage

Liquefied phenol should be stored in a well-closed container which is protected from light. If stored below 4°C, it may deposit crystals. Under such circumstances, it should be completely melted before use.

2. CHOLOROCRESOL

Chlorocresol is a phenol and has the following structure :-

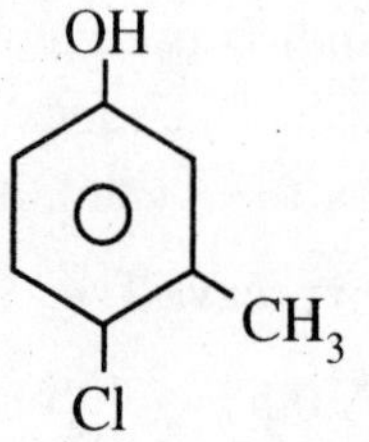

OH

4-chloro-3-methylphenol

In this structure, the chloro and the methyl groups are present at the 4th and the 3rd positions with reference to the position of the hydroxyl group on the benzene nucleus, that is counting from the hydroxyl group as no.1.

Physical Properties

It is a colourless or faintly coloured crystalline powder. It has a characteristic phenolic odour. It is slightly soluble in water (1 in 260 at 20°C). However it is soluble in hot water and more soluble in alcohol. It is freely soluble in other organic solvents such as ether, benzene, chloroform etc. When it is exposed to light and air, the aqueous solution may become slightly yellowish. Chlorocresol is volatile in steam.

Chemical Properties

Since chlorocresol is a phenol, it gives a blue colour with Ferric Chloride T.S. It can be differentiated from non-chlorinated phenols by ignition with sodium carbonate, which will decompose it to sodium chloride. Sodium chloride, thus formed, gives a white precipitate with silver nitrate solution in the presence of dilute nitric acid.

Stability and Storage

Solid chlorocresol is quite stable. It is stored in well closed containers.

Uses

1. Used as a **bactericide**. It is used in 0.2% concentration in the sterilisation of injections by the method of Heating with a Bactericide.

2. Used as a **bacteriostatic preservative** in 0.1% concentration in multidose preparations and aqueous creams for external use.

3. CHLOROXYLENOL

Chloroxylenol has the following structure :-

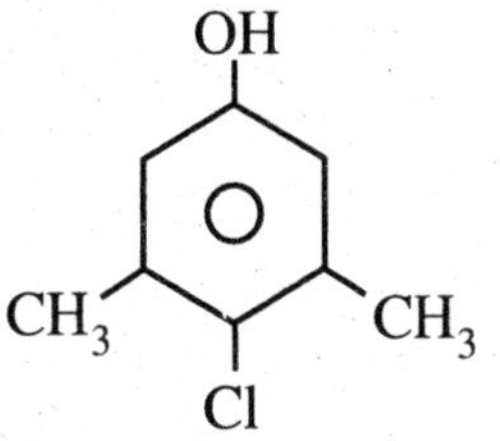

4-chloro-3,5-xylenol

Xylene is a compound in which there are two methyl groups on the benzene nucleus. Since here there is a phenolic -OH group also, it is known as xylenol. Since the two methyl groups are at positions 3 and 5 with reference to the hydroxyl group and there is also a chloro group at the 4th postion, the compound is named as *4-chloro-3,5-xylenol*.

Physical Properties

It consists of white or cream coloured crystals or occurs as a crystalline powder. It has a characteristic odour. It is very slightly soluble in water (1 in 3000) but more soluble in hot water. However it is freely soluble in alcohol, ether, benzene, fixed oils and in solutions of alkali hydroxides. It is volatile in steam.

Chemical Properties

Even though it is also a phenol, it does not give any colour with Ferric Chloride T.S. This distinguishes it from chlorocresol. However when ignited with sodium carbonate, sodium chloride is formed as in the case of chlorocresol and the sodium chloride can be tested with silver nitrate solution in the presence of dilute nitric acid.

Stability and Storage

Chloroxylenol is quite stable. It should be stored in well closed containers.

Uses

Antiseptic and disinfectant. It is used in the form of a 5% solution in castor oil soap solution under the name chloroxylenol solution for skin and wound disinfection.

Official

Chloroxylenol, B.P.

Chloroxylenol Solution, B.P.

Brand Names

Dettol, Roxenol, Benzytol (Chloroxylenol Solution)

4. HEXACHLOROPHENE

Hexachlorophene is a bisphenol which is also known as hexachlorophane. This bisphenol contains two phenols in its structure and each of the phenols contains in addition to the phenolic -OH group three chlorine atoms also (hence the name hexachlorophene). The two phenols are linked by a methylene (-CH$_2$) bridge.

Physical Properties

Hexachlorophene is a white to pale buff crystalline powder with a slight phenolic odour. It is practically insoluble in water and freely soluble in alcohol and ether. It is also soluble in chloroform and being phenolic soluble in solutions of alkalis also. It is stable in air but affected by light.

Chemical Properties

It forms salts with alkalis and alkaline earth metals. Since it is a bisphenol, it gives a transient purple colour when it is suspended in water and ferric chloride solution is added. On heating hexachlorophene in a test tube, a colourless to amber colour liquid is obtained which on further heating turns green, blue and finally purple. When a solution of hexachlorophene in acetone is shaken with titanous chloride, a yellow-orange oil is obtained. This oil is soluble in benzene or chloroform.

Stability and Storage

Even though hexachlorophene is stable in air, it is affected by light So it must be stored in well-closed containers protected from light.

Uses

Local anti-infective. It is a potent antiseptic and it acts by inhibiting bacterial enzymes and in high concentrations causes lysis of the bacterial cells. Its advantages are that it is almost odourless, non-irritating and non-staining. Even though its activity is reduced in the presence of organic matter, it is still active in the presence of soap, so it is used in soaps, creams, dusting powders, ointments etc.

However it has been found that used in a concentration of 3% or more, hexachlorophene is absorbed through the skin and causes brain damage, especially in premature newborn babies. So the use of hexachlorophene in more than 2% concentration in any skin preparation has been banned.

Official

Hexachlorophane, B.P.

Hexachlorophene, I.P.

Hexachlorophane Dusting Powder, B.P.

Brand Names

G-11, Hexachlorophane, Germa-Medica, Dermadex, Surofene, Gamophen.

5. BENZALKONIUM CHLORIDE

Benzalkonium Chloride is not a single substance but a mixture of alkyl benzyldimethyl ammonium chlorides. These are quarternary ammonium salts. Quarternary ammonium salts are highly ionized and have the general formula $R_4N^+X^-$. R represents any alkyl group and X^- may be $-Cl^-$ or $-Br^-$ or $-I^-$.

In the structure of benzalkonium chloride given below, $C_6H_5CH_2-$ is the benzyl group and R may be any alkyl radical having from 8 to 18 carbon atoms.

$$\langle O \rangle - CH_2 - \overset{\overset{\displaystyle CH_3}{|}}{\underset{\underset{\displaystyle CH_3}{|}}{N^+}} - R \cdot Cl^- \qquad R = -C_8H_{17} \text{ to } C_{18}H_{17}$$

BENZALKONIUM CHLORIDE

(Alkylbenzyldimethylammonium chloride)

Physical Properties

Benzalkonium chloride is found as a white or yellowish-white powder or as a thick gel or as gelatinous pieces. It has an aromatic odour and a very bitter taste. It melts to a semisolid mass on heating. It is very soluble in water and alcohol. An aqueous solution is alkaline to litmus and also produces foam on shaking.

Since it is a cationic surface active agent, it is incompatible with anionic agents, that is, detergents like soap which is the sodium or potassium salt of fatty acids. It is also incompatible with nitrates.

Chemical Properties

It can be decomposed by adding either dilute nitric acid or mercuric chloride solution. The white precipitate that is produced is soluble in alcohol.

It can be decomposed and the benzene nucleus from the benzyl part can be nitrated by heating with concentrated sulphuric acid and potassium nitrate. The nitro group can be reduced to the amino group by heating with zinc powder and the amino group can be diazotised with sodium nitrite and acid. When β-naphthol solution is added, an orange red colour is produced since an azo dye is formed.

Stability and Storage

This may be affected by light. So this must be stored in well-closed, light-resistant containers.

Uses

Benzalkonium chloride is used only in the form of a solution. It is used as an **antiseptic detergent** which means that it can be used for cleaning like a soap and also useful as an antiseptic. It is used as a 0.02% solution as an antiseptic detergent for the skin and mucous membrane. As a 0.05%

31

solution it is used for storing surgical instruments. Lozenges and pessaries containing benzalkonium chloride are sometimes used for pharyngeal and vaginal infections. It is also used in aqueous creams containing upto 1%.

Official

Benzalkonium Chloride Solution, I.P.

Brand Names

Germinol, Germital, Drapolex, Droplene, Zephirol, Roccal, Benirol, BTC etc.

BENZALKONIUM CHLORIDE SOLUTION, I.P.

This is a clear, colourless or slightly yellow syrupy liquid with an aromatic odour and a very bitter taste. It is miscible with water and alcohol. It contains about 50% w/v of alkylbenzyldimethylammonium chlorides and also not more than 16% v/v of alcohol. It is stored in tightly-closed, light-resitant containers.

6. CETRIMIDE

Cetrimide is also a quarternary ammonium compound like benzalkonium chloride. It also conforms to the general formula $R_4N^+X^-$. It consists mainly of tetradecyl ($C_{14}H_{29}$) trimethylammonium bromide along with smaller amounts of dodecyl ($C_{12}H_{25}$) and hexadecyl ($C_{16}H_{33}$) trimethylammonium bromides.

$$CH_3 - \overset{\overset{\displaystyle CH_3}{|}}{\underset{\underset{\displaystyle CH_3}{|}}{N^+}} - R . Br^-$$

$R=C_{12}H_{25}$ or $C_{14}H_{29}$ or $C_{16}H_{33}$

CETRIMIDE

32

Physical Properties

Cetrimide is a white to creamy-white, voluminous, freeflowing powder with a slight and characteristic odour and a bitter and soapy taste. It is freely soluble in water, soluble in alcohol and practically insoluble in ether.

Since it is also a cationic surface active agent like benzalkonium chloride, it is incompatible with anionic agents like soap. It is also incompatible with nitrates.

Chemical Properties

Cetrimide solution in water gives a yellow precipitate with potassium ferricyanide solution. With sodium silicate solution, it gives a white, flocculent precipitate. Cetrimide in solution can be decomposed by the addition of dilute nitric acid. The yellow precipitate produced is the basic compound. It may be filtered off and the bromide present in the filtrate gives a yellow precipitate on the addition of dilute nitric acid and silver nitrate solution.

Stability and Storage

The compound is quite stable. It may be stored in well-closed containers.

Uses

Antiseptic detergent. This means that like benzalkonium chloride it can be used for cleaning like a soap and also useful as an antiseptic. It is used in aqueous solutions and creams containing upto 1% of cetrimide. Aqueous solutions may be used for cleaning the skin in any pre-operative procedure and also for disinfecting vessels, utensils, apparatus, surgical instruments etc.

Official

Cetrimide, I.P., B.P.
Cetrimide Cream, B.P.
Cetrimide Emulsifying Ointment, B.P.
Cetrimide Emulsifying Wax, B.P.

Brand Names

Savlon, Cetrimidum.

7. PROFLAVINE

The basic compound in the structure of proflavine is acridine. In the structure of acridine, a pyridine nucleus may be considered to have fused with two benzene rings, one on either side.

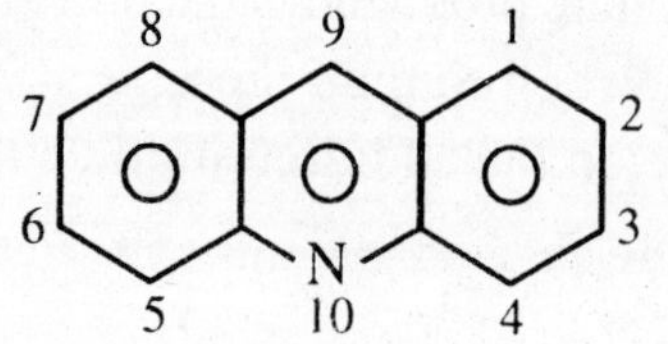

ACRIDINE

Proflavine is *3,6-diaminoacridine*, that is two amino groups are attached to the third and the sixth positions in the acridine nucleus.

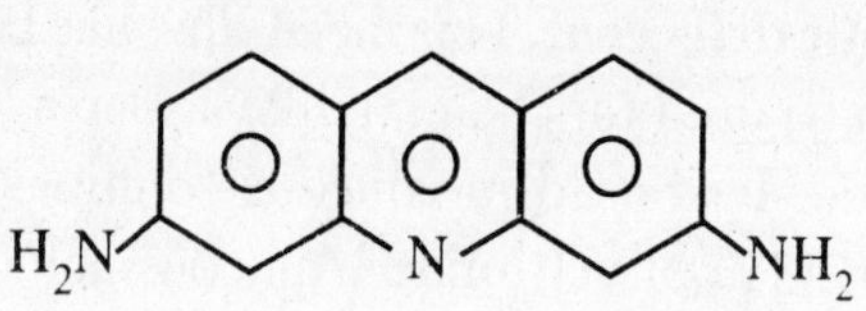

PROFLAVINE
(2 : 6 - Diaminoacridine)

However proflavine is used only as its hemisulphate. A half a molecule of sulphuric acid combines with proflavine to form proflavine hemisulphate.

Physical Properties

Proflavine hemisulphate occurs as an orange to red, crystalline powder. It is odourless with a bitter taste. It is hygroscopic and is also affected by light. It is slightly soluble (1 in 300) in cold water and freely soluble (1 in 1) in hot water. It is practically insoluble in both ether and chloroform.

Chemical Properties

When a dilute solution of proflavine hemisulphate is diluted with a large volume of water, a green fluorescence is produced. When concentrated sulphuric acid is added to a solution of the substance, a bright reddish orange precipitate is immediately formed.

Stability and Storage

Since proflavine is affected by light, it must be stored in well-closed containers protected from light.

Uses

Local antibacterial. It is used as a disinfectant in 0.1 to 1% concentration in the treatment of local wounds.

Official

Proflavine Hemisulphate, I.P. '66.

8. FORMALDEHYDE SOLUTION

Formaldehyde is a gas and it is dissolved in water to form formaldehyde solution. Formaldehyde is the simplest aldehyde and it has the formula HCHO. Formaldehyde solution or

Formalin contains 34 to 38% of formaldehyde with methanol being added as stabilizer. Methanol is added to discourage polymerisation of formaldehyde to solid paraformaldehyde.

Physical Properties

Formaldehyde solution is a colourless liquid with a characteristic pungent and irritating odour and a burning taste. On standing for a long time, a slight white cloudy deposit is formed especially in the cold due to the separation of para-formaldehyde and the solution becomes cloudy. However on warming the solution this white deposit disappears. It is miscible with water and alcohol.

Chemical Properties

Formaldehyde is a powerful reducing agent and is readily oxidized to formic acid.

$$HCHO + O \longrightarrow HCOOH$$

It reduces Fehling's solution, potassium permanganate and ammoniacal silver nitrate. In the last case (that is, reduction of ammoniacal silver nitrate) silver is deposited in the form of a finely divided, grey precipitate or as a bright metallic mirror on the sides of the test tube. A sensitive colour reaction for formaldehyde involves the addition of salicylic acid dissolved in concentrated sulphuric acid and warming gently. A permanent, deep red colour is produced. On evaporation on a water bath, formaldehyde solution leaves a white deposit.

Formaldehyde readily undergoes polymerization. In polymerization, two or more molecules of the substance (in this case formaldehyde) combine together to form another substance. This substance is known as a polymer. For example liquid or gaseous formaldehyde undergoes spontaneous polymerization to produce trioxymethylene.

$$3HCHO \rightleftharpoons (CH_2O)_3$$

When trioxymethylene is strongly heated, it is converted into formaldehyde.

When formaldehyde solution is mixed with ammonia and the liquid is evaporated to dryness on a water bath, hexamine is formed. Hexamine is also known as urotropine.

$$6CH_2O + 4NH_3 \longrightarrow C_6H_{12}N_4 + 6H_2O$$
$$\text{HEXAMINE}$$

Stability and Storage

First, formaldehyde solution is the solution of a gas in water. Secondly when it is stored in the cold, it becomes cloudy due to the formation of paraformaldehyde. So formaldehyde solution or formalin must be stored in well closed containers in a *moderately warm* place.

Uses

Disinfectant. It is mainly used for disinfection of rooms by fumigation and for preserving pathological specimens. It is diluted to 4% and used for hardening and preserving tissues. It acts slowly and denatures proteins. Sometimes it is used for disinfecting instruments and excreta. Even though it has good broad spectrum antimicrobial activity, its use as an antiseptic for human use is restricted by its irritation of the skin and pungent odour. Further it can be used only for surface sterilization since it has poor penetrability. It is also harmful to the tissues and causes allergic reactions.

Official

Formaldehyde Solution, B.P.

Brand Names

Morbicid, Formalin, Formol.

9. NITROFURANTOIN

Nitrofurantoin is not exactly a topical anti-infective but is used as an urinary antiseptic. So in this sense perhaps it is relevant to examine this here. Structurally it is a compound of nitrofuran and imidazolidine.

Physical Properties

Nitrofurantoin consists of lemon yellow crystals or occurs as a fine lemon yellow powder. It is almost odourless with a bitter taste. It is very slightly soluble in water and alcohol and soluble in dimethylformamide. It is discoloured by exposure to light.

Chemical Properties

When nitrofurantoin is treated with a dilute solution of sodium hydroxide, a deep yellow solution is produced which becomes deep red after some time.

Stability and Storage

Since nitrofurantoin is affected by light, store it in tightly closed light-resistant containers in a cool place. Contact with metals other than stainless steel and aluminium should be avoided.

Uses

Urinary antiseptic. It is used for urinary tract infections and is usually effective against common pathogens. Resistance to nitrofurantoin develops slowly. So it may be used in cases where the organism has become resistant to antibiotics.

Official :

Nitrofurantoin, I.P., B.P.

Nitrofurantoin Tablets, I.P., B.P.

Nitrofurantoin Mixture, B.P.

Brand Names

Furadantin, Furachen, Macrodantin, Urantoin, Welfurin.

CHAPTER - 5

ANTIBACTERIAL SULPHONAMIDES

Sulphonamides are antibacterial substances with a sulphonamido ($-SO_2NH_2$) group. Sulphanilamide is the simplest of the sulphonamides.

CHEMISTRY

All sulphonamides may be considered to be derivatives of sulphanilamide which is p-aminobenzene sulphonamide.

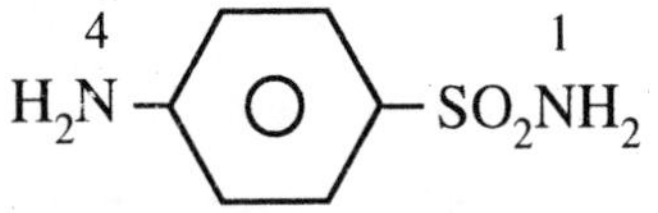

$$H_2N - \overset{4}{\underset{}{\bigcirc}} - \overset{1}{SO_2NH_2}$$

Sulphanilamide

The nitrogen of the sulphonamide group is named as N^1 and the nitrogen of the p-amino group as N^4. Most of the sulphonamides are derived by the substitution of the N^4 nitrogen, that is the sulphonamido group. Except in the case of sulphacetamide and sulphaguanidine, all the others have one heterocyclic nucleus attached to the sulphonamido group. The point of attachement on the heterocyclic nucleus should be specified while describing the structure. For example the thiazole nucleus in sulphathiazole is attached in the second position to the sulphonamido group.

$$H_2N - \bigcirc - SO_2NH - \overset{N}{\underset{S}{\bigsqcup}}$$

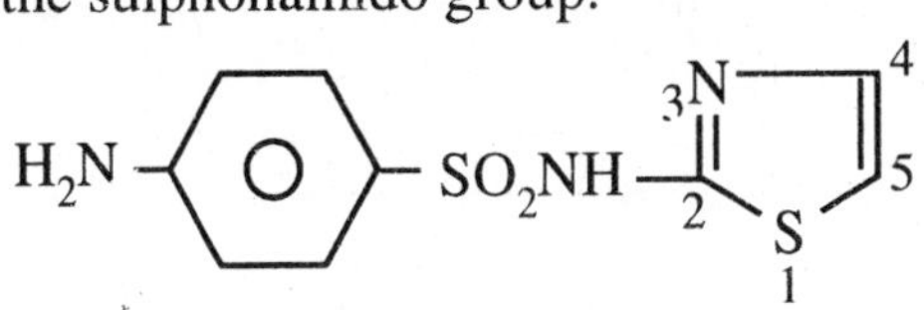

Sulphathiazole
2-(p-aminobenzenesulphonamido)thiazole

39

The free p-amino group in the N^4 nitrogen is not usually substituted, as a free amino group in the para position (N^4) is required for antibacterial activity. However, there are compounds in which the N^4 has been substituted which are still active (eg. phthalyl sulphathiazole or succinylsulphathiazole). This is due to the fact that these compounds are broken down in the colon to the active drugs which now have the free p-amino group. The nature of N^1 substitution is responsible for the solubility, potency and pharmacokinetic properties of the drugs.

CLASSIFICATION

Sulphonamides may be classified in many ways.

1. Chemical Classification

This method of classification is based on the structure of the compounds.

a) **N^1 substitued sulphonamides**

1. Sulphacetamide, 2. Sulphaguanidine, 3. Sulphadiazine, 4. Sulphathiazole, 5. Sulphadimethoxine, 6. Sulphamethoxypyridazine, 7. Sulphaphenazole, 8. Sulphafurazole, 9. Sulphamethoxazole, 10. Sulphamerazine, 11. Sulphamethazine, 12. Sulphasomidine, 13. Sulphadimethoxine, 14. Sulphadoxine.

b) **N^1 and N^4 substituted sulphonamides**
1. Succinylsulphathiazole
2. Phthalylsulphathiazole

c) **N^4 substituted sulphonamide**
Prontosil

d) **Sulphonamide without aromatic amino group**
Mefenide.

2. Pharmacological Classification

Pharmacologically sulphonamides can be classified as antibacterials, eg., sulphadimidine, sulphacetamide etc., as oral hypoglycaemics, eg., tolbutamide, as antidiarroheals, eg., sulphaguanidine, phthalylsulphathiazole, as diuretics, eg., frusemide and as antimalarials, eg., sulphadoxine. However in this chapter our discussion is confined only to sulphonamides acting as antibacterials. They are divided into :-

a) **Sulphonamides useful in intestinal infections**
   1. Sulphaguanidine
   2. Phthalylsulphathiazole
   3. Succinylsulphathiazole

b) **Sulphonamides useful in eye infections**
   Sulphacetamide

c) **Sulphonamides useful in systemic infections**
   1. Sulphadiazine, 2. Sulphathiazole, 3. Sulphadimethoxine, 4. Sulphamethoxypyridazine, 5. Sulphaphenazole, 6. Sulphafurazole, 7. Sulphamethoxazole, 8. Sulphamerazine, 9. Sulphamethazine, 10. Sulphasomidine, 11. Sulphadimethoxine, 12. Sulphadoxine.

d) **Sulphonamides useful in urinary infections**
   1. Sulphafurazole
   2. Sulphaphenazole

3. Classification Based on Duration of Action
a) **Short acting (4 to 8 hours)**
   1. Sulphadiazine
   2. Sulphathiazole
   3. Sulfisoxazole

4. Sulphadiazine

5. Sulphamerazine

6. Sulphamethazine

7. Sulphasomidine

8. Sulphamethizole

b) Intermediate acting (8 to 16 hours)

1. Sulphaphenazole

2. Sulphamethoxazole

c) Long acting (1 - 7 days)

1. Sulphadimethoxine

2. Sulphamethoxypyridazine

MECHANISM OF ACTION

Many bacteria synthesize folic acid, an essential bacterial vitamin required for many reactions in the bacterial cell. To synthesize folic acid, p-aminobenzoic acid, PABA,

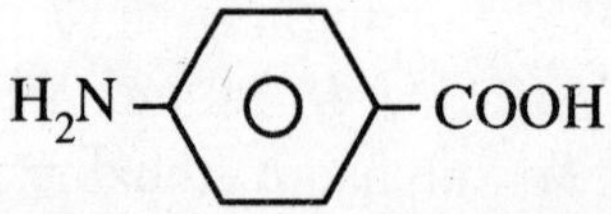

$$H_2N-\langle O \rangle-COOH$$

is required. It is available in the medium (in this case the human body in which the pathogenic bacteria are growing). Sulphonamides, being structural analogues of PABA (this means that they are structurally similar to PABA), inhibit a bacterial enzyme useful for forming folic acid. So folic acid is not formed, Because of this many essential reactions in the bacterial cells do not take place and the cells die. This is known as competitive inhibition or competitive antagonism. This is known as the Woods-Fildes theory.

42

GENERAL PROPERTIES

The sulphonamides are white, crystalline powders which are insoluble in water. They are weakly acidic and form salts with alkalis. The sodium salts are water soluble and form highly alkaline solutions.

METABOLISM AND ADVERSE REACTIONS

The N^1 substituted sulphonamides are quickly and nearly completely absorbed from the gut. Those with N^4 substitution also are not absorbed. After absorption, they are bound to plasma proteins in varying degrees. Generally the sulphas with lower pKa are bound more to the plasma proteins. The highly protein bound sulphas are longer acting.

The sulphonamides are acetylated in the liver and excreted through the kidney. The acetylated sulpha is inactive. Both the free as well as the acetylated compounds are less soluble in acidic urine (the acetylated compound is more insoluble) and may precipitate and cause crystalluria (presence of crystals in the urine) and sometimes haematuria (presence of blood in the urine). This can be prevented by taking plenty of fluids and by alkalinizing the urine by giving alkaline salts such as potassium citrate or sodium bicarbonate. Other adverse reactions are nausea, vomiting and epigastric pain (pain in the upper central region of the abdomen), hyper-sensitivity reactions etc.

ANTIBACTERIAL SPECTRUM

Many Gram positive and Gram negative organisms are sensitive to sulphonamides which are bacteriostatic (preventing the growth of bacteria). The infections are then eliminated by cellular and humoral defence mechanisms.

43

However many bacteria are able to develop resistance to sulphonamides and the usefulness of sulphonamides has come down because of this.

1. SULPHACETAMIDE

Sulphacetamide has the following structure :-

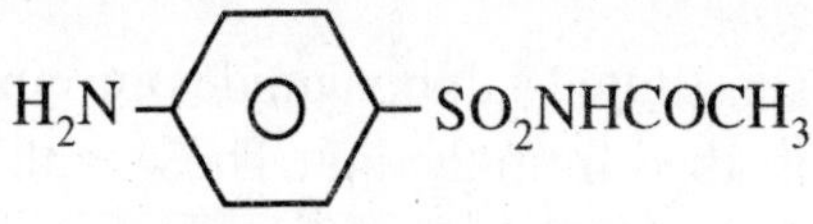

$$H_2N \text{---} \bigcirc \text{---} SO_2NHCOCH_3$$

p-aminobenzenesulphonylacetamide or
N¹-acetylsulphanilamide

CH_3CONH_2 is acetamide. The nitrogen of the acetamide is substituted with a benzenesulphonyl ($C_6H_5SO_2$-) group in which there is also an amino group in the para position. Therefore it is known as paraaminobenzenesulphonylacetamide. Alternatively it can be considered to have an acetyl (CH_3CO-) group attached to N^1 nitrogen of the sulphanilamide. So it can also be termed as N^1-acetylsulphanilamide.

Physical Properties

Sulphacetamide is a white or yellowish-white crystalline powder which is odourless and has an acid and slightly saline taste. It is slightly soluble in cold water and ether, soluble in alcohol and very slightly soluble in chloroform. It is freely soluble in mineral acids and alkali hydroxide solutions. A 10 per cent aqueous solution of sulphacetamide is acid to litmus. It is affected by light.

Chemical Properties

Since sulphacetamide has a free aromatic primary amino group in the para position, it can be diazotised in ice by adding dilute hydrochloric acid and sodium nitrite and the diazo compound coupled with β-naphthol and sodium acetate. An orange azo dye is formed. Sulphacetamide can also be hydrolysed by heating with concentrated sulphuric acid. If some ethyl alcohol is also added, the acetyl group released due to the hydrolysis forms ethyl acetate which can be recognised by its fruity odour. If sulphacetamide is heated gently till it melts and then is boiled, an oily liquid condenses on the walls of the test tube. This oily liquid can be recognised as acetamide by its characteric odour.

Stability and Storage

Sulphacetamide is sensitive to light. So it must be stored in well-closed containers protected from light.

Uses

Antibacterial (ophthalmic). It is used for eye infections in the form of eye ointment or eye drops in concentrations ranging from 10 to 30 per cent. In this concentration it is only mildly irritating to the eye. It is used for eye infections due to susceptible bacteria including ophthalmia neonatorum (severe inflammation of the eyes in the new born baby). Because of its comparatively high water solubility, it is also used in urinary tract infections maintaining high concentration in the urine without the fear of causing any damage to the kidney.

Official

Sulphacetamide, I.P. '66

Brand Names

Albucid, Locula, Acetocid, Urosulfone.

SULPHACETAMIDE SODIUM

Sulphacetamide sodium has the following structure :-

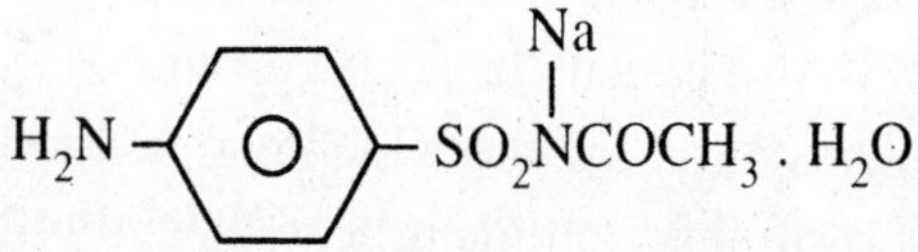

$$H_2N-\!\!\left\langle \bigcirc \right\rangle\!\!-SO_2\overset{\overset{\displaystyle Na}{|}}{N}COCH_3 . H_2O$$

One hydrogen of the acidic sulphonamido group is displaced by the sodium to give sulphacetamide sodium. The structure contains one molecule of water of hydration also. So sulphacetamide sodium is the monohydrate of the sodium salt of N^1-acetylsulphanilamide.

Physical Properties

Sulphacetamide sodium consists of white or yellowish-white crystals or occurs as a microcrystalline powder. It is odourless with a slightly bitter taste. It slowly darkens on exposure to light. It is freely soluble in water, sparingly soluble in alcohol and practically insoluble in organic solvents such as benzene, chloroform and solvent ether. Aqueous solutions are alkaline. A 5% solution has a pH of 8.0 to 9.5.

Chemical Properties

The sulphacetamide base can be released by dissolving the sulphacetamide sodium in water and acidifying the solution with acetic acid. This can be confirmed by finding out the melting point (about 183°C) after washing the white precipitate and drying at 105°C for four hours. This can be diazotised in ice by mixing with dilute hydrochloric acid and sodium nitrite solution and coupled with β-naphthol containing a little sodium acetate to give an orange to orange-red azo dye.

46

As in the case of sulphacetamide, the precipitate (which is nothing but sulphacetamide), when heated with concentrated sulphuric acid and ethyl alcohol, produces ethyl acetate recognised by its characteristic fruity odour.

Stability and Storage

As sulphacetamide sodium slowly darkens on exposure to light, store it in well-closed containers, protected from light.

Uses

Antibacterial (ophthalmic). It is used as an antibacterial in infections of and injuries to the eyes in the form of a 10 per cent ointment or as a 10 to 30 per cent solution. It is also administered orally for urinary tract infections and locally for skin infections as ointment.

Official

Sulphacetamide Sodium, I.P., B.P.

Sulphacetamide Eye Ointment, I.P., B.P.

Sulphacetamide Eye Drops, B.P.

Brand Names

Soluble sulfacetamide, Albucid soluble, Sulamyd sodium, Locula, Op-sulfa.

2. SULPHAGUANIDINE

The structure of sulphaguanidine is equally simple like that of sulphacetamides. In sulphaguanidine a guanyl group

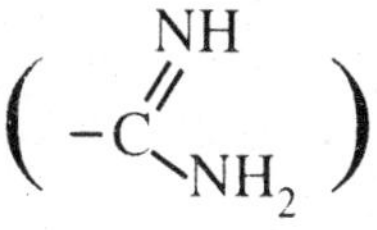

$$\left(-C \underset{\diagdown NH_2}{\overset{\displaystyle \overset{NH}{\|}}{}} \right)$$ is attached to the N^1 nitrogen of the sulphonamido group.

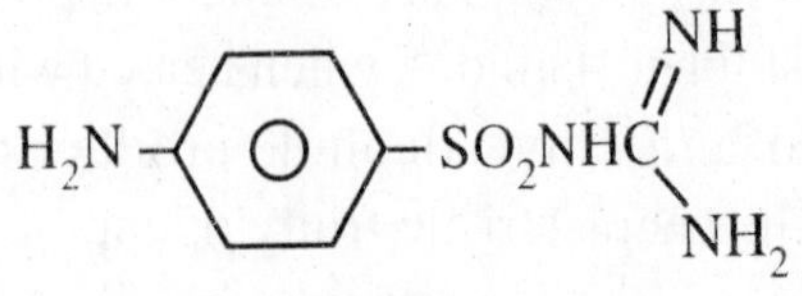

$$H_2N - \langle \bigcirc \rangle - SO_2NHC \overset{NH}{\underset{NH_2}{\overset{\|}{\diagdown}}}$$

N¹-guanylsulphanilamide or
N-p-aminobenzenesulphonylguanidine

The guanyl group is attached to the N^1 nitrogen of the sulphanilamide. So the systematic name for sulphaguanidine is N^1-guanylsulphanilamide. Alternatively guanidine is

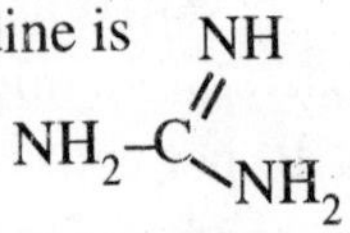

$$NH_2 - C \overset{NH}{\underset{NH_2}{\overset{\|}{\diagdown}}}$$

It is supposed to be attached to the p-amino-benzenesulphonyl group, that is, $H_2N - C_6H_4 - SO_2-$.
So sulphaguanidine can also be described as *N-p-aminobenzenesulphonylguanidine*.

Physical Properties

Sulphaguanidine is a white, needle-like, crystalline powder without any odour and taste. It is slightly soluble in cold water (1 in 1000), soluble in boiling water (1 in 10) and sparingly soluble in alcohol. It is soluble in dilute mineral acids but insoluble in aqueous solutions of alkali hydroxides. It is photosensitive, that is, it slowly darkens on exposure to light.

Chemical Properties

Other sulphonamides such as sulphanilamide, sulphathiazole and sulphadiazine dissolve in cold sodium hydroxide solution and do not evolve ammonia when this solution is heated. But sulphaguanidine does not dissolve in cold sodium hydroxide solution but on boiling it dissolves and also evolves ammonia which can be recognised by its odour. Like sulphacetamide it can also be diazotized in ice with dilute hydrochloric acid and sodium nitrite solution and coupled with β-naphthol solution containing sodium acetate to give an orange azo dye.

Stability and Storage

As sulphaguanidine is photosensitive and slowly darkens on exposure to light, store it in well-closed containers protected from light.

Uses

Antibacterial. It is used for the treatment of intestinal infections, especially in bacillary dysentery. It is also used as intestinal antiseptic before surgical operations of the abdomen. It is very poorly absorbed from the gut.

Official

Sulphaguanidine, I.P. '66
Sulphaguanidine Tablets, I.P. '66

Brand Names

Guanicil, RP2275, Ganidan, Shigatox, Aterian, Sulfaguine etc.

3. SULPHADIAZINE

Sulphadiazine is an example of a sulphonamide in which a heterocyclic nucleus is attached to the N^1 nitrogen (of the sulphonamido group). Here the heterocyclic compound is pyrimidine which is a six-membered ring containing two nitrogens in the 1 and 3 positions. The second position of the pyrimidine ring is linked to the N^1 nitrogen. Therefore the systematic name of sulphadiazine may be given as *2-(p-amino-benzenesulphonamido) pyrimidine*. Alternatively it can also be described as N^1-*2-pyrimidinylsulphanilamide*.

$$H_2N - \langle O \rangle - SO_2NH - \langle N \cdots N \rangle$$

SULPHADIAZINE

Physical Properties

Sulphadiazine occurs as white or yellowish-white or pinkish-white crystals or as a crystalline powder. It is tasteless and almost odourless. It is practically insoluble in water and also in other solvents such as alcohol and acetone. It is freely soluble in dilute mineral acids and in aqueous solutions of alkali hydroxides. It is also photosensitive and darkens slowly when exposed to light.

Chemical Properties

Since it also contains a free primary amino group in the para position of the benzene nucleus, it can also be diazotised in ice cold conditions by mixing with dilute hydrochloric acid and sodium nitrite solution. The diazo salt on coupling with β-naphthol solution containing a little sodium acetate gives an orange precipitate. Sulphadiazine gives an olive-green precipitate on mixing it with decinormal sodium hydroxide solution followed by copper sulphate solution. This olive green precipitate later becomes purple-grey on standing. If

50

sulphadiazine is gently heated in a test tube, a sublimate is obtained. If this sublimate is mixed with a 5% solution of resorcinol in alcohol and mixed, a deep red colour is produced immediately. If this is continuously diluted with a large quantity of ice-cold water and an excess of dilute ammonia solution is added, a blue or reddish-blue colour is produced.

Stability and Storage

Since it is affected by light, store it in well-closed light-resistant containers.

Uses

Antibacterial. Sulphadiazine is quite useful in systemic infections especially meningitis (inflammation of the meninges due to infection by bacteria or viruses. Meninges are the connective tissue membranes enclosing the brain and spinal cord), since it penetrates the cerebrospinal fluid easily. It is also useful in other infections such as pneumonia and influenza. It is rapidly absorbed orally and rapidly excreted. Sulphadiazine sodium dissolves in water easily and yields a highly alkaline solution which is injected intravenously.

Official

Sulphadiazine, I.P., B.P.

Sulphadiazine Tablets, I.P.

Sulphadiazine Injection, B.P.

Brand Names

Eskadiazine, Ultradiazine, Sterazine, Sulfolex, Pyrimal etc.

4. SULPHAMETHOXAZOLE

Sulphamethoxazole has a structure in which an isoxazole is attached to the N^1 nitrogen of the sulphonamido group in the 3rd positon. There is also a methyl group in the 5th position of the isoxazole, therefore the name sulphamethoxazole.

Physical Properties

Sulphamethoxazole is a white or yellowish-white, crystalline powder with a slightly bitter taste and almost without odour. It is very slightly soluble in water but slightly soluble in alcohol. It is soluble in dilute mineral acids and solutions of alkali hydroxides. It is affected by light.

Chemical Properties

Since it also contains a primary aromatic amino group, it can also be diazotised and coupled with β-naphthol to give an orange or orange-red azo dye. When it is dissolved in sodium hydroxide solution, heated to boiling, cooled and chlorinated soda solution is added, a golden yellow colour is immediately produced.

Stability and Storage

Since it is affected by light, store it in well-closed, light-resistant containers.

Uses

Antibacterial. It is used in urinary tract infections. It is combined with trimethoprim and used for antibacterial action. This combination is known as co-trimoxazole.

Official

Sulphamethoxazole, I.P., B.P.
Trimethoprim and Sulphamethoxazole Tablets, I.P.
(Co-trimoxazole Tablets, B.P.)

Co-trimoxazole Injection, B.P.
Co-trimoxazole Oral Suspension, B.P.
Paediatric Co-trimoxazole Oral Suspension, B.P.
Dispersible Co-trimoxazole Tablets, B.P.
Paediatric Co-trimoxazole Tablets, B.P.

Brand Names

Gantanol, Sinomin, Sulphamethizole, Bactrim, Septran, Bactromin, Linaris etc.

5. SULPHADIMETHOXINE

Sulphadimethoxine has a structure which is very similar to that of sulphadiazine, in that there is a pyrimidine attached to the sulphonamido group as in sulphadiazine. However the difference is that the pyrimidine is attached to the sulphonamido group not in the 2nd position but in the 4th position. Further the pyrimidine has two methoxy groups in the 2nd and the 6th positions. This is the reason behind the naming of the compound as sulphadimethoxine.

Physical Properties

Sulphadimethoxine occurs as a white or creamy-white, crystalline powder. It is tasteless and almost odourless. It is very slightly soluble in water and slightly soluble in alcohol. It is soluble in dilute mineral acids and in solutions of carbonates and alkali hydroxides. It is affected by light.

Chemical Properties

Since there is a primary aromatic amino group in the para position in this compound also, it can be diazotised and coupled with β-naphthol to give an orange-red azo dye. Further the copper sulphate and sodium hydroxide test applied to sulphadimethoxine gives a yellow colour.

Stability and Storage

Since sulphadimethoxine is affected by light, store it in well-closed containers which are light-resistant.

Uses

Antibacterial. It is used for the treatment of bacterial infections. Since it is highly plasma protein bound and also slowly excreted, it is a long acting sulphonamide. Its duration of action is for 1-2 days.

Official

Sulphadimethoxine, I.P.

Sulphadimethoxine Tablets, I.P.

Brand Names

Madribon, Agribon, Radonin, Metoxidan, Diasulfyl, Bactrovert, Roscosulf etc.

6. SULPHAMETHOXYPYRIDAZINE

Even though the structure of sulphamethoxypyridazine appears to resemble that of sulphadimethoxine, two differences can be seen on closer examination. The first difference is that a pyrazine nucleus is attached to the sulphonamido group in sulphamethoxypyridazine in place of the pyrimidine nucleus found in the structure of sulphadimethoxine. Pyrazine differs from pyrimidine in having the two nitrogens in the ring in the 1 and 2 positions compared to the 1 and 3 positions in pyrimidine and it is attached to the N^1 nitrogen in the 3rd postion. Secondly there is only one methoxy group in the 6th position in sulphamethoxypyridazine compared to two methoxy groups in sulphadimethoxine. Considering the methoxy group and the pyridazine in the structure, the compound has been aptly named as sulphamethoxypyridazine.

Physical Properties

It occurs as a white or yellowish-white, crystalline powder which is bitter in taste and is odourless. It is very slightly soluble in water but soluble in dilute mineral acids and in alkali hydroxide solutions. It is affected by light.

Chemical Properties

Its chemical properties resemble those of sulphadimethoxine almost. It also has a primary aromatic amino group which can be diazotised and coupled with β-naphthol to give an orange red azo dye.

Stability and Storage

Since it is affected by light, store it in well-closed, light-resistant containers.

Uses

Antibacterial. It is a long-acting sulphonamide. Duration of action is 1 - 2 days. It is bound to plasma proteins strongly and is also lipid (fat) soluble. It is also excreted very slowly, all these contributing to the long duration of action. It is used usually for long term treatment of infection of the urinary tract.

Official

Sulphamethoxypyridazine, B.P.'88.

Sulphamethoxypyridazine Tablets, B.P.'88.

Brand Names

Lederkyn, Petrisol, Depovermil, Midicel, Myasul, Sulfalex, Lentac etc.

7. CO-TRIMOXAZOLE

Co-trimoxazole is a combination of trimethoprim, an effective antibacterial with sulphamethoxazole. Trimethoprim is a diaminopyrimidine derivative structurally related to the antimalarial drug pyrimethamine. In the synthesis of folic acid from paraaminobenzoic acid (PABA) in the bacterial cell, trimethoprim inhibits the conversion of PABA into dihydrofolic acid (DHFA). The conversion of DHFA into tetrahydrofolic acid (THFA) is inhibited by sulphamethoxazole. This is known as sequential block. Since the biosynthesis of folic acid from PABA available in the medium is prevented at two stages in the pathway by the two drugs, the organisms become more susceptible to the combination and the usually individually bacteriostatic drugs become bactericidal in the combination. The combination also becomes more broad spectrum in activity including more Gram positive and Gram negative organisms in its fold. Since sulphamethoxazole has the same half-life as trimethoprim, it is preferred to other sulpha drugs. Resistance to this combination develops only slowly. All adverse effects of sulphonamides may be produced by co-trimoxazole also. Trimethoprim and sulphamethoxazole are present in co-trimoxazole in a ratio of 5 : 1 for effective action. Another combination used similarly is that of trimethoprim and sulphadiazine known as **co-trimazine.** It has actions and uses similar to that of co-trimoxazole.

Uses

Antibacterial. Co-trimoxazole is used mainly in urinary tract infections, respiratory tract infections and other systemic infections. It is also useful in bacterial diarrhoeas and dysenteries.

Official

Trimethoprim and Sulphamethoxazole Tablets, I.P.
(Co-trimoxazole Tablets, B.P.)
Co-trimoxazole Injection, B.P.
Co-trimoxazole Oral Suspension, B.P.
Paediatric Co-trimoxazole Oral Suspension, B.P.
Dispersible Co-trimoxazole Tablets, B.P.
Paediatric Co-trimoxazole Tablets, B.P.

Brand Names

Septran, Bactrim, Septrim, Gantaprim, Uro-septra etc.

8. SUCCINYLSULPHATHIAZOLE

Succinylsulphathiazole is a compound in which both the N^1 and N^4 nitrogens, that is both the primary amino group in the para position of the benzene ring and the sulphonamido group have been substituted. Thiazole, a heterocyclic compound, is attached to the sulphonamido group. Thiazole is a 5-membered fully unsaturated compound in which one sulphur atom and one nitrogen atom are present in the 1st and 3rd positions. It is attached to the sulphonamido group in its 3rd postion. Succinic acid is a dicarboxylic acid with the formula $HOOC-CH_2-CH_2-COOH$. The acyl group of succinic acid, that is succinyl radical ($HOOC-CH_2-CH_2-CO-$) is attached to the nitrogen in the primary aromatic amino group. Thus for the first time we see a compound in which the primary amino group has also been substituted. This substitution has conferred very low solubility on the compound, so it is not absorbed from the gut and so is useful only as an intestinal antiseptic.

Physical Properties

Succinylsulphathiazole consists of white or yellowish-white crystals or powder with a slightly bitter taste and without odour. It is very slightly soluble in water and practically insoluble in organic solvents such as chloroform. However, it is soluble in alkali hydroxide solutions and also sodium bicarbonate solution evolving carbon dioxide. It is affected by light.

Chemical Properties

The sulphathiazole portion in the compound can be precipitated by heating it with dilute sodium hydroxide solution at about 100°C, then cooling and diluting and neutralising with dilute hydrochloric acid. The plate-like crystals may be washed and dried. They melt at 198°C - 203°C. Since the primary aromatic amino group is not free, it can be released by hydrolysis with dilute hydrochloric acid. It can be diazotised by treating it with dilute hydrochloric acid and sodium nitrite in ice-cold conditions and then coupled with β-naphthol solution containing a little sodium acetate to give an orange azo dye.

Stability and Storage

Since it is affected by light, store it in well-closed containers resistant to light.

Uses

Antibacterial. It is initially inactive in the gut due to the N^4 substitution which is, however, split off in the colon by the bacteria to release sulphathiazole which acts as an antibacterial in the colon. It is used for bacillary dysentery and diarroheas and also for cleaning up the bowel before colonic surgery.

Official

Succinylsulphathiazole, I.P., B.P.
Succinylsulphathiazole Tablets, I.P.

Brand Names

Sulfasuxidine, Sulfenterone, Thiacyl etc.

9. PHTHALYLSULPHATHIAZOLE

Phthalylsulphathiazole resembles succinylsulphathiazole fully, in that both the N^1 and N^4 nitrogens have been substituted. The only difference in the structure is that at the N^4 nitrogen the acyl group present is the phthaloyl group instead of the succinoyl group as in succinylsulphathiazole. That is why the compound is named as phthalysulphathiazole. The phthaloyl group is derived from phthalic acid which is a benzene ortho-dicarboxylic acid. Because of this substitution, the compound has become practically insoluble in water. So it is not absorbed from the gut and is useful only as an intestinal antiseptic like succinylsulphathiazole.

Physical Properties

It consists of white or yellowish-white crystals or occurs as a crystalline powder. It is almost odourless with a slightly bitter taste. It is practically insoluble in water, ether and chloroform.

It is soluble in strong alkalies including ammonia and strong acids. It liberates carbon dioxide from a solution of sodium bicarbonate. It is affected by light.

Chemical Properties

As in the case of succinylsulphathiazole, the basic compound can be released by hydrolysis with dilute sodium hydroxide solution and adding dilute hydrochloric acid. When the solution is neutralised with enough of dilute sodium hydroxide solution, a white precipitate is formed. This can be washed and dried at 105°C. It melts between 200 and 203°C. It also yields the reaction given by primary aromatic amines, that is, after diazotisation with dilute hydrochloric acid and sodium nitrite and coupling with β-naphthol, it gives an orange azo dye. The sulphur in the sulphonamido group may be converted into hydrogen sulphide by boiling phthalylsulphathiazole with dilute sulphuric acid and zinc powder. The hydrogen sulphide evolved turns lead acetate paper black.

The phthalic acid portion of the molecule can be tested by heating the substance with resorcinol and concentrated sulphuric acid and the mixture poured into very dilute sodium hydroxide solution. An intense green fluorescence is formed due to the formation of fluorescein. The fluorescence disappears when acid is added but reappears when it is made alkaline.

Stability and Storage

This is just like any other sulpha drug. Since it is affected by light, store it in containers protected from light.

Uses

Antibacterial. All other details are the same as given under succinylsulphathiazole.

Official

Phthalylsulphathiazole, I.P. / B.P.

Phthalylsulphathiazole Tablets, I.P.

Brand Names

Thalazole, Intestiazol, Talidine, Ftalazol, Entero-sulfina etc.

Other sulphonamides clinically used are *sulphamerazine, sulphamethazine, sulfisoxazole, sulphasomidine, sulpha-methizole, sulphaphenazole, sulphadimethoxine, sulphadoxine, sulphamethopyrazine, sulphasalazine, mafenide, silver sulphadiazine etc.*

CHAPTER 6

ANTIBIOTICS

Antibiotics are chemical substances produced by various microorganisms such as fungi, actinomycetes and bacteria. They eliminate the other microorganisms by either killing them outright (in which case they are referred to as being bactericidal or fungicidal etc.) or by inhibiting or preventing the growth of microorganisms (in which case they are referred to as being bacteriostatic or fungistatic etc.,). However other compounds which are purely synthetic products made as structural analogs (that is, compounds having almost the same structure) of known antibiotics can also be used in a similar way against micro organisms.

Often they are selectively toxic to the microorganisms while even in large doses they may not harm the host. They are effective in low concentrations. Most of the antibiotics are manufactured by fermentation while some like chloramphenicol may also be made by synthesis. Some antibiotics such as the tetracyclines and chloramphenicol are known as broad spectrum antibiotics since they are active against a wide variety of microorganisms such as Gram positive and Gram negative bacteria and viruses etc., whereas antibiotics such as penicillin-G, bacitracin, nystatin etc. are called as narrow spectrum antibiotics since they are highly specific and are active against only a specific group of organisms.

MECHANISM OF ACTION

Antibiotics act through various mechanisms which are listed below :-

a) **By interfering with cell wall synthesis :**

e.g: Penicillins, Cephalosporins, Bacitracin, Cycloserine etc.

b) **By promoting leakage from cell membranes :**

e.g: Colistin, Polymyxins, Nystatin, Hamycin, Amphotericin B etc.

c) **By interfering with protein synthesis in ribosomes in the cells of the organisms :**

e.g: Chloramphenicol, Tetracyclines, Erythromycin, Lincomycins, Aminoglycoside antibiotics such as streptomycins, gentamicin, neomycin etc.

d) **By interfering with DNA and m-RNA synthesis :**

e.g: Actinomycin, Griseofulvin etc.

e) **By interfering with DNA function :**

e.g: Rifampin.

CLASSIFICATION

The classification is based on chemical structure.

a) **β-lactam antibiotics :**

Penicillins, Cephalosporins

b) **Tetracyclines :**

Chlortetracycline, Oxytetracycline etc.

c) **Nitrobenzene derivative :**

Chloramphenicol

d) **Polypeptide antibiotics :**

Bacitracin, Polymyxin-B, Colistin, Tyrothricin

e) Aminoglycosides :

Streptomycin, Neomycin, Gentamicin etc.

f) Macrolide antibiotics :

Erythromycin, Oleandomycin etc.

g) Polyene antibiotics :

Nystatin, Hamycin, Amphotericin - B etc.

h) Miscellaneous :

Rifampicin, Lincomycin, Sodium fusidate, Cycloserine, Griseofulvin etc.

A. THE PENICILLINS

The penicillins and the cephalosporins are beta-lactam antibiotics. They contain in common in their structure a beta-lactam ring. If this ring is opened by acid or enzymatic hydrolysis, these compounds lose activity.

Penicillins are a group of antibiotics produced by the growth of the moulds *Penicillium notatum, Penicillium chrysogenum* etc. in artificial culture media. They are of two types :- 1. Natural penicillins, 2. Semisynthetic penicillins. First the mould produces the compound 6-aminopenicillanic acid whose structure is given below :-

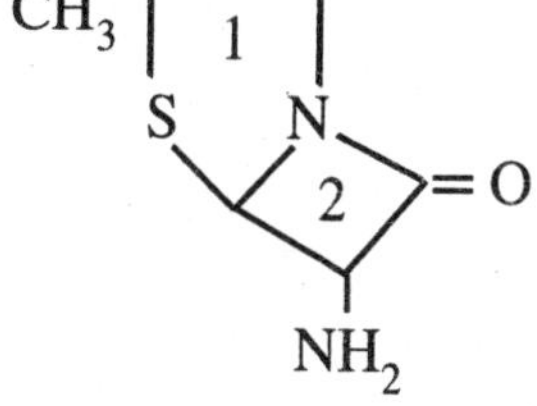

This compound has a thiazolidine ring (1) fused with a beta-lactam ring (2). If suitable substances known as 'precursors' are availabe in the medium, the mould adds them to the amino group in the beta-lactam ring. The compounds now made are known as natural penicillins. For example if phenylacetic acid ($C_6H_5CH_2COOH$) is available in the medium, the mould acylates the amino group with the phenylacetyl group ($C_6H_5CH_2CO-$) and thus makes benzylpenicillin. Over 30 different penicillins have been made like this.

However if no precursor is available in the medium, only 6-aminopenicillanic acid is formed. 6-Aminopenicillanic acid can also be produced by hydrolysing benzylpenicillin or any other penicillin with a bacterial or fungal enzyme. If the 6-aminopenicillanic acid is acylated with any acid by chemical means, we get a series of penicillins which are known as semisynthetic penicillins. The most important natural penicillins are benzylpenicillin and phenoxymethylpenicillin.

Benzylpenicillin is used as either the sodium or potassium salt. They are soluble in water, absorbed easily from the site of injection and excreted rapidly. Benzylpenicillin also forms a salt with procaine and the product procaine penicillin is only slightly soluble in water, absorbed slowly from the site of injection and excreted slowly. Similarly the salt of benzylpenicillin with the base benzathine is very slightly soluble in water and lasts for a longer time in the body. They are known as *repository or depot* preparations. Phenoxymethylpenicillin and phenoxymethylpenicillin potassium are given orally because they are acid resistant and so are not affected by the gastric acid. Benzylpenicillin is, however, administered parenterally since it is easily hydrolysed by the acid in the stomach.

Some bacteria have the capacity to produce an enzyme known as penicillinase which hydrolyses and breaks open the beta-lactarn ring in the penicillin structure. Because of this the affected penicillin loses activity. However, semisynthetic penicillins which are resistant to penicillinase have been developed.

The most important semisynthetic penicillins are given below :-

1) Phenethicillin
2) Cloxacillin
3) Flucloxacillin
4) Ampicillin
5) Amoxycillin
6) Carbenicillin
7) Methicillin

Phenoxymethyl penicillin and phenethicillin are acid resistant and can be given orally. Cloxacillin and flucloxacillin are resistant to both acid and penicillinase. Ampicillin is resistant to acid but not to penicillinase but has extended spectrum or broad spectrum activity. Amoxycillin is both acid and penicillinase-resistant and also has broad spectrum activity. Carbenicillin is comparatively unstable in acid and also is inactivated by penicillinase. However, it has good broad spectrum activity. It is always given by intramuscular or intravenous injection. Methicillin is not acid-resistant but is highly penicillinase-resistant. It is given by injection only.

1. BENZYLPENICILLIN (PENICILLIN G)

Benzylpenicillin is manufactured by a submerged culture technique using *P.chrysogenum* in a sterile medium consisting mainly of corn steep liquor, several inorganic salts and lactose. It is extracted by butyl or amyl acetate after acidification of the medium. It is then concentrated, extracted with a buffer solution and re-extracted with chloroform. It may be isolated as a sodium or potassium salt or as a salt with an organic base such as cyclohexylamine and purified.

Physical Properties

It is a white, amorphous powder, sparingly soluble in water but soluble in organic solvents such as methanol, ethanol, ether, benzene and chloroform. When heated, it loses its potency. It is stable in powder form and is stored in airtight containers below 30°C. The aqueous solutions are unstable unless stored at a temperature of 4°C when they are stable for 3 days. It is destroyed by the acid of the stomach and cannot be administered orally. It is given only by injection. It is effective against most of the Gram positive organisms.

2. BENZYLPENICILLIN, I.P.

The benzylpenicillin of the I.P. is *either the sodium or potassium salt of 6 - (2 - phenylacetamido) penicillanic acid*. It has the following structure :-

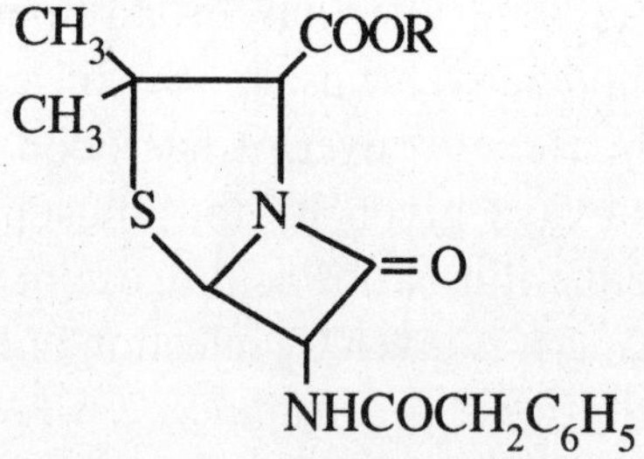

R = Na or K

The 6-amino group of the 6-aminopenicillanic acid has been acylated with phenylacetic acid ($HOOCCH_2C_6H_5$). The carboxyl group in the 3rd position has also been converted into either the sodium or the potassium salt. The structure of 6-aminopenicillanic acid is given below :-

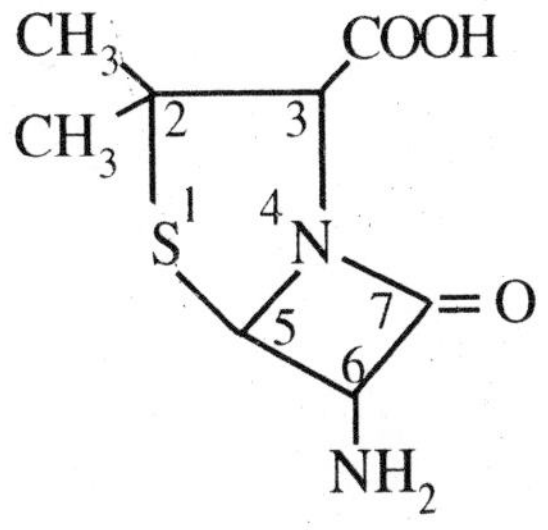

Physical Properties

It is a fine, white, crystalline powder which is almost odourless. It is very soluble in water, soluble in alcohol and almost insoluble in organic solvents such as chloroform and ether, fixed oils and liquid paraffin. It has a potency of not less than 1500 units and not more than 1750 units per mg if it is the sodium salt or not less than 1440 units and not more than 1680 units per mg if it is the potassium salt. One I.U. (International Unit) is equal to 0.6 microgram of sodium benzylpenicillin.

Chemical Properties

Some of the penicillins (and the cephalosporins) give distinct colours when they are moistened with a little water and treated with sulphuric acid (96% w/w) or with sulphuric acid - formaldehyde reagent. Both benzylpenicillin sodium and potassium do not give any colour either with sulphuric acid (96% w/w) or with sulphuric acid-formaldehyde reagent. However a reddish-brown colour is obtained when after the addition of formaldehyde-sulphuric acid reagent, the mixture is heated for one minute by immersion in a boiling water bath. Both the sodium and potassium salts of benzyl penicillin answer this reaction and give the same colour.

Stability and Storage

It is stable in powder form. So is must be stored in sterile well-closed, dry containers in a cool, dry place. If it is to be used for parenteral administration, store in sealed containers to exclude micro-organisms.

Uses

Antibiotic. Penicillin G is the drug of choice in infections caused by organisms susceptible to it. It is used in streptococcal infections, pneumococcal infections, meningococcal infections, gonorrhoea, syphilis, diphtheria, tetanus, gas gangrene, actinomycosis, trench mouth, rat bite fever etc.

Official

Benzylpenicillin, I.P.
Benzylpenicillin Injection, I.P., B.P.
Benzylpenicillin Potassium, B.P.
Benzylpenicillin Sodium, B.P.
Fortified Procaine Penicillin Injection, B.P.

Brand Names

a) **For Benzylpenicillin Sodium**
Sodium penicillin G,
Penicillin G Sodium,
Nalpen G,
Penilarin,
Novacillin,
Venticillin etc.

b) **For Benzylpenicillin Potassium**
Crystalline penicillin G,
Penicillin G potassium,
Penicillin

3. PHENOXYMETHYLPENICILLIN, B.P.
(PENICILLIN V)

Phenoxymethylpenicillin is 6-(2-phenoxyacetamido) penicillanic acid.

$$CH_3$$ $$CH_3$$ COOR S N $$= O$$

NHCOCH$_2$OC$_6$H$_5$

The amino group in the 6th position of the 6-amino-penicillanic acid has been acylated with phenoxyacetic acid (HOOCCH$_2$OC$_6$H$_5$) to give phenoxymethylpenicillin.

This acylation can be done either by supplying the precursor, that is, phenoxyacetic acid in the medium in which the mould *P.Chrysogenum* is growing so that phenoxymethyl penicillin can be made biosynthetically or it can be done in the laboratory by chemical means (semisynthetic method).

Physical Properties

Phenoxymethyl penicillin is official in B.P. It is white, crystalline powder which is very slightly soluble in water, freely soluble in ethanol (96%) and practically insoluble in fixed oils and liquid paraffin. It is stable in the presence of acid upto a pH of 1.8. The dextrorotatory D-form is the biologically active compound. The L-form is not active. Its biological activity is 1696 units per mg.

Chemical Properties

Phenoxymethylpenicillin gives a reddish brown colour when treated with formaldehyde - sulphuric acid reagent. This colour changes to dark reddish brown when the mixture is heated at 100°C in a water bath for one minute. A test for purity for phenoxyacetic acid (TLC method) is given in the B.P.

Stability and Storage

It is quite stable. It should be stored in an airtight container.

Uses

Antibiotic. Since it is acid-resistant, it can be administered orally in the form of tablets or capsules. It dissolves in the duodenum and produces higher plasma concentrations than the same quantity of Penicillin G given orally. It acts against the same infections as benzylpenicillin. It can't be used for serious infections and is used usually for sinusitis, otitis media, streptococcal pharyngitis, prophylaxis of rheumatic fever etc.

Official

Phenoxymethylpenicillin, B.P.

Brand Names

Penicillin V, Aciperi V, Distaquaine V, Oracillin, V-cillin etc.

4. PHENOXYMETHYL PENICILLIN POTASSIUM

Phenoxymethylpenicillin potassium is the potassium salt of phenoxymethylpenicillin.

Physical Properties

It is white crystalline powder. It may have a slight characteristic odour and has a slighly bitter taste. It is freely soluble in water and practically insoluble in chloroform and ether and in fixed oils and liquid paraffin.

Chemical Properties

It reacts in the same way as phenoxymethyl penicillin with formaldehyde-sulphuric acid reagent giving a reddish brown colour in the cold and a dark reddish brown colour after the mixture is heated for one minute at 100°C in a boiling water bath. A test for purity for phenoxyacetic acid is prescribed for this substance also.

Stability and Storage

It is stable and is stored in airtight containers.

Uses

Antibiotic. It is used in the same way as phenoxymethylpenicillin.

Official

Phenoxymethylpenicillin Potassium, I.P., B.P.
Phenoxymethylpenicillin Potassium Tablets, I.P.
Phenoxymethylpenicillin Capsules, B.P.
Phenoxymethylpenicillin Oral Solution, B.P.
Phenoxymethylpenicillin Tablets, B.P.

Brand Names

Crystapen V, Fenocyn, Oracyn, Beromycin, Distacillin V-K, Ledercillin V-K, Pfizerpen V-K etc.

5. BENZATHINE PENICILLIN

This is nothing but the benzathine salt of benzyl-penicillin. Benzathine is a base and is, structurally, N,N'-dibenzylethylenediamine. Benzathinepenicillin is acid resistant and so can be given orally as tablets. It is only very slightly soluble in water and so can be used as a repository or depot preparation.

Physical Properties

It is a white, crystalline powder without odour. It is very slightly soluble in water. It is, however, freely soluble in formamide and dimethylformamide, sparingly soluble in alcohol and practically insoluble in chloroform and ether.

Chemical Properties

Benzathine penicillin can be decomposed by adding sodium hydroxide solution. The benzathine part can be extracted with ether, ether removed by evoporation and the benzathine obtained as a residue. When it is dissolved in glacial acetic acid and potassium dichromate solution is added, a golden yellow precipitate is formed.

If the residue is dissolved in alcohol 50%, treated with picric acid solution, heated for about 5 minutes and allowed to cool slowly, a precipitate is formed.

Benzathine penicillin gives a reddish brown colour when treated with formaldehyde - sulphuric acid reagent and heated at 100°C for one minute in a water bath.

Stability and Storage

It should be stored in an airtight container at a temperature less than 30°C. If it is to be used for parenteral administration, the container should be sterile and sealed to exclude micro-organisms. It is affected by light, moisture and high temperature.

Uses

Antibiotic. It is well absorbed orally when given as tablets. It is not affected by the gastric acidity. Since it is very slightly soluble in water, it has long duration of action. So it is mainly used in the treatment of syphilis and streptococcal infections particularly of the upper respiratory tract.

Official

Benzatthine Penicillin, I.P., B.P.
Benzathine Penicillin Injection, I.P.
Fortified Benzathine Penicillin Injection, I.P.
Benzathine Penicillin Tablets, I.P.

Brand Names

Penidure-A, Longacillin, Diapen, Beacillin, Bicillin, Dibencillin etc.

6. AMPICILLIN

Ampicillin is a semisynthetic penicillin and is prepared by artificial means. If has the following structure :-

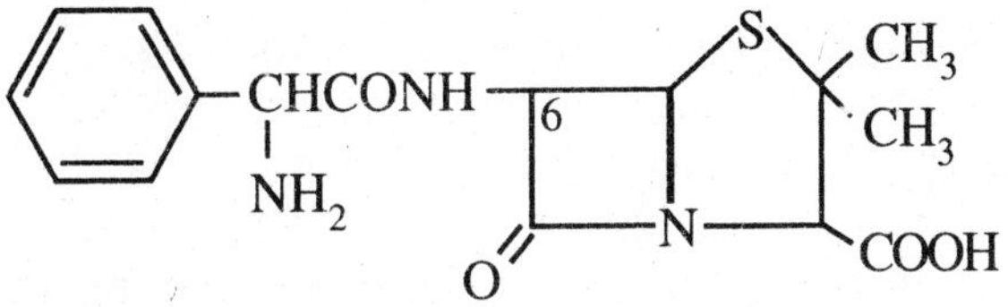

As can be seen there is an α-phenyl-α-amino-acetamido group attached to the 6th position. In the acetyl group (CH_3CO-) attached to the amino group in the 6th position of the 6-aminopenicillanic acid the α-carbon (CH_3–) carries one phenyl group and one amino group. So ampicillin is 6-(α-amino-α-phenyl) acetamidopenicillanic acid.

Physical Properties

Ampicillin is a white, microcrystalline powder. It is odourless or almost odourless with a bitter taste. It is slightly soluble in water and practically insoluble in alcohol and in organic solvents like chloroform and solvent ether and also in fixed oils. However it dissolves in dilute solutions of acids and alkali hydroxides.

Chemical Properties

Ampicillin gives a dark yellow colour when treated with formaldehyde-sulphuric acid reagent and heated at 100°C for one minute in a boiling water bath.

Stability and Storage

May be affected by high temperature. So it should be stored in an airtight container at a temperature not exceeding 30°C.

Uses

Broad spectrum antibiotic. It is active against Gram positive bacteria like benzylpenicillin and also is active against many gram negative bacilli. It is acid resistant and so may be given orally but it is not resistant to penicillinase.

7. AMPICILLIN SODIUM

Ampicillin sodium is the sodium salt of ampicillin.

Physical Properties

It is a white, crystalline powder which is hygroscopic. It tastes bitter but is odourless. It is freely soluble in water, slightly soluble in chloroform but practically insoluble in solvent ether, liquid paraffin and fixed oils.

Chemical Properties

As given under Ampicillin.

Stability and Storage

Since it is hygroscopic, it should be stored in tightly-closed containers protected from moisture and also in a cool place. If it is meant for parenteral administration, it should be stored in sterile containers which are sealed to exclude microorganisms.

Uses

See under Ampicillin. Since it is freely soluble in water, it is used to prepare Ampicillin Injection.

8. AMPICILLIN TRIHYDRATE

Ampicillin trihydrate has three molecules of water of crystallization combined with ampicillin.

Physical Properties

It is a white, crystalline powder. It is odourless and the taste is bitter. It is slightly soluble in water and practically insoluble in alcohol, chloroform, solvent ether and fixed oils. However it dissolves in dilute solutions of acids and alkali hydroxides.

Chemical Properties

As given under Ampicillin.

Stability and Storage

Should be stored in an airtight container at a temperature not exceeding 30°C.

Uses

See Ampicillin.

Official

Ampicillin, I.P., B.P.
Ampicillin Sodium, I.P., B.P.
Ampicillin Trihydrate, I.P., B.P.
Ampicillin Capsules, I.P., B.P.
Ampicillin for Oral Suspension, I.P.
(Ampicillin Oral Suspension, B.P.)
Ampicillin Injection, I.P., B.P.

Brand Names

Ampicillin, Roscillin, Dynacil, Polycillin, Totacillin etc.

9. CLOXACILLIN SODIUM

In the structure of cloxacillin there is an isoxazolyl group attached to the 6-amino group through a carboxylic acid group. The isoxazole carries a chlorophenyl group. Because of this the antibiotic has been named as cloxacillin.

Physical Properties

Cloxacillin is a white or almost white crystalline powder. It is odourless and hygroscopic. It is freely soluble in water and alcohol and slightly soluble in chloroform. Aqueous solutions of cloxacillin are stable for 24 hours at 25°C and for about 72 hours at 5°C.

Chemical Properties

It gives a slightly greenish-yellow colour when reacted with formaldehyde-sulphuric acid reagent. If the mixture is heated at 100°C for one minute in a boiling water bath, the colour becomes yellow.

Stability and Storage

Since the substance is hygroscopic, it must be kept in an airtight container and stored at a temperature not exceeding 25°C. If it is meant for parenteral administration, the container should be sterile and also sealed in such a way as to exclude micro-organisms.

Uses

Antibiotic. It is mainly used to treat infections due to staphylococci resistant to benzylpenicillin. It is usually used in combination with ampicillin. It is resistant to both acid and penicillinase.

Official

Cloxacillin Sodium, I.P., B.P.
Cloxacillin Capsules, I.P., B.P.
Cloxacillin Injection, I.P., B.P.
Cloxacillin Oral Solution, B.P.

Brand Names

Klox, Cloxacillin, Cloxapen, Ekvacillin, Tegopen etc.

10. CARBENICILLIN SODIUM

Carbenicillin is a semisynthetic penicillin in which the acylation of the 6-amino group has been carried out using α-carboxyphenylacetic acid. It is used as the disodium salt. It carries an α-carboxy group in the structure.

Physical Properties

It occurs as a white, hygroscopic powder. It is odourless and has a bitter taste. It is freely soluble in water, soluble in ethanol and practically insoluble in chloroform and ether. Aqueous solutions of carbenicillin are stable at room temperature for 24 hours.

Chemical Properties

When it is heated at 100°C in a boiling water bath for 3 minutes in a sealed container, it is decomposed. A drop of phenolphthalein solution (already made alkaline) introduced into the container is decolourized.

Stability and Storage

Since it is hygroscopic, it must be stored in a well-closed container at a temperature not exceeding 5°C. The container should be sterile and sealed to exclude microorganisms.

Uses

Antibiotic. This is a good broad spectrum antibiotic and is mainly used in infections due to pseudomonas and proteus bacteria. It is comparatively unstable in acid and is also inactivated by penicillinase. It is inactive orally and is given only by injection.

Official

Carbenicillin Sodium, B.P.
Carbenicillin Disodium, I.P.
Carbenicillin Injection, I.P., B.P.

Brand Names

Pyopen, Carbenicillin Sod., Carbelin, Carbapen, Microcillin, Pyopen etc.

B. THE CEPHALOSOPORINS

The cephalosporins are a group of antibiotics, derived from 'Ceplalosporin - C' which was obtained from a culture of a fungus *Cephalosporium* by Brotzu in 1945. They are chemically related to the penicillins. They have a β-lactam ring fused to a dihydrothiazine ring (instead of a thiazolidine ring present in penicillin). In the structure of cephalosporins there is a side chain at position 7 and a side chain at position 3 is also present.

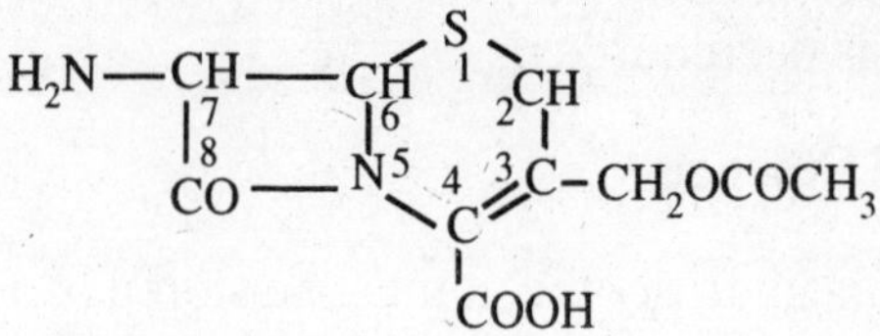

7-AMINOCEPHALOSPORANIC ACID

The removal of the side chain at position 7 gives the 7-Aminocephalosporanic acid (just like 6-APA in penicillin). By introducing a different side chain at position 7 (by acylating the amino group) or at position 3, many cephalosporins have been synthesised. By this way the spectrum of activity and the pharmacokinetics of the compounds have been altered. The cephalosporins are bactericidal and just like penicillins they kill the bacteria through inhibition of cell wall synthesis.

11. CEPHALEXIN

Cephalexin is a first generation cephalosporin and is one of the most commonly used cephalosporins. In the structure of cephalexin, there is an α-amino-α-phenylacetamido group at position 7 and a methyl group at position 3 of 7-amino-cephalosporanic acid. It is orally effective.

Physical Properties

Cephalexin is a white or almost white, crystalline powder. It has a characteristic odour. It is slightly soluble in water and practically insoluble in ethanol (95%), chloroform and ether. It is resistant to acid.

Chemical Properties

When cephalexin is treated with concentrated sulphuric acid, initially there is no colour produced. But on heating at 100°C for one minute, a pale yellow colour is produced. A similar pale yellow colour is produced when cephalexin is treated with formaldehyde - sulphuric acid reagent. The colour deepens when the mixture is heated at 100°C for one minute.

Stability and Storage

Since it is affected by light, it may be stored in well-closed, light-resistant containers in a cool place.

Uses

Antibiotic. It is orally administered and is used mainly in respiratory and urinary tract infections and in otitis media (ear infection). It is well absorbed orally.

Official

Cephalexin, I.P., B.P.
Cephalexin Capsules, I.P., B.P.
Cephalexin Oral Suspension, I.P., B.P.
Cephalexin Tablets, I.P., B.P.

Brand Names

Cephacillin, Alcephin, Cephaxin, Sporidex, Larixin, Mamalexin, Oracocin etc.

12. CEPHALORIDINE

Cephaloridine is also a first generation cephalosporin. It is not resistant to acid and must be injected. It is also very susceptible to β-lactamases of certain bacterial organisms. It is also the most nephrotoxic (toxic to the nephrons of the kidneys) cephalosporin.

Cephaloridine contains a pyridinomethyl group at position 3 of 7-ACA and also a thienylacetylamino group at postion 7.

Physical Properties

Cephaloridine is a white or almost white, crystalline powder with an odour which is slight and resembles that of pyridine. It is soluble in water, slightly soluble in ethanol (95%) and practically insoluble in ether and chloroform. It deteriorates rapidly in aqueous solution and should be used within 24 hours after storing at 2°C in a refrigerator.

80

Chemical Properties

Cephaloridine gives a yellow colour when treated with sulphuric acid. However after cephaloridine is kept at 100°C for one minute, if sulphuric acid is now added, there is no colour. Cephaloridine gives a red colour with formaldehyde - sulphuric acid reagent. However if cephaloridine is heated at 100°C for one minute and the reagent is added, a brownish red colour is produced.

Stability and Storage

Since it is decomposed easily by heat and light, store it in tightly closed, light-resistant containers at a temperature between 8° and 15°C in a sterile, tamper proof and sealed container.

Uses

Antibiotic. It has activity similar to cephalothin. However its use now has been discontinued due to its toxicity.

Official

Cephaloridine, I.P., B.P.
Cephaloridine Injection, I.P., B.P.

Brand Names

Ceporan, Cephlodine, Sporidine, Floridin, Loridin, Cepalorin etc.

13. CEPHALOTHIIN SODIUM

This contains the usual acetoxymethyl group at postion 3 and the α-thienylacetamido group at postion 7 of the 7-ACA. It is not absorbed orally. Since i.m.injection is very painful, it is always injected intravenously.

Physical Properties

It is a white or almost white, crystalline powder. It is freely soluble in water, slightly soluble in ethanol (96%) and practically insoluble in chloroform and ether. The aqueous solution may darken when stored at room temperature.

Chemical Properties

When cephalothin sodium is treated with 80% sulphuric acid containing a little dilute nitric acid, an olive green colour is produced. It changes to reddish brown.

Stability and Storage

Cephalothin sodium should be kept in a well-closed container at a temperature not exceeding 25°C. The sterile material should be kept in a sterile, tamper-proof and sealed container.

Uses

Antibiotic. It is mainly active against penicillin-G sensitive organisms including those producing penicillinase. It is highly resistant to staphylococcal β-lactamase and so its main use is in the treatment of penicillinase-producing staphylococcal infections.

Official

Cephalothin Sodium, B.P.
Cephalothin Injection, B.P.

Brand Names

Cefalotin, Ceporacin, Keflin, Synclotin etc.

14. CHLORAMPHENICOL

This antibiotic was isolated in 1947 by Burkholder from a culture of *Streptomyces venezuelae*. It is unique because of three reasons :-

1. It is a naturally occuring nitro compound, that too an aromatic nitro compound.
2. It is active against viruses and bacteria.
3. It is the first antibiotic to be synthesized on a large scale.

Structure

$$O_2N-\underset{}{\bigcirc}-\overset{\overset{H}{|}}{\underset{\underset{OH}{|}}{C}}-\overset{\overset{NHCOCHCl_2}{|}}{\underset{\underset{H}{|}}{C}}-CH_2OH$$

It is a propanediol structure containing two asymmetric carbon atoms. The first carbon atom carries a p-nitrophenylgroup and the second carbon atom the dichloroacetamido group (-$NHCOCHCl_2$). The configuration of the groups at the carbon atoms is that of D-threose. So the systematic name for chloramphenicol is *D-threo-2-dichloroacetamido-1-p-nitrophenyl-1, 3-propanediol.*

Physical Properties

Chloramphenicol is a white to greyish-white or yellowish-white, fine, crystalline powder or consists of fine crystals, needles or elongated plates. It is odourless and disagreeably bitter. It melts between 149 and 153°C and sublimes in high vacuum. It is slightly soluble in water (1 in 400), freely soluble in ethanol (95%) (1 in 2.5), in propylene glycol (1 in 7) and also freely soluble in acetone, ethyl acetate, butanol and methanol. It is affected by light. Otherwise it is quite stable.

Since chloramphenicol is very bitter, efforts were made to prepare derivatives to make it more palatable. Chloramphenicaol palmitale is a tasteless (bland), insoluble ester of chloramphenicol. This ester is inactive by itself but is hydrolysed in the intestine by the pancreatic lipase and absorbed as free chloramphenicol. Chloramphenicol succinate is freely soluble in water and the solution may be injected intramuscularly or intravenously. It is hydrolysed in the tissues to free chloramphenicol.

Chemical Properties

The aromatic nitro group behaves in a characteristic way. It can, for example, be reduced, diazotised and coupled with β-naphthol to form a red azo dye. The molecule can be disintegrated by boiling with alcoholic potash on a water bath. The resulting solution will give the reactions of chlorides.

Stability and Storage

Since it is affected by light, store it in tightly-closed, light-resistant containers. If it is to be used for the preparation of sterile preparations such as injection or eye drops etc., the container in which it is stored should be sterile, tamper-proof and sealed to exclude micro-organisms.

Uses

Antibiotic. The clinically unseful preparations are the capsules, dry syrup and oral suspension which are used for systemic treatment and the ear drops, eye drops and eye ointments which are used topically. Its adverse effects have severely limited its uses. It causes bone marrow depression, hypersensitivity effects etc. It has been used in the treatment of typhoid (enteric fever) but ciprofloxacin and other such compounds have replaced it. It is useful against many other infections, being a broad spectrum antibiotic. However it should not be used for minor infections and should be used with great caution. It is very useful in the treatment of eye and ear infections.

Official

Chloramphenicol, I.P., B.P.
Chloramphenicol Capsules, I.P., B.P.
Chloramphenicol Eye Drops, I.P., B.P.
Chloramphenicol Eye Ointment, I.P., B.P.
Chloramphenicol Palmitate, I.P., B.P.
Chloramphenicol Sodium Succinate, I.P., B.P.
Chloramphenicol Sodium Succinate Injection, I.P., B.P.
Chloramphenicol Ear Drops, B.P.

Brand Names

Chloromycetin, Enteromycetin, Paraxin, Chlorocid, Ciplamycetin, Novamycetin, Synthomycetine, Phenimycin, Vanmycetin, Lykacetin etc.

C. THE TETRACYCLINES

The antibiotics included in this group are made from acetate or propionate units in their biosynthesis by the organisms. The tetracyclines are derivatives of octa-hydronaphthacene, Napthacene is an aromatic hydrocarbon consisting of four benzene rings fused together. The important tetracyclines are tetracycline, oxytetracycline, chlortetracycline, demeclocycline, methacycline, doxycycline and rollitetracycline. They are active against a wide range of Gram positive and Gram negative bacteria, rickettsiae, some of the larger viruses, some of the intestinal amoebae etc., and hence are known as broad spectrum antibiotics. They can be administered orally.

The structure of tetracycline is given below. The structures of other tetracyclines are similar with minor differences :-

85

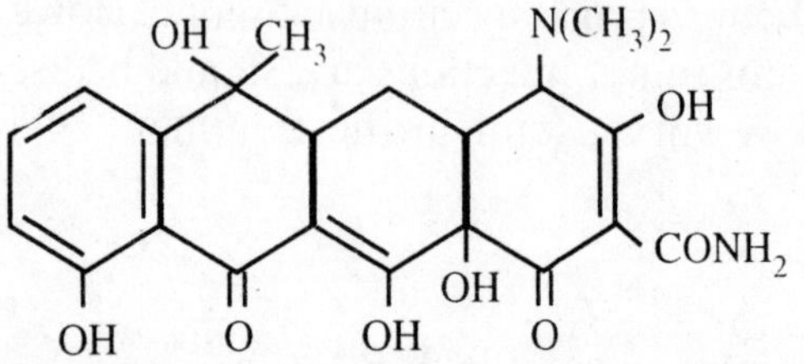

TETRACYCLINE

The structures of the other tetracyclines are given below:-

General Formula

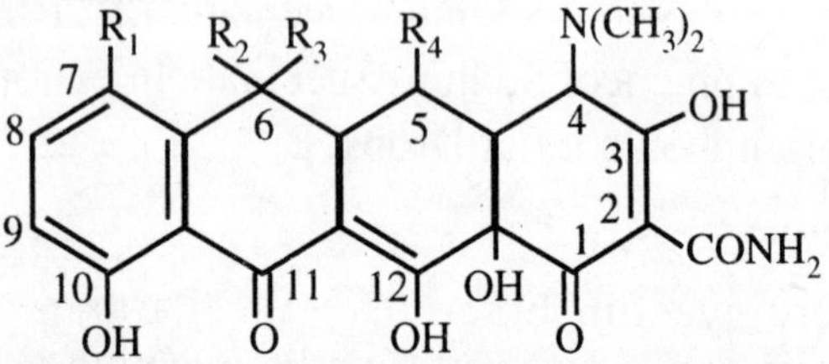

ANTIBIOTIC	R1	R2	R3	R4
7-Chlortetracycline	Cl	OH	CH_3	H
5-Oxytetracycline	H	OH	CH_3	OH
Demeclocycline (6-Demethyl-7-chlor-tetracycline)	Cl	OH	H	H
Doxycycline	H	H	CH_3	OH
Minocycline	$N(CH_3)_2$	H	H	H
Rollitetracycline (Pyrrolidinomethyl-tetracycline)	H	OH	CH_3	H

(in addition at C_2-

86

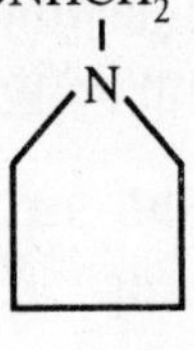

The tetracyclines are slightly bitter and are slightly soluble in water. They are amphoteric and form salts with acids and bases. The hydrochlorides are more soluble in water and are used to prepare injections. They are most stable in acid and very much less stable in alkali. All have almost the same antimicrobial activity but there may be minor differences. The latest members such as minocycline, doxycycline etc. have high lipid solubility and greater potency.

Tetracyclines form stable chelates with polyvalent metals such as iron, aluminium, calcium and magnesium. These complexes are insoluble and are not absorbed from the gut. So simultaneous administration of milk (containing calcium), iron preparations and nonsystemic antacids will reduce the absorption of tetracyclines from the gut.

15. TETRACYCLINE

Tetrecycline is manufactured by the fermentation of mutant strains of *Streptomyces* or by the catalytic hydrogenolysis of 7-chlortetracycline in which the chlorine atom present at position 7 is replaced by hydrogen.

Physical Properties

It is a yellow, crystalline powder melting at 170-175°C. It is stable in air but when it is exposed to strong sunlight in a moist condition, it darkens. It is stable in neutral, alkaline and acid solution (pH above 2). It is very slightly soluble in water (1 in 2500) and soluble in ethanol (95%) (1 in 50) and in methanol. It is slightly soluble in chloroform and practically insoluble in ether. It dissolves in dilute acids and alkalis.

Chemical properties

A reddish-violet colour is produced when concentrated sulphuric acid is added to tetracycline. When water is added to it, the colour changes to yellow.

Stability and Storage

Since it is affected by light, store it in well-closed, light-resistant containers.

Uses

Antibiotic. See the introduction for the details of the organisms against which it is active.

Official

Tetracycline, I.P., B.P.
Tetracycline Hydrochloride, I.P., B.P.
Tetracycline Hydrochloride Capsules, I.P
Tetracycline Hydrochloride Eye Ointment, I.P.
Tetracycline Oral Suspension, B.P.
Tetracycline Capsules, B.P.
Tetracycline Intravenous Infusion, B.P.
Tetracycline Tablets, B.P.

Brand Names

Achromycin, Alcycline, Idilin, Subamycin, Supramycin, Unicin, Unimycetin etc.

16. CHLORTETRACYCLINE

Chlortetracycline was isolated from the culture filtrates of *Streptomyces aureofaciens* by Duggar in 1948

Physical Properties

Chlortetracycline occurs in yellow crystals having no odour. It is slightly soluble in water and ethanol (96%). It is soluble in solutions of alkali hydroxides and carbonates. It is practically insoluble in chloroform, acetone, ether and dioxan. When heated, it decomposes above 210°C. It is affected by exposure to light.

Chemical Properties

When it is dissolved in 0.1M sodium hydroxide, the solution is yellow. It gives a blue fluorescence when examined under ultraviolet light with a wave length of 365 nm. When concentrated sulphuric acid is added to chlortetracycline, a deep blue colour changing to bluish green is produced. When this solution is added to water, a brownish colour is produced.

Stability and Storage

It should be kept in a well closed container protected from light. The sterile material should be kept in a sterile, tamper-proof and sealed container.

Uses

Antibiotic. For further details see the introduction to these antibiotics.

Official

Chlortetracycline Hydrochloride, B.P.
Chlortetracycline Capsules, B.P.
Chlortetracycline Eye Ointment, B.P.
Chlortetracycline Ointment, B.P.

Brand Names

Aureomycin, Biomycin, Isphamycin, Biomitsin.

17. OXYTETRACYCLINE

Oxytetracycline was isolated from the culture filtrates of *Streptomyces rimosus* in 1950.

Physical Properties

It is a yellow, crystalline powder without odour which loses its activity in solutions of pH below 2 and in alkali hydroxides. It is very sparingly soluble in water and slightly soluble in ethanol. It is readily soluble in dilute acid. Oxytetracycline hydrochloride is a yellow, crystalline substance with a bitter taste. It is hygroseopic and melts at 180°C with decomposition. It dissolves easily in water but is easily hydrolysed, the solution becoming turbid due to the liberation of the base. It is practically insoluble in chloroform and ether. It is an amphoteric substance.

Chemical Properties

When conc.sulphuric acid is added to it, a red colour is produced. When this is added to water, the colour changes to yellow. When diazotised sulphaniclic acid is added to oxytetracycline dissolved in a dilute solution of sodium carbonate, an orange red to brownish red colour is produced.

Stability and Storage

It may be kept in well closed light-resistant containers. The sterile material should be kept in sterile, tamper-proof and sealed containers.

Uses

Antibiotic. For further details see the introduction to these antibiotics.

Official

Oxytetracycline, I.P., B.P.
Oxytetracycline Injection, I.P., B.P.
Oxytetracycline Hydrochloride, I.P., B.P.
Oxytetracycline Hydrochloride Capsules, I.P.
(Oxytetracycline Capsules, B.P.)
Oxytetracycline Hydrochloride Eye Ointment, I.P.
Oxytetracycline Hydrochloride Injection, I.P.
Oxytetracycline Tablets, B.P.
Oxytetracycline Calcium, B.P.

Brand Names

Terramycin,Oxysteclin,Oxybiocycline,Oxycyclin,Riomycin HCl etc.

18. DEMECLOCYCLINE

Demeclocycline is *6-demethyl-7-chlortetracycline*.It has the same structure as chlortetracycline except for the fact that there is no methyl group at the 6th position. Due to this change, it has acquired enhanced stability towards acid and alkali. Because of high plasma protein binding and slower renal excretion, its plasma half-life (plasma t½) is enhanced to 16-18 hours so that it can be administered (orally) twice a day only.

Physical Properties

Demeclocycline hydrochloride is a yellow, crystalline powder without odour. It is soluble to sparingly soluble in water, slightly soluble in ethanol, very slightly soluble in acetone and chloroform and practically insoluble in ether. It dissolves in solutions of alkali hydroxides and carbonates. pH of a 1% solution in water is 2 to 3. It is affected by exposure to light.

Chemical Properties

When concentrated sulphuric acid is added to demeclocyline, a violet colour is produced. When this solution is added to water, the colour changes to yellow.

Stability and Storage

It should be kept in well closed containers protected from light.

Uses

Antibiotic. For futher details, see the introduction to these antibiotics.

91

Official

Demeclocycline Hydrochloride, B.P.
Demeclocyline Capsules, B.P.

Brand Names

Ledermycin, Declomycin, Bioterciclin, Deganol etc.

D. THE MACROLIDE ANTIBIOTICS

These are a group of antibiotics containing a large macrocyclic non-planar strainless lactone ring. In addition they contain an aminosugar linked glycosidically to the nucleus and also a neutral sugar similarly linked either to the nucleus or to the aminosugar. These sugars are all 6-deoxypyranosides.

These are produced by various strains of *Streptomyces* and many other compounds with almost similar structures and similar activities known as congeners are also produced along with the antibiotics. The principal macrolide antibiotics are erythromycin, carbomycin, oleandomycin and the spiramycins. They are mainly active against Gram positive bacteria but also act against a few Gram negative organisms such as the Haemophilus-Brucella group. The most important of these antibiotics is erythromycin.

19. ERYTHROMYCIN

Erythromycin was isolated in 1952 from the culture filtrates of *Streptomyces erythreus* by Mcguire and co-workers. In this fermentation erythromycin A is the main component accompanied by congeners erythromycin B and erythromycin C. The congeners have activity similar to that of erythromycin A which is simply known as erythromycin.

92

Physical Properties

Erythromycin consists of colourless or slightly yellow crystals or it may be a white or slightly yellow powder which is slightly hygroscopic. When heated, it melts at 135-140°C, resolidifies and melts again at 190-193°C. It is slightly soluble in water, freely soluble in ethanol (95%) and soluble in methanol and chloroform. It dissolves in hydrochloric acid. It is unstable at a pH of 4 or below. An aqueous solution of the substance has a pH of 8 to 10.5. Since erythromycin is very bitter, it is administered as film or enteric coated tablets or as capsules. It is stable at a pH which is almost neutral.

Chemical Properties

Derivatives have been prepared to overcome the bitter taste of erythromycin and also to improve its water solubility. Since it is a monacid base and contains a dimethylamino group in its structure, two types of salts have been prepared. One type of derivatives are salts formed by the acids such as the glucoheptonate or gluceptate, stearate and lactobionate. The other type is produced by esterification of the hydroxyl group present in the desosamine part such as the ethyl carbonate, ethyl succinate and lauryl sulphate of the propionate (erythromycin estolate).

Since the gluceptate and the lactobionate are water soluble, they are administered parenterally. The stearate is water insoluble and tasteless and so is used in the form of tablets and suspensions. The ethyl carbonate, another insoluble salt, is similarly used for children.

When erythromycin is mixed with a solution of xanthydrol in hydrochloric acid and acetic acid and heated on a water bath, a red colour is produced. When erythromycin is dissolved in 7M hydrochloric acid and allowed to stand for 20 minutes, a yellow colour is produced.

Stability and Storage

Since it is affected by light and is also slightly hygroscopic, keep it in well closed light-resistant containers in a cool place.

Uses

Antibiotic. It is used normally as an alternative to penicillin to treat infections caused by penicillinase-producing organisms and in penicillin-allergiç patients such as streptococcal pharyngitis, tonsillitis etc and respiratory infections caused by pneumococci. It is used in diphtheria along with antitoxin. It is also used in penicillin-resistant staphylococcal infections. However many organisms have acquired resistance to erythromycin and this has limited its use.

Official

Erythromycin, I.P., B.P.
Erythromycin Tablets, I.P., B.P
Erythromycin Estolate, I.P., B.P.
Erythromycin Estolate Tablets, I.P.
Erythromycin Estolate Capsules, B.P.
Erythromycin Stearate, I.P., B.P.
Erythromycin Stearate Tablets, I.P., B.P.
Erythromycin Ethyl Succinate, B.P.
Erythromycin Lactobionate, B.P.
Erythromycin Lactobionate Intravenous Infusion, B.P.

Brand Names

Erythromycin A,
Erythromycin stearate —Erythrocin, Etrocin and Eryster.
Erythromycin estolate —Althrocin, E-mysin
Erythromycin ethylsuccinate - Erynate

E. THE AMINOGLYCOSIDE ANTIBIOTICS

The aminoglycoside antibiotics include gentamicin, neomycin and streptomycin. These have compounds with amino groups linked glycosidically to two or more sugar or aminosugar residues. They are produced by soil actinomycetes and are used as sulphates. They are also very water-soluble and the solutions are quite stable. They are bactericidal and are very active in alkaline pH. They are broad spectrum antibiotics but mainly active against Gram negative organisms. They have a low margin of safety compared to other antibiotics. The aminoglycoside antibiotics produce ototoxicity(damage to the ear) and nephrotoxicity (damage to the kidney).

20. GENTAMICIN

Gentamicin is a mixture of antibiotics produced by fermentation of *Micromonospor purpurea*. It consists of three closely related compounds, gentamicins C_1, C_2 and C_{1a} and gentamicin A. It occurs as a white powder which is freely soluble in water, soluble in methanol, ethanol and acetone and practically insoluble in chloroform and benzene. It forms salts with acids and the sulphate is being used clinically.

GENTAMICIN SULPHATE

Properties

This is a mixture of the sulphates of the antibiotics present in gentamicin. It is a white or almost white powder and it is hygroscopic. It is freely soluble in water and practically insoluble in ethanol (95%), ether and chloroform.

Stability and Storage

Store in well closed containers. The containers should be sterile and sealed to exclude microorganisms if it is to be used for manufacturing injections or eye drops.

Uses

Antibiotic. It is a very potent and powerful broad spectrum antibiotic, useful especially against gram negative organisms. It is the cheapest aminoglycoside antibiotic. It is used to treat critically ill patients and also burns, urinary tract infections, septicaemia, osteomyelitis, ear infection etc. It is used to treat endocarditis due to streptococci, enterococci etc. It is also used to treat a variety of skin infections. It is especially valuable in treating patients with impaired host defence such as those receiving anticancer drugs or high doses of corticosteroids and also those being treated for AIDS.

Official

Gentamicin Sulphate, I.P., B.P.
Gentamicin Sulphate Eye Drops, I.P., B.P.
Gentamicin Sulphate Injection, I.P., B.P.
Gentamicin Cream, B.P.
Gentamicin Ointment, B.P.

Brand Names

Garamycin, Gentasporin, Genticin, Refobacin etc.

21. NEOMYCIN SULPHATE

Neomycin is a mixture of three substances, Neomycin A, B and C and was isolated in 1949 from the culture of *Streptomyces fradiae*. Neomycin A is nothing but a basic disaccharide (neomine)which is present in Neomycin B and C. Neomycins B and C contain four carbohydrate units and they differ from each other only in the configuration of the aminomethyl group in the neosamine ring attached to the ribose. Neomycin sulphate is a mixture of the sulphates of the substances obtained by the growth of certain selected strains of *Streptomyces fradiae*.

Physical Properties

It is a white or yellowish white powder without odour. It is hygroscopic and its solution darkens on exposure to light. It is freely soluble in water, very slightly soluble in ethanol (95%) and practically insoluble in acetone, chloroform and ether.

Chemical Properties

When pyridine and ninhydrin are added to an aqueous solution of the substance and heated on a water bath at 70°C for 10 minutes, a deep violet colour is produced.

Stability and Storage

Since it is hygroscopic and is also affected by light, store it in tightly closed, light-resistant containers in a cool place.

Uses

Antibiotic. It is a broad spectrum antibiotic active against a wide range of Gram negative bacilli and some Gram positive cocci. It is poorly absorbed from the gut and is also very toxic to the kidney. Therefore it is used only locally and not systemically. It is used topically in superficial infections and orally for suppression of bacterial flora in intestine especially for preoperative preparation of the bowels. It is used to treat infected wounds, ear infections, eye infections such as conjunctivitis, ulcers, burns etc.

Official

Neomycin Sulphate, I.P., B.P
Neomycin Sulphate Eye Drops, I.P.
(Neomycin Eye Drops, B.P.)
Neomycin Sulphate Eye Ointment, I.P.
(Neomycin Eye Ointment, B.P)
Hydrocortisone and Neomycin Cream, B.P.
Hydrocortisone and Neomycin Ear Drops, B.P.

Hydrocortisone and Neomycin Eye Drops, B.P.
Hydrocortisone and Neomycin Eye Ointment, B.P.
Neomycin Oral Solution, B.P.
Neomycin Tablets, B.P.

Brand Names

Neomycin Sulphate, Nepodex Eye/Ear, Nebasulf, Polybiotic cream, Mycifradin, Neobiotic.

22. STREPTOMYCIN SULPHATE

Waksman and others disconvered streptomycin in 1944 produced by a culture of *Streptomyces griseus*. Structurally it consists of three units, that is streptidine, N-methyl-L-glucosamine and streptose linked glycosidically. This is an antibiotic with broad spectrum activity especially against *Mycobacterium tuberculosis*. It forms salts with acids. The sulphate is official.

Physical properties

Streptomycin sulphate is a white or almost white powder. It has no odour and is hygroscopic. It is very soluble in water, slightly soluble in ethanol (95%) and practically insoluble in chloroform and ether. When stored at a low temperature, aqueous solutions are stable at a pH of 5 to 6.5. It is decomposed by acids, alkalis and oxidising and reducing agents. Streptomycin is very much ionized in the gastrointestinal tract. It is neither absorbed nor destroyed in the gastrointestinal tract.

Chemical Properties

Streptomycin is hydrolysed by both acid and alkali. Alkaline hydrolysis produces maltol which is formed by the rearrangement of streptose molecule. The following colour reactions are due to the formation of maltol :-

a) When to an aqueous solution of the substance 1M sodium hydroxide is added and heated on a water bath for 4 minutes and a slight excess of 2M hydrochloric acid and ferric chloride solution are added, a violet colour is produced.

b) When to an aqueous solution of the substance are added sodium hydroxide solution, 1-naphthol solution and sodium hypochlorite solution, a red colour is produced.

Stability and Storage

Since it is hygroscopic, store in tightly closed containers in a cool, dry place. If it is is meant for preparing injections, the container should be sterile and sealed to exclude micro-organisms.

Uses

Antitubercular antibiotic. It is useful in the treatment of tuberculosis. However it must be used along with other drugs. Otherwise resistance develops rapidly. It is the drug of choice in plague. In other infections such as urinary tract infection, septicaemia, peritonitis etc., other aminoglycoside antibiotics such as gentamicin have replaced it.

Official

Streptomycin Sulphate, I.P., B.P.
Streptomycin Sulphate Injection, I.P., B.P.
Streptomycin Sulphate Tablets, I.P.

Brand Names

Ambistryn-S, Streptonex, Comycin-S.

F. ANTIFUNGAL ANTIBIOTICS

Some of the antifungal antibiotics are amphotericin B, candicidin, griseofulvin, nystatin and hamycin.

23. GRISEOFULVIN

Griseofulvin was isolated by Raistrick in 1939 from *Penicillium griseofulvum*. However it received no attention because it had no antibacterial activity. Its clinical utility as an antifungal agent was discovered only around 1960. Chemically it is spiran.

Physical Properties

Griseofulvin is a white or yellowish white powder. The particle size should be as far as possible below 5 millimicrons. Howerver larger particles which may occassionally exceed 30 millimicrons may also be present. It is almost odourless. It is practically insoluble in water, soluble in acetone and chloroform and slightly soluble in ethanol (95%). It is freely soluble in dimethylformamide. In dry state it is stable for at least twenty months.

Chemical Properties

When griseofulvin is dissolved in concentrated sulphuric acid and powdered potassium dichromate is added to it, a wine red colour is produced.

Stability and Storage

Since it is quite stable, store it in well closed containers.

Uses

Antifungal antibiotic. It is active against certain fungi which actively concentrate it. Because of its low water solubility, its absorption is irregular. Absorption can be enhanced by taking it along with fats or by reducing the particle size to millimicron levels. It gets deposited in skin, hair and nails. The deposition is more when they are infected with tinea. It is, therefore used against tinea (ring worm) infestation of the hair, skin and nails. It is administered orally in tablets and is ineffective topically.

Official

Griseofulvin, I.P., B.P

Griseofulvin Tablets, I.P., B.P.

Brand Names

Grisovin-FP, Idifulvin, Grifulvin, Lamoryl, Spirofulvin Etc.

Other antibiotics clinically used are *flucloxacillin, phenethicillin, methicillin, dicloxacillin, nafcillin, bacampicillin, pivampicillin, hetacillin, amoxycillin, carbenicillin indanyl, carbenicillin phenyl, ticarcillin, clavulanic acid, sulbactam, cephapirin, cefazolin, cefotaxime, lymecycline, doxycycline, minocycline, rollitetracycline, kanamycin, bacitracin, tyrothricin, amphotericin B, nystatin, hamycin etc.*

CHAPTER - 7

ANTITUBERCULAR DRUGS

Tuberculosis is a disease primarily caused by *Mycobacterium tuberculosis.* In India about 140 lakhs of people are affected by tuberculosis of which 5 lakhs die every year. AIDS affected people are easily affected by tuberculosis and this is a dangerous new dimension added to the AIDS problem. Remarkable progress has been made in the treatment of tuberculosis in the last 50 years and multidrug therapy for 4-9 months has produced good results.

CLASSIFICATION

1) **Synthetic Drugs**
   Isoniazid
   PAS
   Ethambutol
   Thiacetazone
   Ethionamide
   Pyrazinamide

2) **Antibiotics**
   Streptomycin
   Rifampicin
   Cycloserine

In the case of synthetic drugs, isoniazid, pyrazinamide and ethionamide are pyridine derivatives.

1. ISONIAZID (INH)

Isoniazid is an excellent antitubercular drug which is also the cheapest. It is a pyridine derivative and has a simple structure. It is the hydrazide (hydrazine derivative) of isonicotinic acid.

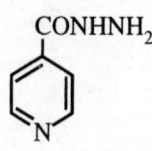

Physical Properties

It consists of colourless crystals or it is a white, cystalline powder without odour. It melts at 171.4°C. It is freely soluble in water, sparingly soluble in ethanol (95%) slightly soluble in chloroform and very slightly soluble in ether. It is affected by light.

Chemical Properties

When a warm solution of vanillin is added to a solution of isoniazid, allowed to stand and the inside of the container scratched with a glass rod, a yellow precipitate is produced.

Stability and Storage

Since it is affected by light, store in well closed, light-resistant containers.

Uses

Antitubercular drug.

Official

Isoniazid, I.P., B.P.
Isoniazid Tablets, I.P., B.P.
Isoniazid Injection, B.P.

Brand Names

INH, Isocid, Isonex, Nydrazid, Hydrazid etc.

2. PARA AMINO SALICYLIC ACID

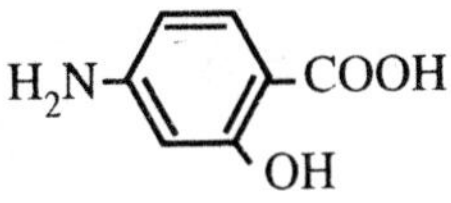

This is 4-aminosalicylic Acid

Physical Properties

It is a microcrystalline powder without odour or with a slight acetous odour. It melts at 150-151°C and darkens on exposure to air and light. It is slightly soluble in water and more soluble in alcohol. It is readily decarboxylated at temperatures above 40°C.

Chemical Properties

It gives a reddish-brown colour with ferric chloride solution. Since it has an armatic primary amino group, it can be diazotised and coupled with β-naphthol to give an orange red azo dye.

Stability and Storage

Since it is decarboxylated if stored at temperatures over 40°C, store it at a temperature below 30°C well protected from light.

Uses

Antitubercular drug. It is tuberculostatic and is one of the least active drugs. It only delays development of resistance by the tubercular organisms to other drugs. It is used now adays only as calcium aminosalicylate or sodium aminosalicylate. The latter is official in I.P

SODIUM AMINOSALICYLATE

This is the sodium salt of paraaminosalicylic acid.

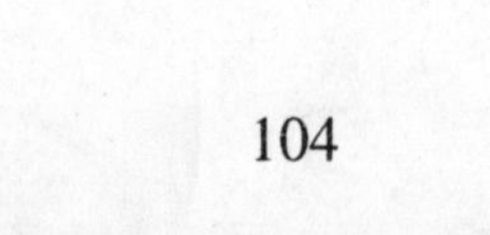

Physical Properties

It is a white to cream-coloured powder without odour and with a bitter sweet taste. It is hygroscopic. It is freely soluble in water and sparingly soluble in ethanol. Its aqueous solutions slowly darken in colour. It is affected by light.

Chemical Properties

When an aqueous solution of the sample is treated with ferric chloride test solution, a purple red colour is produced. It does not disappear even on the addition of alcohol or acetic acid. When it is diazotised and coupled with 1-naphthylamine in ethanol, a red colour is produced. It changes to orange when sodium hydroxide solution is added to it.

Stability and Storage

Store in well closed, light-resistant containers in a cool place.

Uses

Antitubercular drug.

Official

Sodium Aminosalicylate, I.P.
Sodium Aminosalicylate Granules, I.P.
Sodium Aminosalicylate Tablets, I.P.

Brand Names

Aminox, Parnisyl sodium, PAS sodium, dihydrate, Aminosalicylate sodium, Sodium PAS, Pasara sodium etc.

3. ETHAMBUTOL HYDROCHLORIDE

It is the hydrochloride of an aliphatic diamine. The dextroisomer is more potent than the laevo or meso isomer.

Physical Properties

It is a white, crystalline powder which is almost odourless. It is freely soluble in water and soluble in ethanol (95%). It melts at 87-89°C.

Chemical Properties

When to an aqueous solution of ethambutol hydrochloride are added cupric sulphate solution and sodium hydroxide solution, a blue colour is produced.

Stability and Storage

Store in well closed containers.

Uses

Antitubercular drug. It is a good antitubercular drug which is selectively tuberculostatic. Resistance to this drug develops slowly and it is used in combination with INH.

Official

Ethambutol Hydrochloride, I.P., B.P.
Ethambutol Hydrochloride Tablets, I.P.
(Ethambutol Tablets, B.P.)

Brand Names

Sural, Ebutol, Dadibutol, EMB etc.

4. ETHIONAMIDE

Ethionamide is a substituted thioamide of isonicotinic acid. It is actually 2-ethylpyridine-4-carbothioamide. It contains one ethyl group in the second position and carbothioamide ($-CSNH_2$) in the fourth position of the pyridine ring.

Physical Properties

It consists of small, yellow crystals or occurs as a yellow, crystalline powder without odour. It melts at 164 to166°C. It darkens on exposure to light acquiring a slight, sulphur-like odour. It is practically insoluble in water, soluble in methanol and sparingly soluble in ethanol (95%). It is slightly soluble in chloroform and ether.

Chemical Properties

When Silver nitrate solution is added to a solution of the substance in methanol, a dark brown precipitate is produced.

Stability and Storage

Since it is affected by light, store it in tightly-closed, light-resistant containers.

Uses

Antitubercular drug. It is a drug of moderate efficacy. It is not very much used, only in case of development of resistance to other drugs.

Official

Ethionamide, I.P., B.P.
Ethionamide Tablets, I.P.

Brand Names

Amidazine, Ethimide, Iridocin, Tiomid etc.

5. PYRAZINAMIDE

Pyrazinamide is derived from pyrazine.It is the 3-carboxamide of pyrazine.

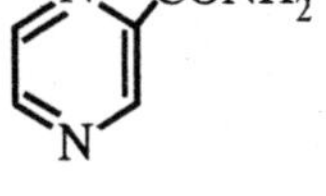

PYRAZINAMIDE

Physical Properties

It is a white or almost white, crystalline powder which has almost no odour. It melts between 188 and 191°C. It is sparingly soluble in water and chloroform, slightly soluble in ethanol (95%) and very slightly soluble in ether.

Chemical Properties

When it is boiled with sodium hydroxide solution, ammonia is evolved. It can be recognised by its smell and other reactions.

Stability and Storage

Store it in well-closed containers.

Uses

Antitubercular drug. It is toxic to the liver. Eventhough it is quite a good drug, resistance to it develops quite rapidly, especially if used alone.

Official

Pyrazinamide, I.P., B.P.
Pyrazinamide Tablets, I.P., B.P.

Brand Names

Unipyramide, Zinamide, pirilene, addinamide etc.

6. THIACETAZONE

Thiacetazone is a thiosemicarbazone.It is derived from an aldchyle which has condensed with thiosemicarbazide and formed the thiosemicarbazone. It is actually the thiosemi-carbazone of p-acctylaminobenzaldehyde.

Physical Properties

It consists of pale yellow crystals or occurs as a pale yellow, crystalline powder which has almost no odour. It melts from 225 to 230°C (dec). It darkens on exposure to light. It is very slightly soluble in water, slightly soluble in ethanol (95%) and practically insoluble in acetone, benzene, chloroform and other organic solvents.

Chemical Properties

Since it is the thiosemicarbazone of acetylamino-benzaldehyde, it can be hydrolysed with hot hydrochloric acid to release the primary amino group in the para position of the benzene nucleus of the aldehyde. This primary aromatic amino group can be diazetised by adding sodium nitrite and coupled with 2-naphthol to give a red azo dye.

Stability and Storage

Since it is affected by light, store it in well-closed, light-resistant containers.

Uses

Antitubercular drug. It is a convenient, low-cost drug. Its efficacy is low but it delays resistance to other drugs. It is used in combination with other drugs.

Official

Thiacetazone, I.P.
Thiacetazone and Isoniazid Tablets, I.P.

Brand Names

Thiacetazone, Thizone, Tebalon, Myvizone, Livazone etc.

7. STREPTOMYCIN

See Chapter 6.

8. RIFAMPICIN

Rifampicin is a cyclic polypeptide antibiotic which is obtained from *Streptomyces mediterranei.*

Physical Properties

It is a brick-red to reddish-brown, crystalline powder without odour. It melts at 183-188°C (dec). It is very slightly soluble in water, acetone and ethanol (95%) and soluble in chloroform and methanol. When exposed to atmosphere, it is affected by oxygen. It is also affected by light.

Chemical Properties

When ammonium persulphate solution in phosphate buffer pH 7.4 is added to the filtrate of a suspension of the substance in water, and shaken for a few minutes, the orange-yellow colour of the solution changes to violet-red without the formation of a precipitate.

Stability and Storage

Since it is affected by oxygen of the air and light, store it in tightly-closed, light-resistant containers in an atmosphere of nitrogen and in a cool place.

Uses

Antitubercular drug. Rifampicin is bactericidal to M.tuberculosis and also to many other Gram positive and Gram negative organisms. It is as effective as INH in tuberculosis and is used along with INH. It is also used in the treatment of leprosy, meningitis etc.

Official

Rifampicin, I.P., B.P.
Rifampicin Capsules, I.P., B.P.
Rifampicin Oral Suspension, B.P.

Brand Names

Rifampin, Rifadin, Rifaldine, Rifa etc.

9. CYCLOSERINE

Cycloserine has a very simple structure. It is a derivative of isooxazolidine. It is obtained from the cultures of *Streptomyces garyphalus, S.lavendulae and S.orchidaceus.* It is a ketone which exists in equilibrium with its enolic form. It exists as a zwitterion and forms stable salts with strong acids and bases.

Physical Properties

It is a white or pale yellow, crystalline powder which is hygroscopic. Its racemic mixture is more active than the dextro or laevo form. It is freely soluble in water, very slightly soluble in ethanol (95%) and practically insoluble in chloroform and ether. The neutral and acid solutions are unstable.

Chemical Properties

When the substance is dissolved in sodium hydroxide solution and dilute acetic acid and a mixture of freshly prepared sodium nitroprusside and sodium hydroxide solutions are added, a blue colour is produced slowly.

Stablility and Storage

It may be stored in well-closed containers in a cool place.

Uses

Antitubercular drug. It is rarely used now-a-days and used only in cases resistant to other drugs.

Official

Cycloserine, I.P.
Cycloserine Capsules, I.P.
Cycloserine Tablets,I.P.

Brand Names

Seromycin, D-cycloserin, Cycloserina etc.

Other antitubercular drugs are *kanamycin, amikacin, capromycin and ciprofloxacin.*

CHAPTER - 8

ANTILEPROTIC DRUGS

Hansen's disease or leprosy is common in India, especially south India and is caused by *Mycobacterium leprae*. It produces characteristic lesions in the skin and peripheral nerves. Leprosy can be divided into six different types based on the immunological response.

CLASSIFICATION

1) **Sulfones :**
   Dapsone, Solapsone

2) **Phenazine derivative :**
   Clofazimine

3) **Disubstited thiourea :**
   Thiambutosine

1. DAPSONE (DDS)

Dapsone is derived from diphenylsulphone and is actually bis (4-aminophenyl) sulphone.

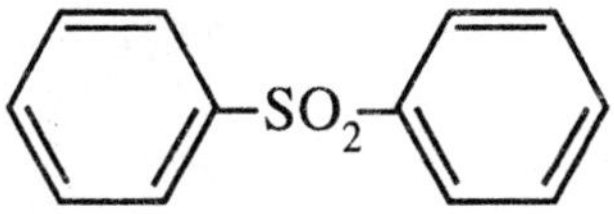

DIPHENYLSULPHONE

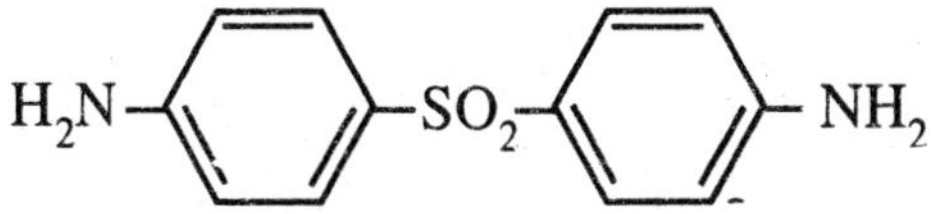

DAPSONE

It is the cheapest drug used in the treatment of leprosy.

Physical Properties

It is a white or creamy - white, crystalline powder which is very slightly soluble in water. It is freely soluble in ethanol (95%) and acetone. It is soluble in dilute mineral acids. It melts at 175-176°C. In the presence of traces of impurities it becomes photosensitive and is discolourized.

Chemical Properties

Since it contains two aromatic primary amino groups, it can be diazotised by treatment with HCl and sodium nitrite and the resulting compound coupled with β-naphthol to give an orange red azo dye.

Stability and Storage

Since it is affected by light, store it in well-closed light-resistant containers.

Uses

Antileprotic drug. It is the simplest, cheapest and most active antileprotic drug. All other sulphones are found to be converted to dapsone in the body. It is also used in combination with pyrimethamine in the treatment of chloroquine-resistant malaria.

Official

Dapsone, I.P., B.P.

Dapsone Tablets, I.P., B.P.

Brand Names

Dapsone, DDS, Avlosulphone, Novophone, Diphenasone etc.

2. SOLAPSONE

Solapsone is the tetrasodium sulphonate derivative of dapsone. It is also used in the treatment of leprosy but is considered to be less potent.

Properties

It is a white powder soluble in water. It is practically insoluble in alcohol. Acid-catalysed hydrolysis decomposes solapsone giving cinnamaldehyde, sulphurous acid and a dapsone salt. Due to the presence of cinnamaldehyde and sulphurous acid, the resulting solution answers the reactions of unsaturated compounds.

Stability and Storage

Store it in a well-closed container.

Uses

Antileprotic drug. It is less potent than dapsone and is used when there is gastric intolerance to dapsone.

Brand Names

Sulphetrone, Solusulfone, Salapsone etc.

3. CLOFAZIMINE

This is an iminophenazine dye which is used as an antileprotic agent.

Physical Properties

It consists of dark red crystals or it is a reddish-brown, fine powder without odour. It is practically insoluble in water but soluble in chloroform, dioxan and dimethylformamide. It is slightly soluble in ethanol (95%) and very slightly soluble in ether.

Chemical Properties

When it is dissolved in water and hydrochloric acid is added, an intense violet colour is produced. If sodium hydroxide solution is added to this, the colour changes to orange-red.

Stability and Storage

Store in well-closed containers.

Uses

Antileprotic drug. It is orally active and is used as a component of multidrug therapy of leprosy. It is also used as a second line drug in dapsone-resistant cases. It has anti-inflammatory action also.

Official

Clofazimine, I.P., B.P.
Clofazimine Capsules, I.P., B.P.

Brand Names

Lamprine, Clofozine, Hansepran.

4. THIAMBUTOSINE

As already mentioned, thiambutosine is a thiourea derivative. It is also a phenolic ether and a tertiary aromatic amine.

Properties

It is a white powder which almost insoluble in water. It is odourless and has a bitter taste. It is practically insoluble in water but soluble in chloroform and ether.

Stability and Storage

Store in well-closed containers.

Uses

Antileprotic drug.

Brand Names

Cibe-1906, DPT, Su-1906.

Other antileprotic drugs in clinical use are *acedapsone(DA-DDS), rifampin, ethionamide, thiacetazone, sulfadoxine and ofloxacin.*

CHAPTER - 9

ANTIFUNGAL DRUGS

There are two types of antifungal drugs, that is, drugs used to treat infections caused by fungi. They are a) drugs used for treating local infections such as those infecting hair, mucous, membranes, nails or skin. They are used in the form of ointments, creams, liniments, lotions, suspensions, solutions etc. and b) drugs used for treating systemic infections. In persons afflicted with AIDS since host defence mechanisms break down, fungi easily invade and cause infections. Antifungal agents may be classified as a) antibiotics, and b) chemical antifungal agents.

CLASSIFICATION

Chemical Antifungal Drugs

1. Tolnaftate
2. Undecylenic acid

Antibiotics

1. Amphotericin
2. Nystatin
3. Hamycin

1. TOLNAFTATE

Tolnaftate is a naphthalene derivative and a thiocarbamate.

Properties

Tolnaftate occurs as a white to creamy white powder. It is almost odourless. It is practically insoluble in water, freely soluble in acetone and chloroform and sparingly soluble in ether. It melts at 110°-112°C. It is applied externally in fungal infections as a 1% solution in propylene glycol.

Stability and Storage

Store in well-closed containers.

Uses

Antifungal drug. It is used topically as an 1% cream or lotion or as powder in the treatment of tinea infections such as *T.cruris* and *T.corporis*. It can be used with salicylic acid.

Official

Tolnaftate, B.P.

Brand Names

Tinaderm, Tolnaderm, Tonofal etc.

2. UNDECYLENIC ACID

This is an unsaturated long chain fatty acid with one double bond and 11 carbon atoms.

$$CH_2 = CH\text{-}(CH_2)_8\ COOH$$

It is prepared by distilling castor oil in vacuum. The ricinoleic acid in the castor oil is converted to undecylenic or undecenoic acid.

Properties

It is a white or very pale yellow, crystalline mass or a pale yellow liquid. It has a characteristic odour. It is practically insoluble in water but freely soluble in chloroform, ethanol, ether and in fixed and volatile oils. Since it is unsaturated, it decolourises acidified potassium permanganate solution.

Stability and Storage

Since undecenoic acid is unsaturated, it will be affected by oxygen of the atmosphere and also by light. This is catalysed by the presence of some metals. So it must be stored in a well-closed, nonmetallic container, protected from light and at a temperature between 8 and 15°C.

Uses

Antifungal drug. It is a fungistatic agent. Both undecenoic acid and its zinc salts are used in the treatment of *T.pedis, T.cruris* and nappy rash in the form of creams, ointments or as powders. They are also used as capsules to cure psoriasis.

Official

Undecenoic Acid, B.P.

Brand Names

Tineafax, Declin, Renselin, Sevinon etc.

3. AMPHOTERICIN

Amphotericin is an antifungal antibiotic obtained from *Streptomyces nodosus*. It is a mixture of two substances, amphotericins A and B. The B compound is more active. Amphotericin B is a polyene antibiotic because it contains several double bonds. Its structure contains a macrocyclic ring. One side of this ring has seven conjugated double bonds. The other side contains several hydroxyl groups. At one end of the macrocyclic ring is attached a polar aminosugar (mycosamine) and also a carboxylic acid group. As its name implies, amphotericin is amphoteric.

Physical Properties

Amphotericin B is a yellow to orange powder without any odour. It decomposes gradually around 170°C. The solid and its solutions are stable between pH 4 and 10 when stored at a cold temperature without being exposed to light and air. Even when it is not exposed to light, it is gradually decomposed when the humidity is high. It is also decomposed faster at higher temperatures. At low pH values and in the presence of light, it is inactivated in solution. It is practically insoluble in water, ether, ethanol (95%) and benzene. It is soluble in dimethyl sulphoxide and slightly soluble in methanol and dimethyl formamide.

Chemical Properties

When phosphoric acid is added to a solution of the substance in dimethyl sulphoxide to form a lower layer, a blue ring is immediately formed at the interface, that is, at the junction of the two liquids. When it is mixed, the mixture becomes intensely blue. If water is added and mixed, the solution gets a pale straw colour.

Stability and Storage

For the reasons mentioned under "Physical Properties", store amphotericin B in tightly-closed, light-resistant containers in a cold place.

Uses

Antifungal drug. It is not absorbed when given orally. However it is given orally for intestinal candidiasis without systemic toxicity. It is also administered intravenously. It is also applied locally. It is a toxic drug.

Official

Amphotericin, B.P.
Amphotericin Lozenges, B.P.

Brand Names

Mysteclin (amphotericin B with tetracycline),
Fungizone otic (ear drops),
Fungizone intravenous

4. NYSTATIN

Nystatin is an antifungal antibiotic obtained from *S. noursei*. Like amphotericin, it is also a polyene antibiotic containing a macrocyclic ring. It has a conjugated tetraene system and also a diene. The polar aminosugar attached to the ring is mycosamine as in amphotericin.

Physical Properties

It is a yellow to slightly brown powder with a characteristic odour. It is hygroscopic. When heated, it decomposes above 160°C without melting. It has strong reducing properties. It is very slightly soluble in water and freely soluble in dimethyl formamide. It is slightly soluble in methanol and insoluble in chloroform, ether and ethanol (95%). It is affected by light, heat and moisture and also when exposed to air. Aqueous suspensions are not stable and start deterioriting soon after preparation. Its solutions are also inactivated by acids and bases.

Chemical Properties

With hydrochloric acid, it gives a brown colour. With sulphuric acid also a brown colour is produced but it becomes violet on standing. It gives a green colour when its aqueous solution is shaken with a solution of sodium molybdo-phosphotungstate. When its aqueous solution is shaken with decolourised magenta solution containing a little pyrogallol dissolved in it, a dark pink colour is produced. Even after standing for one hour, the colour is retained.

Stability and Storage

Since it is hygroscopic and is also affected by light, heat and moisture, it should be stored in tightly-closed, light-resistant containers in a cool place.

Uses

Antifungal antibiotic. Because of higher systemic toxicity, it is used only locally. It is the drug of choice in monilial diarrhoea. It is also very effective in monilial vaginitis and oral thrush. Also it is used for corneal, conjunctival and cutaneous candidiasis in the form of an ointment.

Official

Nystatin, I.P., B.P.
Nystatin Ointment, I.P., B.P.
Nystatin Pessaries, I.P., B.P.
Nystatin Tablets, I.P., B.P.
Nystatin Oral Suspension, B.P.

Brand Names

Mycostatin
Nystin Eye (Eye ointment)
Fungicidin
Candex, etc.

5. HAMYCIN

Hamycin is an antifungal antibiotic isolated from the culture filtrate of *S. pimprina* at Pimpri, near Pune. It is a polyene compound like amphotericin and nystatin. Hamycin is a mixture of components A, B, C and D.

Properties

It is a yellow amorphous compound. When heated, it decomposes at about 160°C. It is very slightly soluble in water, ethanol, methanol, benzene, chloroform etc. It is soluble in aqueous alcohols and basic solvents like pyridine. It is amphoteric. It gives a blue colour with concentrated sulphuric acid. Compared to nystatin it is more water-soluble.

Uses

Antifungal antibiotic. It is used topically only in the treatment of oral thrush, cutaneous candidiasis and monilial and trichomonal vaginitis.

Brand Names

Hamycin
Imprima
Primamycin

Other antifungal drugs in clinical use are *griseofulvin* (see the chapter on "antibiotics"), *flucytosine, clotrimazole, econazole, miconazole, ketoconazole, fluconazole, itraconazole, benzoic acid, quiniodochlor, buclosamide, sodium thiosulphate* etc.

CHAPTER - 10

ANTIAMOEBIC DRUGS AND ANTHELMINTICS

This chapter can be divided into two parts: 1. antiamoebic drugs and 2. anthelmintics. They are taken together here since some of the antiamoebic drugs are also anthelmintics.

A. ANTIAMOEBIC DRUGS

Antiamoebics are drugs used in the treatment of *amoebiasis* caused by the protozoa *Entamoeba histolytica*. It is endemic in many parts of India where sanitation is poor. It is spread by faecal contamination of food and water by amoebic *cysts*. The cysts after reaching the intestine get changed into what are known as *trophozoites*. They either cause *acute dysentery* with blood and mucus appearing in the stools or cause vague abdominal symptoms leading to chronic *intestinal amoebiasis*. They may also form cysts (which can be detected by a microscopic examination of the stools) which are passed out into the stools serving to contaminate others. Sometimes trophozites reach the liver through the portal vein and produce amoebic liver abscess. Rarely other organs like kidney, lung, spleen and brain may be affected. This is known as *extraintestinal amoebiasis*. In the colon the amoebae live in symbiosis with the colonic bacteria. Therefore a reduction of the colonic bacteria indirectly brings down the number of amoebae also.

CLASSIFICATION

I. Synthetic Drugs

a) **Nitroimidazole :**
   Metronidazole

b) **Halogenated hydroxyquinolines :**
(1) Clioquinol
(2) Diiodohydroxyquinoline

c) **Amide :**
Diloxanide furoate

II. Natural Alkaloid
Emetine

1. METRONIDAZOLE

Metronidazole is a derivative of imidazole. It contains one hydroxyethyl ($HOCH_2CH_2-$) group in the first position, a methyl group in the second position and a nitro group in the fifth position. So it is *1-(2-hydroxyethyl)-2-methyl-5-nitroimidazole.*

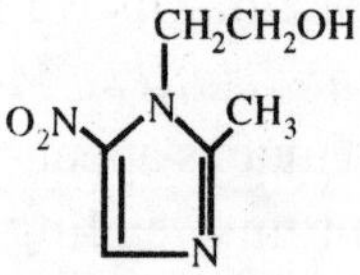

$$CH_2CH_2OH$$
$$O_2N \quad N \quad CH_3$$
$$N$$

METRONIDAZOLE

Physical Properties

It is a white or yellowish, crystalline powder melting between 159 and 163°C. Though it is stable in air, it darkens on exposure to light. It is slightly soluble in water, ethanol (95%) and acetone. It is very slightly soluble in ether.

Chemical Properties

By heating metronidazole with zinc and hydrochloric acid, it is possible to reduce the nitro group to an amino group which now answers the reactions of primary aromatic amines, that is, it can be diazotised by adding sodium nitrite and coupled with 2-naphtol to give an orange or red azo dye.

126

Stability and Storage

Since it is affected by light, store it in well-closed, light-resistant containers.

Uses

Amoebicide. It is a very effective amoebicide and is used in all types of amoebiasis. It is also used in the treatment of *giardiasis, Trichomonas vaginitis, ulcerative gingivitis and trench mouth, guinea worm infestation and anaerobic infections.*

Official

Metronidazole, I.P., B.P.
Metronidazole Tablets, I.P.
Metronidazole Benzoate, I.P.
Metronidazole Benzoate Oral Suspension, I.P.
Metronidazole Suppositories, B.P.

Brand Names

Flagyl, Metrogyl, Unimezol, Danizol etc.

2. CLIOQUINOL

Clioquinol is a quinoline derivative and contains a chloro group in the 5th position, an iodo group in the 7th position and a hydroxy group in the 8th position of the quinoline nucleus. So it is *5-chloro-7-iodo-8-hydroxyquinoline.*

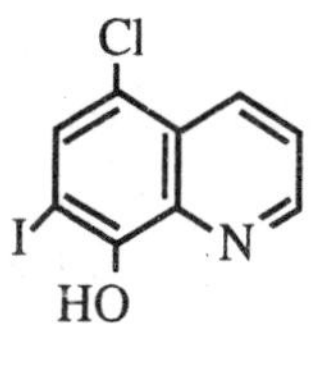

CLIOQUINOL

Physical Properties

Clioquinol is a yellowish white to brownish yellow, voluminous powder It has a faint but characteristic odour. It melts at 178 - 180° (dec). It is affected by light and darkens on exposure to light. It is practically insoluble in water and ethanol (96%) and freely soluble in pyridine and dimethylformamide. It is also soluble in boiling acetic acid and hot ethyl acetate.

Chemical Properties

If the molecule is disintegrated by using oxygen-flask combustion technique, both the chlorine and iodine atoms are released and absorbed in sodium hydroxide solution. By adding silver nitrate, a yellow precipitate is produced (due to silver iodide). Now ammonia is added, shaken well and filtered. The filtrate is acidified with nitric acid. A white precipitate (due to silver chloride) is produced.

Stability and Storage

Since clioquinol is affected by light, store it in well-closed containers, protected from light.

Uses

Antiamoebic drug. Topical and intestinal antiseptic. It has antibacterial and antifungal activity in addition to antiamoebic activity. It is used in creams and ointments for the treatment of skin infections. It is also used along with corticosteroids in infections accompanied by inflammation of the skin.

Note

Since it is found to cause neuritis and optic damage, fixed dose combinations of clioquinol except those used for diarrhoea, dysentery and for external application are banned in India. A caution that it should not be used for more than 14 days should be given on the label.

Official

Quiniodochlor, I.P.
Quiniodochlor Tablets, I.P.
Clioquinol, B.P.
Clioquinol Cream, B.P.
Hydrocortisone Acetate and Clioquinol Ointment, B.P.
Zinc Paste, Calamine and Clioquinol Bandage, B.P.

Brand Names

Enteroquinol, Clioquinol, Enterovioform, Chinioform etc

3. DIIODOHYDROXYQUINOLINE

This is the *5,7-diiododerivative of 8-hydroxyquinoline.*

DIIODOHYDROXYQUINOLINE

Physical Properties

It is a light yellowish to yellowish-brown, microcrystalline powder without odour or with a faint odour only. It is practically insoluble in water and sparingly soluble in ethanol (95%) and ether. It is affected by light.

Chemical Properties

Violet vapours of iodine are evolved when a few crystals of the substance are heated with concentrated sulphuric acid.

Stability and Storage

Since it is affected by light, store in well-closed, light-resistant containers in a cool place.

Uses

Antiamoebic. It can be used in chronic intestinal amoebiasis. It can eradicate cysts from asymptomatic carriers. It is totally useless in the treatment of extraintestinal amoebiasis.

Caution : The caution given earlier under clioquinol applies to this drug also with equal force.

Official

Diiodohydroxyquinoline, I.P.
Diiodohydroxyquinoline Tablets, I.P.

Brand Names

Diodoquin, Iodoquinol, Diiodohydroxyquin etc.

4. DILOXANIDE FUROATE

Diloxanide furoate is the ester of an aromatic alcohol with 2-furoic acid.

Physical Properties

It is a white or almost white, crystalline powder. It melts between 114° and 116°C. It is very slightly soluble in water and slightly soluble in alcohol and ether. It is freely soluble in chloroform.

Chemical Properties

The aromatic alcohol part in the structure of diloxanide furoate contains a dichloroacetamido group. When diloxanide furoate is burnt by the oxygen-flask method using sodium hydroxide solution, the molecule is disintegrated and the chlorine is converted to sodium chloride. The solution gives a white precipitate (of silver chloride) when it is treated with nitric acid and silver nitrate solution.

Stability and Storage

Since it is affected by light, store it in well-closed, light-resistant containers.

Uses

Antiamoebic drug. It is a very effective luminal amoebicide. It eliminates trophozoites which produce cysts.

Official

Diloxanide Furoate, I.P., B.P.
Diloxanide Furoate Tablets, I.P.
(Diloxanide Tablets, B.P.)

Brand Names

Furamide, Histamibal, Miforan.

5. EMETINE

Emetine is an alkaloid obtained by extraction from *Cephaelis ipecacuanha*. It contains a variable amount of water of hydration and forms emetine hydrochloride with two equivalents of hydrochloric acid and seven molecules of water $(E,2HCl,7H_2O)$ Emetine is a white, amorphous powder melting at 74°C. It is affected by light and heat and turns yellow. It is sparingly soluble in water but freely soluble in ethanol, methanol, acetone and chloroform. The following are the properties and other details of emetine hydrochloride which is clinically used.

Physical Properties

Emetine hydrochloride is a white or very slightly yellowish, crystalline powder without odour. It turns a faint yellow on exposure to light. It contains 7 molecules of water of crystallization and the anhydrous salt melts between 235 and 255°C. The solid as well as the aqueous solution turn yellow on exposure to light. It is freely soluble in water and ethanol.

Chemical Properties

If a small quantity of the substance is added to a solution of ammonium molybdate in concentrated sulphuric acid, a bright green colour is formed.

Uses

Antiamoebic drug. Emetine is a very potent amoebicide. It kills trophozoites but does not clear cysts. It is highly effective in curing liver abscess also. It cannot be given orally since it induces vomiting or emesis. So it is always given by s.c. or i.m. injection only. Emetine is very toxic. So the use of emetine has been discontinued and metronidazole is used in its place.

Official

Emetine Hydrochloride, I.P., B.P.
Emetine Hydrochloride Injection, I.P.
Emetine Hydrochloride Pentahydrate, B.P.

B. ANTHELMINTICS

Anthelmintics are drugs which are used for killing or expelling worms. Those which kill the worms are known as *vermicides* and those which expel are known as *vermifuges*. The worms which are parasites are known as helminths. They infect the alimentary canal or other tissues of the host. They can be spread by mosquito bites or by coming into contact with infected animals or infected animal or human excreta or infected water or by eating infected meat. They enter the body in the form of eggs or larvae. Harm is caused to the host by depriving him of food or by injuring the organs or by causing blood loss or by causing obstruction of lympatic system or intestine or by secreting toxins. The usual parasitic worms are *tape worms, round worms, thread worms, hook worms, guinea worms and filarial worms.*

132

The most important anthelmintics are:-

1. Piperazine
2. Diethylcarbamazine citrate (D.E.C.)
3. Mebendazole
4. Paramomycin

1. PIPERAZINE

Piperazine has the following structures:-

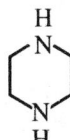

It is official in the I.P. in the form of piperazine adipate, piperazine citrate, piperazine hydrate and piperazine phosphate.

Physical Properties

Piperazine adipate is a white, crystalline powder which is stable to heat and air. It has a pleasant, slightly acid taste. It melts at about 250°C with decomposition. It is soluble in water and practically insoluble in ethanol. It is the neutral salt of adipic acid and piperazine.

Chemical Properties

If an aqueous solution of piperazine adipate is treated with sodium bicarbonate, freshly prepared potassium ferricyanide solution and mercury and shaken vigorously and allowed to stand for 20 minutes, a reddish colour slowly develops.

Stability and Storage

Store in well-closed containers.

User

Anthelmintic. It is used to treat infections caused by round worms and pin worms. It is highly active and gives almost 100% cure.

Official

Piperazine Adipate, I.P., B.P.
Piperazine Adipate Tablets, I.P.
Piperazine Citrate, I.P., B.P.
Piperazine Citrate Syrup, I.P.
Piperazine Hydrate, I.P., B.P.
Piperazine Phosphate, I.P., B.P.
Piperazine Phosphate Tablets, I.P.
Piperazine Citrate Elixir, B.P.

Brand Names

Antepar (citrate with sennosides), Helmacid (phosphate with sennosides).

2. DIETHYLCARBAMAZINE CITRATE

This compound has the following structure:-

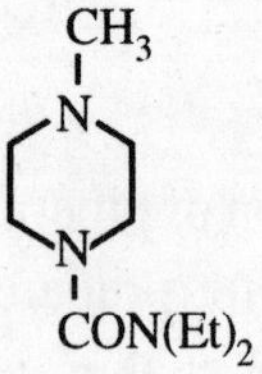

It has the basic structure of piperazine and has a diethylcarbamoyl (-CONEt$_2$) group in the first position and a methyl group in the fourth position. So the systematic name for diethylcarbamazine is *1-diethylcarbamoyl-4-methylpiperazine*.

Physical Properties

It is a white, crystalline powder without odour. It is slightly hygroscopic. It melts at about 138°C with decomposition. It is very soluble in water, soluble in ethanol and practically insoluble in acetone, chloroform and ether.

Chemical Properties

An aqueous solution of the substance gives the reactions of citrates.

Stability and Storage

Since the drug is quite stable to air and moisture, it is enough if it is stored in well-closed containers.

Uses

Anthelmintic. It is the only drug available for the treatment of filariasis. It also produces dramatic cure of tropical eosinophilia.

Official

Diethylcarbamazine Citrate, I.P., B.P.
Diethylcarbamazine Citrate Tablets, I.P.

Brand Names

Hetrazan; Banocide, Caricide etc.

3. MEBENDAZOLE

Mebendazole, structurally, is a benzimidazole derivative.

Physical Properties

Mebendazole is a white to slightly yellow, amorphous powder which is without odour. It melts at about 290°C. It is practically insoluble in water and also in other solvents such as ethanol, ether, chloroform and dichloromethane. It is also insoluble in dilute mineral acids. However it is freely soluble in formic acid. It is affected by light.

Chemical Properties

An intense yellow colour is produced when ethanol, dinitrobenzene solution and sodium hydroxide solution are added to mebendazole.

Stability and Storage

Since it is affected by light, store it in well-closed, light resistant containers.

Uses

Anthelmintic. This is a broad spectrum anthelmintic. It is used mainly to treat infections caused by round worms, thread worms, hook worms and whip worms.

Official

Mebendazole, I.P.
Mebendazole Tablets, I.P.

Brand Names

Mebex, Mendazole, Telmin, Vermirax etc.

4. PAROMOMYCIN

Paramomycin is an aminoglycoside antibiotic which has a structure very similar to that of neomycin. It is actually a mixture of two substances, paramomycins I and II. It is a white, amorphous powder soluble in water. It is used as the sulphate which is very soluble in water. It is stored in well-closed containers. Paramomycin was formerly used for tape worm infestation. It is no longer used for this purpose.

Other anthelmintics which are clinically used are *albendazole, pyrantel pamoate, levamisole, tetramisole, bephenium hydroxynapthoate, thiabendazole, niclosamide, praziquantel etc.*

CHAPTER - 11

ANTIMALARIALS

Malaria is caused by species of *Plasmodium* which are protozoan parasites.

There are two hosts for all species of Plasmodium, man and mosquito. The mosquito bites and gives the infection to man. Through the bite sporozoites are injected into the circulation. They grow, multiply and form spores in the liver. This is the preerythrocytic stage and the organisms are known as merozoites. They are released from the liver and infect the red blood cells, where the merozoites grow and divide. The red blood cells then burst and release the merozoites into the blood where they will infect more red blood cells. At this stage only chillness and fever are felt by the affected man. Some of the merozoites develop into male and female gametocytes. When mosquito bites the man, the gametocytes enter the gut of the female mosquitoes and undergo sporogony to form sporozoites and the cycle is repeated.

The drugs used in malaria are of different types. Some like quinine and chloroquine are used to kill the erythrocytic form in the blood and reduce the fever. They are known as suppressives. Drugs like primaquine kill the gametocytes and tissue forms so that further spread of infection and reinfection are prevented. They may be given along with a suppressive drug.

CLASSIFICATION

They can be classified as below:

(a) **Quinine salts :** like quinine hydrochloride, quinine dihydrochloride, quinine sulphate etc.

(b) 4-Aminoquinolines
  (1) Chloroquine
  (2) Amodiaquine.

(c) 8-Aminoquinolines
  Primaquine

(d) Biguanides
  Proguanil hydrochloride

(e) Diaminopyrimidines
  (1) Pyrimethamine
  (2) Trimethoprim.

1. QUININE

Quinine is an alkaloid extracted from the barks of plants belonging to the species of *Cinchona*. These plants are native to South America but are also cultivated in India (in the Nilgiris in Tamilnadu and in Bengal) and in Java. *Cinchona ledgeriana* is rich in quinine yielding about 6 to 10% of the alkaloid. About 35 different alkaloids and organic bases have been isolated from cinchona. The most abundant and the most important cinchona alkaloids are quinine, quinidine, cinchonine and cinchonidine. Structurally, quinine is made up of one quinoline ring and one quinuclidine ring linked by a –CHOH group. The structure of quinidine is given in the chapter on "Antiarrhythmic Agents". It may be taken as the structure of quinine also, sine both are stereoisomers.

Physical Properties

Quinine crystallises with 3 molecules of water and melts at 57°C. This compound is efflorescent or loses water when exposed to the atmosphere. When it is heated, all 3 water molecules are lost at 110°C. The anhydrous quinine melts at 172.8°C. It has an intensely bitter taste. It is very sparingly soluble in water but readily soluble in common organic solvents. It is also soluble in aqueous ammonia.

Quinine forms two series of salts, that is, the neutral salt and the acid salt. The monacid or neutral salts are much less soluble in water than the diacid or acid salts. Thus quinine sulphate is much less soluble in water (1 in 810) than quinine bisulphate. Similarly quinine hydrochloride is soluble 1 in 23 and the dihydrochloride is soluble 1 in 0.5. Quinine forms various other salts such as phosphate, salicylate, hydrobromide, glycerophosphate etc.

Chemical Properties

If quinine or any of its salts is dissolved in a hydroxy acid such as sulphuric, tartaric or phosphoric acid, it exhibits a strong blue fluroescence. If any quinine salt is dissolved in water and saturated bromine water and enough dilute ammonia to make it distinctly alkaline are added to the solution, an emerald green colour is produced. This is known as the Thalleioquin test.

Stability and Storage

Quinine and its salts should be stored in well-closed, light-resistant containers, since they are affected by light.

Uses

Antimalarial. It is an erythrocytic schizontocide for all types of Plasmodium species, acting as a suppressive. It is especially useful for the treatment of resistant falciparum malaria and it is the drug of choice for cerebral malaria.

Official

Quinine Bisulphate, I.P., B.P.
Quinine Bisulphate Tablets, I.P., B.P.
Quinine Dihydrochloride, I.P., B.P.
Quinine Dihydrochloride Injection, I.P.
Quinine Sulphate, I.P., B.P.
Quinine Sulphate Tablets, I.P., B.P.
Quinine Hydrochloride, B.P.

Brand Names

Quinine Sulphate, Quininga, Quinine Di HCl etc.

2. CHLOROQUINE

Structurally chloroquine is a 4-aminoquinoline derivative.

4-Aminoquinolines : Quinoline, a heterocyclic compound, has the structure and numbering given below:

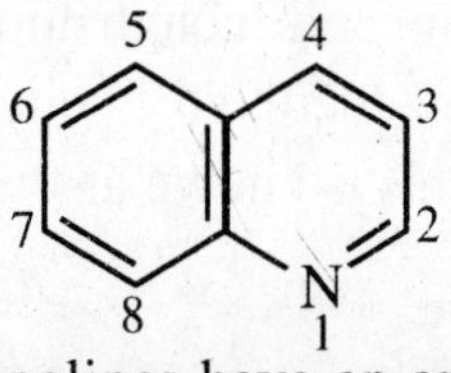

The 4-aminoquinolines have an amino group in the 4th position of the quinoline nucleus and this amino group is substituted.

For ex: in chloroquine 1-methylbutyamine

$$\begin{matrix} CH_3 & & & & \\ | & & & & \\ -\underset{1}{CH} & \underset{2}{CH_2} & \underset{3}{CH_2} & \underset{4}{CH_2} & NH_2 \end{matrix}$$

is substituted in the 4-amino group. In addition the amino group attached to the 4th carbon atom in this 1-methylbutylamine is also substituted with two ethyl groups, so that the group now becomes 4-diethylamino-1-methylbutyl group.

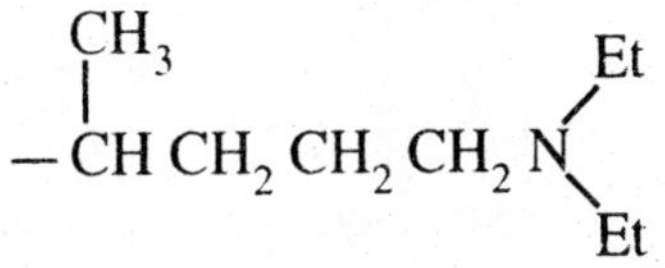

$$\overset{\overset{\displaystyle CH_3}{|}}{-CH}\ CH_2\ CH_2\ CH_2\ N\overset{\nearrow Et}{\underset{\searrow Et}{}}$$

Chloroquine has also a chlorine at the 7th position of the quinoline nucleus. Therefore chloroquine has the structure and systematic name shown below:

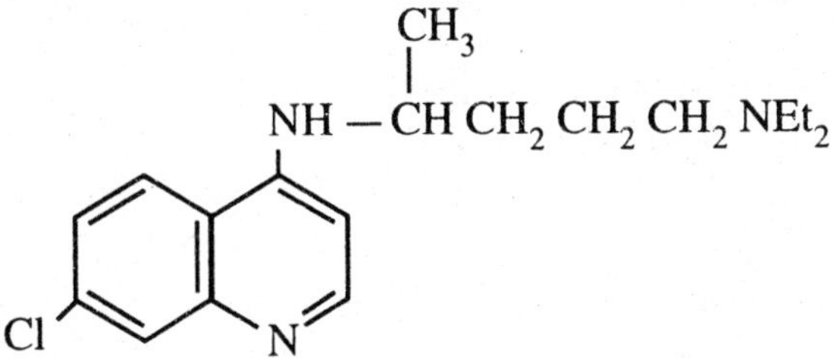

$$NH-\overset{\overset{\displaystyle CH_3}{|}}{CH}\ CH_2\ CH_2\ CH_2\ NEt_2$$

CHLOROQUINE

7-chloro-4-(4-diethylamino-1-methylbutylamino) quinoline.

Physical Properties

Chloroquine is a white or slightly yellow, odourless, crystalline powder. It is odourless and has an intensely bitter taste. It is soluble in water, ether and chloroform. It is used as chloroquine phosphate and as chloroquine sulphate.

Chloroquine phosphate is a white or almost white, crystalline powder which has no odour. It is affected by light and slowly gets discoloured. It exists in two polymorphic forms. One of these forms melts at 195°C and the other form melts at 218°C. It is freely soluble in water and very slightly soluble in ethanol, ether, chloroform and methanol.

141

Chemical Properties

Chloroquine phosphate, on treatment with picric acid, forms chloroquine picrate which, after thorough washing with water, ethanol and ether and drying, melts at a temperature between 205°C and 210°C. It also answers the test for phosphates. In this test the substance is treated with sodium hydroxide solution and extracted with chloroform to remove the chloroquine base. The aqueous layer which contains only the phosphate is neutralised with nitric acid, ammonium molybdate solution is added and warmed. A yellow precipitate is produced.

Stability and Storage

Since it is affected by light, store it in well-closed, light-resistant containers.

Uses

Antimalarial. It is a suppressive in malaria and is the drug of choice in all types of malaria. It is also used in the treatment of lupus erythematosus, rheumatoid arthritis and extraintestinal amoebiasis. It is well absorbed by the oral or parenteral route.

Official

Chloroquine Phosphate, I.P., B.P.
Chloroquine Phosphate Injection, I.P., B.P.
Chloroquine Phosphate Tablets, I.P., B.P.
Chloroquine Sulphate, I.P., B.P.
Chloroquine Sulphate Injection, I.P., B.P.
Chloroquine Sulphate Tablets, I.P., B.P.
Chloroquine Syrup, I.P.

Brand Names

Nivaquine, Lariago, Resochin, Avlochlor, Ciplaquine, Miniquin etc.

3. AMODIAQUINE

Amodiaquine is also a 4-aminoquinoline derivative. Amodiaquine is official as the hydrochloride. Actually it is a dihydrochloride.

Physical Properties

Amodiaquine hydrochloride is a yellow, crystalline powder with almost no odour. It is soluble in water, sparingly soluble in ethanol and practically insoluble in chloroform and ether. It melts at about 158°C.

Chemical Properties

When cobalt thiocyanate solution is added to an aqueous solution of the substance, a green precipitate is produced.

Stability and Storage

Since it is fairly stable in air, store it in tightly closed containers.

Uses

Antimalarial. It is also a suppressive drug used in the same way as chloroquine. WHO recommended in 1990 that it should not be used, since it is toxic to liver and bone marrow.

Official

Amodiaquine Hydrochloride, I.P.
Amodiaquine Hydrochloride Tablets, I.P.

Brand Names

Camoquin, Basoquin, Flavoquine, Miaquine etc.

4. PRIMAQUINE

Primaquine is an 8-aminoquinoline derivative which means that the aminoalkylamino group is present at the 8th position of the quinoline nucleus. Actually it is official as the diphosphate which is clinically used.

Physical Properties

Primaquine phosphate is an orange, crystalline powder. It has no odour. It melts at about 200°C. It is soluble in water and practically insoluble in ethanol and ether. It is affected by light.

Chemical Properties

As in the case of chloroquine phosphate, this substance also can be decomposed with sodium hydroxide solution and the liberated primaquine base extracted with chloroform. The aqueous layer can be acidified with nitric acid, ammonium molybdate solution added and warmed. A yellow precipitate is produced. Here the phosphate component of the substance answers the test.

Stability and Storage

Since it is affected by light, store it in well-closed, light-resistant containers.

Uses

Antimalarial. It is now used only for the radical cure of relapsing malaria.

Official

Primaquine Phosphate, I.P., B.P.
Primaquine Phosphate Tablets, I.P.
(Primaquine Tablets, B.P.)

Brand Names

Primaquine, Primachin phosphate, SN-13, 272 etc.

5. PROGUANIL HYDROCHLORIDE

Proguanil is a biguanide derivative.

Physical Properties

Proguanil hydrochloride is a white, crystalline powder which has no odour. It is slightly soluble in water and soluble in ethanol. It is practically insoluble in chloroform and ether.

Chemical Properties

If potassium ferrocyanide solution is added to a saturated solution of the substance, a white precipitate is produced. It dissolves on adding a few drops of dilute nitric acid. If a small quantity of the substance is dissolved in a warm solution of cetrimide and sodium hydroxide and bromine solutions are added, a deep red colour is produced.

Stability and Storage

Since it is affected by light, store it in well-closed, light-resistant containers.

Uses

Antimalarial. It is a slow suppressive and acts also on gametocytes and tissue forms.

Official

Proguanil Hydrochloride, I.P., B.P.
Proguanil Hydrochloride Tablets, I.P.
(Proguanil Tablets, B.P.)

Brand Names

Paludrine, Proguanide hydrochloride, SN-12, 837 etc.

6. PYRIMETHAMINE

Pyrimethamine belongs to the series of compounds known as 2, 4-diamino-5-arylpyrimidines.

Diaminopyrimidines : Pyrimethamine is a derivative of pyrimidine which is a six-membered ring with two nitrogens in the 1 and 3 positions. It has two amino groups in the 2nd and 4th positions, one 4-chlorophenyl group in the 5th position and one ethyl group in the 6th position.

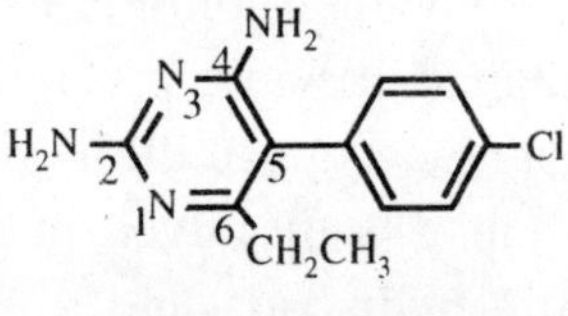

PYRIMETHAMINE
[2, 4 –Diamino –5–(4–chlorophenyl) –6–ethyl pyrimidine]

Properties

Pyrimethamine occurs as colourless crystals or as an almost white, crystalline powder. It has no odour. It melts at 239° to 243°C. It is practically insoluble in water, slightly soluble in chloroform and ethanol and very slightly soluble in ether. It is soluble in boiling ethanol. It is affected by light.

Stability and Storage

Since it is affected by light, store it in well-closed, light-resistant containers.

Uses

Antimalarial. It is a slowly acting *erythrocytic schizontocide*. It functions as a casual prophylactic for falciparum malaria. For vivax malaria it is a suppressive prophylactic. It is nowadays used in combination with a sulphonamide such as sulfadoxine or sulfomethopyrazine or dapsone. This combination is more potent.

Official

Pyrimethamine, I.P., B.P.
Pyrimethamine and Sulphadoxine Tablets, I.P.
Pyrimethamine Tablets, B.P.

Brand Names

Daraprim, Pyridex (Pyrimethamine)

Malocide, Malarprim, Croydoxin-FM, Rimodar, Fancidar (Pyrimethamine + sulfadoxine)

Metakelfin (Pyrimethamine + sulfamethopyrazine)

Maloprim (Pyrimethamine+dapsone)

7. TRIMETHOPRIM

Trimethoprim is also a pyrimidine derivative with a trimethoxybenzyl in the 5th position and two amino groups in the 2nd and the 4th positions.

Physical Properties

It is a white or yellowish-white powder without odour or almost without odour. It melts between 199° and 203°C. It is very slightly soluble in water, slightly soluble in ethanol, sparingly soluble in chloroform and practically insoluble in ether.

Stability and Storage

Store in well-closed containers.

Uses

Antimalarial. It is mainly an antibacterial but has some antimalarial action also. It is used in combination with a sulphonamide such as sulphamethoxazole which is known as cotrimoxazole.

Official

Trimethoprim, I.P., B.P.
Trimethoprim Tablets, I.P., B.P.
Trimethoprim and Sulphamethoxazole Oral
                          Suspension, I.P.
(Co-trimoxazole Oral Suspension, B.P.)
Trimethoprim and Sulphamethoxazole Tablets, I.P.
(Co-trimoxazole Tablets, B.P.)
Co-trimoxazole Injection, B.P.
Paediatric Co-trimoxazole Oral Suspension, B.P.
Dispersible Co-trimoxazole Tablets, B.P.
Paediatric Co-trimoxazole Tablets, B.P.

Brand Names

Septran, Bactrim, Septrim, Gantaprim, Teleprim etc.

Other antimalarials clinically used are *hydroxy-chloroquine, mefloquine, mepacrine, cycloguanil pamoate etc.*

CHAPTER - 12

CENTRAL NERVOUS SYSTEM STIMULANTS

Central nervous system stimulants are drugs which stimulate and increase the activity of some parts of brain and spinal cord. Since they are not very selective in action, they are therapeutically not so useful as, for example, hypnotics and sedatives. Moreover excessive stimulation is followed by depression. Some of these drugs which directly stimulate the C.N.S. including the respiratory centre are known as analeptics. They are able to reverse the respiratory depression caused by carbon dioxide accumulation due to respiratory disease or post-surgical respiratory depression. Those which stimulate the sensory areas of the brain increase mental alertness and delay fatigue and drowsiness and this produces a state of wakefulness.

CLASSIFICATION

They can be classified into drugs of natural origin and synthetic compounds.

I. Naturally occuring

1. Caffeine
2. Theophylline $\left.\right\}$ xanthine derivatives

II. Synthetic

1. Nikethamide (coramine)
2. Dextroamphetamine (dexedrine)

1. CAFFEINE

Caffeine is *1,3,7-trimethylxanthine*. Three methyl groups are substituted at positions 1, 3 and 7 in xanthine which is the basic compound.

CAFFEINE

(1,3,7-trimethylxanthine)

Caffeine occurs in coffee (1 to 1.5%), tea (1 to 4.8%), mate (1.24 to 2%), guaraña (3.1 to 5%) and kola (2.7 to 3.6%). It also occurs in a small quantity along with theobromine in cocoa. It is usually extracted from damaged tea or tea dust. It is also synthesised from uric acid which occurs in abundant quantities in guano.

Physical Properties

Caffeine consists of silky white crystals or white glistering needles or occurs as a white, crystalline powder. It is odourless. Caffeine, I.P. is either the anhydrous substance or the monohydrate. After drying the substance at 100°C, it melts at 234-239°C. It is sparingly soluble in cold water (1 in 60) and ethanol and freely soluble in hot water and chloroform. It is slightly soluble in ether. It is soluble in concentrated solutions of and forms water-soluble complexes in benzoates, citrates, cinnamates and salicylates. Since it is a weak base, it readily forms salts. Its aqueous solutions are neutral to litmus. As already stated, its salts are readily soluble in water but when more water is added, they undergo hydrolysis with separation of caffeine. About 60 mg of caffeine are present in a cup of tea or coffee.

Chemical Properties

When caffeine is treated with hydrochloric acid and potassium chlorate (concentrated nitric acid also can be used in place of HCl and potassium chlorate), evaporated to dryness on a water bath and the residue exposed to the vapours of dilute ammonia solution (or one drop of dilute ammonia may be added to the residue), a purple colour is produced. The colour disappears on the addition of dilute sodium hydroxide solution. Caffeine also gives a white precipitate of caffeine tannate when treated with tannic acid solution. Caffeine tannate dissolves when excess of tannic acid solution is added. Caffeine is not precipitated by iodine in neutral solution. But when a few drops of dilute hydrochloric acid are added, a brown precipitate is formed. It dissolves on neutralisation with sodium hydroxide solution.

Stability and Storage

Since caffeine is slightly efflorescent, store it in tightly-closed containers.

Uses

Central nervous system stimulant. It is usually used as a stimulant in combination with an analgesic like aspirin. It has no analgesic action itself. It is also used to treat migraine in combination with ergotamine.

Official

Caffeine, I.P.
Aspirin and Caffeine Tablets, I.P., B.P.
Caffeine, B.P. (Anhydrous Caffeine)
Caffeine Hydrate, B.P.

Brand Names

Guaranine, Thein, Coffeine
Cafergot (Caffeine + ergotamine)
Micropyrin (Caffeine + aspirin)

151

2. THEOPHYLLINE

Theophylline is also a xanthine derivative like caffeine. In the structure of theophylline there are only two methyl groups present at positions 1 and 3. There is no methyl group at position 7 as in caffeine. So theophylline is *1, 3–dimethylxyanthine* (see the structure of caffeine).

Physical Properties

Theophylline is a white, odourless, crystalline powder. It melts at 270-274°C. It is slightly soluble in water and chloroform, sparingly soluble in ethanol and very slightly soluble in ether. It is soluble in mineral acids, aqueous solutions of alkali hydroxides and ammonia.

Chemical Properties

If to an aqueous solution of theophylline, mercuric acetate solution is added and allowed to stand, a white, crystalline precipitate is produced. It also answers the reaction of xanthines. In this reaction, theophylline is mixed with hydrogen peroxide solution and dilute hydrochloric acid and heated to dryness on a water bath until a yellowish-red residue is produced. If dilute ammonia is added to the residue, the colour of the residue changes to reddish-violet.

Stability and Storage

Store in well-closed containers.

Uses

Central nervous system stimulant. It is more useful as a bronchodilator and diuretic than as a C.N.S. stimulant. It is mostly used in combination with ethylenediamine (aminophylline) in severe bronchial asthma especially in status asthmaticus. It is also used to relieve apnoea (suspended respiration or temporary cessation of breathing due to any cause) in premature infants.

Official

Theophylline, I.P., B.P.
Theophylline Injection, I.P.
Aminophylline, I.P.
Aminophylline Injection, I.P., B.P.
Aminophylline Tablets, I.P.

Brand Names

Theolong, Theosal, Theocontin etc.,
Aminophylline (Theophylline+ethylenediamine),
Deriphylline (Hydroxyethyltheophylline) and
Choliphylline (Choline theophyllinate).

3. NIKETHAMIDE OR CORAMINE

Nikethamide is the *diethylamide of nicotinic acid*. It is derived from the amide of nicotinic acid, nicotinamide.

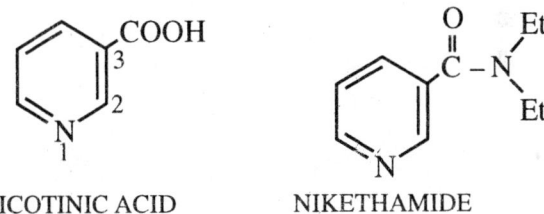

NICOTINIC ACID   NIKETHAMIDE

Physical Properties

It is a colourless or slightly yellowish, oily liquid or crystalline mass depending on the temperature. It has a slight, characteristic odour and a faintly bitter taste which is accompanied by a sensation of warmth. It melts at 24-26°C and boils at 296-300°C. It is miscible with water, ethanol, ether and chloroform.

153

Chemical Properties

When nikethamide is heated with dilute sodium hydroxide solution, diethylamine is evolved and it can be recognised by its odour and the fumes also turn red litmus blue. A yellow colour is produced when an aqueous solution of nikethamide is mixed with cyanogen bromide solution and aniline.

Stability and Storage

Store in well-closed containers.

Uses

C.N.S. stimulant. It was formerly used to counteract the respiratory depression caused by depressants such as barbiturates. Now it is no longer used.

Official

Nikethamide, I.P., B.P.
Nikethamide Injection, I.P., B.P.

4. DEXTROAMPHETAMINE

Dextroamphetamine is the dextro isomer of amphetamine which is a racemic mixture of dextro and laevo isomers. It is prepared by resolution of the racemic mixture by fractional crystallization of the D-tartrates. Structurally amphetamine is 2-aminopropylbenzene. Dexamphetamine is official as the sulphate.

Physical Properties

Dexamphetamine sulphate is a white or almost white, crystalline powder. It is odourless. It is freely soluble in water, slightly soluble in ethanol and practically insoluble in ether.

Chemical Properties

Dexamphetamine can be benzoylated by treatment with dilute sodium hydroxide solution and benzoyl chloride. The benzoyl derivative is precipitated. After recrystallisation from ethanol, it melts at about 157°C. If dexamphetamine is dissolved in water and dilute hydrochloric acid, diazotised nitroaniline solution, dilute sodium hydroxide solution and n-butanol are added, shaken and allowed to separate, a red colour is produced in the butanol layer.

Stability and Storage

Keep it well-closed containers.

Uses

C.N.S. stimulant. It acts centrally and produces increased alertness, increased concentration, increased work capacity and euphoria. It is used to stimulate the C.N.S. in narcolepsy (tendency to fall asleep) and in treating certain psychogenic depressive conditions. It is also used in the management of obesity (accumulation of excess fat in the body.) It is also used as an anorexic (agent causing loss of appetite).

This is *a drug of abuse and a dangerous drug of addiction.* Excessive use of the drug may produce tolerance and physical dependence.

Official

Dexamphetamine Sulphate, B.P.
Dexamphetamine Tablets, B.P.

Brand Names

Dexedrine, Dexamphetamine sulphate, Dexampex, Dexten etc.

CHAPTER - 13

Central Nervous System Depressants

GENERAL ANAESTHETICS

General anaesthetics are depressants of the central nervous system. They are supposed to particularly depress the ascending reticular activating system in the brain which is responsible for maintaining a state of wakefulness. Therefore they produce a total or partial insensibility to pain and also temporary loss of consciousness. This is known as anaesthesia. It is necessary to produce anaesthesia for certain surgical operations to be carried out.

CLASSIFICATION

I. Volatile Anaesthetics or Inhalation Anaesthetics.

1. Diethyl ether
2. Cyclopropane
3. Trichloroethylene
4. Halothane

II. Non-volatile Anaesthetics or Intravenous Anaesthetics

1. Thiopentone sodium
2. Methohexital sodium

1. ETHER (DIETHYL ETHER)

Ether has the structure $C_2H_5-O-C_2H_5$. There are two types of ether, that is solvent ehter and anaesthetic ether. Only anaesthetic ether is used as a general anaesthetic.

Properties

Ether is a clear, colourless, volatile and very mobile liquid with a characteristic odour. It has a sweet, burning taste. It is highly inflammble. Particular care has to be taken to keep it away from naked flame, since it is highly inflammable. It is very volatile at room temperature and boils at 35°C. When exposed to air, moisture or light, it forms explosive peroxides. It is soluble in water and miscible with alcohol, chloroform, benzene, petroleum ether and with fixed and volatile oils.

Peroxides should not be allowed to be formed in anaesthetic ether since they are poisonous. Addition of aromatic amines, aminophenols, polyphenols and naphthols is required to promote the stability of ether and prevent the formation of peroxides. Usually a non-volatile substance such as hydroquinone or propyl gallate in a concentration not exceeding 0.002% is used as the preservative. If peroxides are already present in a sample of ether, they can be removed by shaking the ether with a solution of a reducing agent in water such as ferrous sulphate or sodium hydrosulphite or catechol. They can also be removed by filtering through activated alumina.

The identification tests given for anaesthetic ether in B.P. are its distillation range and relative density. The distillation range of ether is a good index of its purity. Common impurities such as alcohols and acetone raise the upper limit of its distillation range. Pure anaesthetic ether is required to distil between 34°C and 35°C. Precautions should be taken to avoid using naked flame for heating ether. The relative density of anaesthetic ether is required to be between 0.714 and 0.716.

Stability and Storage

It should be kept in a securely closed, airtight, dry container, protected from light and stored in a cool place at a temperature of 8°C to 15°C. Contents in a partially filled or partly used container may deteriorate rapidly. The label must state the nature and the concentration of any added non-volatile antioxidant.

Uses

General Anaesthetic. It is a potent general anaesthetic producing good analgesia and good muscular relaxation. Even though induction is prolonged and unpleasant and recovery is slow with complications like nausea and vomiting, it is still preferred for use in poor developing countries since it is cheap and can be administered by even inexperienced staff.

Other uses of ether include its use as a solvent for alkaloids, fats, oils, waxes, gums etc., and as a reagent in organic syntheses. It is also used in the isolation and extraction of many natural products such as alkaloids etc., from their natural sources.

Official

Anaesthetic Ether, I.P., B.P.

Brand Names

Ether, Sulphuric ether, Anaesthetic ether, Ethyl oxide.

2. CYCLOPROPANE

Cyclopropane is cyclic trimethylene.

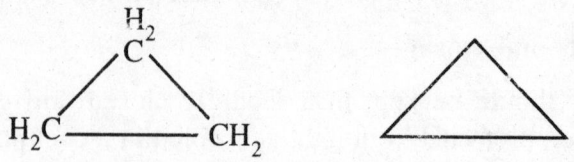

Properties

Cyclopropane is a colourless gas with a characteristic odour. It has a pungent taste. It is freely soluble in water (1 in 2.85) and very soluble in ethanol, ether and chloroform. It is absorbed by concentrated sulphuric acid readily. Mixtures of cyclopropane with air or oxygen in concentrations ranging from 3 to 8.5% of oxygen are explosive.

Stability and Storage

It is stored under pressure in metal cylinders in a cool place. The cylinder should be painted orange and either the name of the gas cyclopropane or its symbol C_3H_6 should be stencilled on the cylinder.

Uses

Genereral Anaesthetic. It is now no longer used.

Official

Cyclopropane, I.P.

3. TRICHLOROETHYLENE

Trichloroethylene is 1-chloro-2, 2-dichloroethylene.

$$HCCl = CCl_2$$

Properties

It is clear, colourless or pale blue liquid which is mobile and non-inflammable. It has an odour which is very much like that of chloroform. It boils at 88°C. It is decomposed by light especially when moisture is present and hydrochloric acid is produced. It is practically insoluble in water but miscible with alcohol, chloroform and ether. Thymol (0.001%) and ammonium carbonate are used as preservatives for trichloro-ethylene. When trichloroethylene and bromine water are shaken together for one hour in a stoppered glass cylinder at intervals of fifteen minutes, a white turbid solution is formed in the lower layer. This is a test to distinguish trichloroethylene from other halohydrocarbons such as chloroform and carbon tetrachloride which remain clear.

Stability and Storage

It should be stored in tightly-closed, light-resistant containers in a cool place.

Uses

General anaesthetic. It is no longer used.

Official

Trichloroethylene, I.P.'85.

Brand Names

Trilene, Gemalgene, Trichloran etc.

4. HALOTHANE.

Its structure is CF_3-CHBrCl. It is a derivative of ethane CH_3-CH_3. The three hydrogen atoms at the first carbon atom are replaced by three fluorine atoms. Two hydrogen atoms at the second carbon atom are displaced by one bromine atom and one chlorine atom. Therefore halothane is *2-bromo-2-chloro-1, 1,1-trifluoroethane*.

Properties

Halothane is a clear, colourless, mobile, heavy, highly volatile liquid. It is non-inflammable. It has a characteristic odour very much like that of chloroform. It boils at 50°C. In the presence of moisture it reacts with many metals. It is slightly soluble in water but miscible with other liquids like chloroform, absolute alcohol, ether, trichloroethylene and fixed oils.

Stability and Storage

It should be kept in an airtight container which should be protected from light and kept at a temperature below 25°C. It should not be stored in a container made of any metal with which it may react.

Uses

General anaesthetic. At present it is a popular anaesthetic since it is non-irritant, non-inflammable, pleasant and rapidly acting. However, it is not a good analgesic or muscle relaxant. It also causes profound hypotension and is toxic to the liver.

Official

Halothane, B.P.

Brand Names

Fluothane, Bromochlorotrifluoroethane, Rhodialothan.

5. THIOPENTONE SODIUM

Thiopentone is a short-acting barbiturate. It is used in the form of thiopentone sodium. For detailed explanation of general structure, refer Hypnotics and Sedatives. Thiopentone has one ethyl group and one 1-methylbutyl group at the 5th position. In addition the oxygen at the 2nd position is replaced by a sulphur atom. Therefore thiopentone is *5-ethyl-5-(1-methylbutyl)-2-thiobarbiturate*. It is official as the sodium salt.

$$S=C \begin{array}{c} N = C \cdot ONa \\ \diagdown \\ NH \longrightarrow C \\ \parallel \\ O \end{array} \begin{array}{c} CH_2CH_3 \\ C \\ \diagdown \\ CHCH_2CH_2CH_3 \\ \mid \\ CH_3 \end{array}$$

THIOPENTONE SODIUM

(Sodium 5-ethyl-5-(1-methylbutyl)-2-thiobarbiturate)

Actually thiopentone or thiopental has the same structure as pentobarbitone. The only difference is that thiopentone has a sulphur atom in place of the oxygen atom at position 2.

Physical Properties

Thiopentone sodium is a white to yellowish-white powder with an alliaceous odour faintly resembling the odour of garlic. It is hygroscopic. It is freely soluble in water, partly soluble in ethanol and practically insoluble in benzene, ether and petroleum ether. Aqueous solution of thiopentone sodium is alkaline to litmus. The aqueous solution slowly decomposes and deposits thiopentone on boiling. Carbon dioxide also causes precipitation of thiopentone. Thiopentone Sodium, I.P. is a mixture of thiopentone and anhydrous sodium carbonate. It is affected by light.

Chemical Properties

Thiopentone base may be precipitated by acidifying an aqueous solution of thiopentone sodium with dilute acetic acid. The precipitate may be filtered, recrystallised from water and dried at 70°C. The crystals melt at about 160°C. The thiopentone crystals may be dissolved in dilute sodium hydroxide solution and to the solution are added sodium nitroprusside and after 15 minutes, dilute hydrochloric acid. A reddish violet colour is produced.

Stability and Storage

It should be stored in tightly closed, light-resistant. containers.

Uses

General anaesthetic. Thiopentone is a non-irritant, ultrashort acting thiobarbiturate. Even though it induces anaesthesia quickly, it is a poor analgesic and a poor muscle relaxant. So an opiod or nitrous oxide should also be administered. It can be used as a simple anaesthetic for painless, short operations. Thiopentone is commonly used as the inducing agent for general anaesthesia.

Official

Thiopentone Sodium, I.P., B.P.
Thiopentone Sodium Injection, I.P.
(Thiopentone Injection, B.P.)

Brand Names

Pentothal, Intraval sodium, Nesdonal sodium, Thionembutal etc.

6. METHOHEXITAL SODIUM

Methohexitone sodium or methohexital sodium contains an allyl group and a 1-methyl-2-pentynyl group in the 5th position and a methyl group in the 1st postion. It is not a thiobarbiturate.

Properties

It is a white, hygroscopic powder without odour. It is soluble in water and insoluble in organic solvents. It melts at 92-96°C. It is affected by moisture, carbon dioxide and light. It is used in the form of an intravenous injection and solution is made in carbon dioxide-free water immediately before injection.

Stability and Storage

Since it is affected by moisture, carbon dioxide and light, it must be stored in tightly-closed, light-resistant containers.

Uses

General anaesthetic. It is like thiopentone but is 3 times more powerful and also has quicker and more brief action. It is not official in I.P. or B.P.

Brand Names

Brevital sodium, Brietal sodium, Brevimytal sodium etc.

Other general anaesthetics clinically used are *methoxy-flurane, enflurane, isoflurane, nitrous oxide, propofol, etomidate, diazepam, lorazepam, midazolam, ketamine, fentanyl, droperidol etc.*

CHAPTER - 14

Central Nervous System Depressants

HYPNOTICS AND SEDATIVES

Hypnotics are drugs which produce sleep and so are used in cases of insomnia (sleeplessness). Sedatives are drugs which reduce excitement and cause sedation. The same drug may act as a hypnotic or sedative or both depending upon the dose. Hypnotics and sedatives depress the central nervous system for producing sleep and sedation.

CLASSIFICATION

a) Cyclic ureides or barbiturates
1. Phenobarbitone
2. Butobarbitone
3. Cyclobarbitone

b) Aldehyde
Paraldehyde

c) Benzodiazepine
Nitrazepam

d) Miscellaneous
1. Methyprylone
2. Glutethimide
3. Triclofos sodium

a) Barbiturates : Barbiturates are further subdivided into (1) long-acting. (2) intermediate-acting and (3) ultra-short acting barbiturates. The first two are used as sedatives and hypnotics and the last, viz, ultra-short acting barbiturates are useful as general anaesthetics (eg:thiopentone). The sodium salts of barbiturates are freely soluble in water.

Structures : The points to be noted are : (1) The substituents at position 5, (2) in the case of sodium salts, enolization and formation of the sodium salt at position 4.

Long-acting barbiturates

Barbitone is 5,5-diethyl bartituric acid.

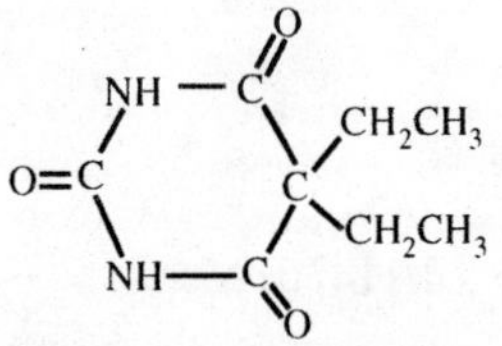

BARBITONE

Barbitone sodium is the *sodium salt of 5,5-diethylbarbituric acid.*

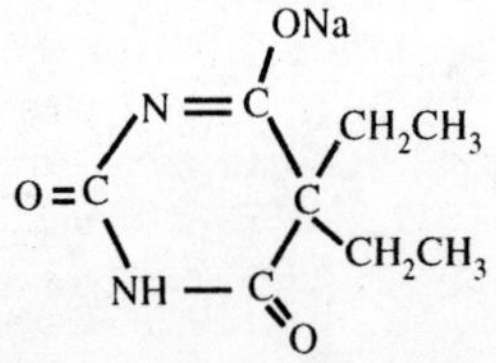

BARBITONE SODIUM

The hydrogen atom has migrated from position 3 to postion 4 forming an enolic –OH which is converted into a sodium salt –ONa by sodium hydroxide. In the process, a double bond is also created between 3 and 4.

166

Phenobarbitone

This differs from barbitone in having one phenyl group at position 5. The othe group remains as ethyl.

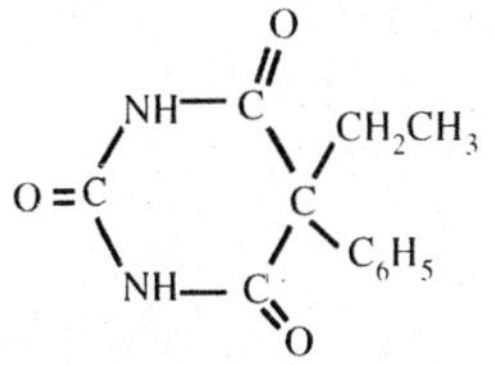

PHENOBARBITONE 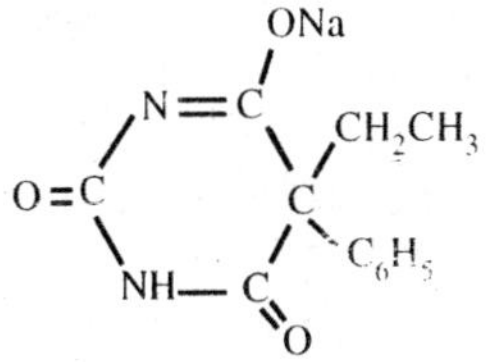   PHENOBARBITONE SODIUM

1. PHENOBARBITONE

Phenobarbitone is a long acting barbiturate. It is a derivative of barbituric acid and its structure has been explained above.

Physical Properties

It consists of colourless crystals or occurs as a white, crystalline powder. It has no odour. It is very slightly soluble in water. It is soluble in ethanol and ether and sparingly soluble in chloroform. It is soluble in aqueous solutions of alkali hydroxides and alkali carbonates.

Phenobarbitone sodium is a white, hygroscopic, bitter, crystalline powder or it may occur as crystalline granules or flaky crystals. It is freely soluble in carbon dioxide-free water, soluble in ethanol and practically insoluble in ether. Aqueous solution of phenobarbitone sodium is alkaline to phenolphthalein and litmus.

Chemical Properties

When phenobarbitone is dissolved in ethanol and one drop of cobalt chloride solution and one drop of dilute ammonia

167

solution are added, a violet colour is produced. If pheno-barbitone or phenobarbitone sodium is dissolved in methanol and a mixture of cobaltous chloride and calcium chloride solutions is added to this solution and then after mixing and shaking, dilute sodium hydroxide solution is added, a violet-blue colour and a precipitate are produced.

Stability and Storage

Since the compound may be affected by carbon dioxide of the atmosphere (especially phenobarbitone sodium), store them in tightly closed containers.

Uses

Sedative, hypnotic and anticonvulsant. Pheno-barbitone is mainly used as an anticonvulsant and seldom used as sedative and hypnotic nowadays. It is a valuable antiepileptic drug. It is used to treat grand mal and status epilepticus.

Official

Phenobarbitone, I.P., B.P.
Phenobarbitone Tablets, I.P., B.P.
Phenobarbitone Sodium, I.P., B.P.
Phenobarbitone Sodium Injection, I.P.
(Phenobarbitone Injection, B.P.)
Phenobarbitone Sodium Tablets, I.P., B.P.
Phenobarbitone Elixir, B.P.

Brand Names

For phenobarbitone : Gardenal, Luminal, Dormiral, Euneryl, Somonal etc.

For phenobarbitone sodium : Gardenal sodium, Luminal sodium, Sol Phenobarbitone etc.

2. BUTOBARBITONE

This compound has the same structure as barbitone but differs from it in having a n-butyl group in place of one of the ethyl groups at the 5th position. So it is *5-ethyl-5-n-butylbarbituric acid.*

Physical Properties

Butobarbitone consists of colourless crystals or occurs as a white, crystalline powder. It is practically odourless. It is slightly soluble in water, soluble in ether and freely soluble in ethanol and in chloroform. It dissolves in and forms water-soluble compounds with alkali hydroxides and alkali carbonates and also with ammonia.

Chemical Properties

If butobarbitone is dissolved in methanol and a mixture of cobaltous chloride and calcium chloride solutions is added to this solution and then after mixing and shaking, dilute sodium hydroxide solution is added, a violet-blue colour and a precipitate are produced.

Stability and Storage

Store in well-closed containers.

Uses

Sedative and hypnotic.

Official

Butobarbitone, B.P.

Brand Names

Soneryl, Neonal, Etoval, Butobarbital etc.

3. CYCLOBARBITONE

Cyclobarbitone contains in addition to the ethyl group, a cyclohexenyl group. So it is *5-ethyl-5-cyclohex-1-enylbarbituric acid.*

Physical Properties

Cyclobarbitone is met with in the form of shiny crystals with a bitter taste and melting at 171° - 174°C. It is very slightly soluble in cold water, more soluble in hot water, alcohol and ether. It is official as its calcium salt

Cyclobarbitone calcium is a white or slightly yellowish, crystalline powder. It is slightly soluble in water, very slightly soluble in absolute alcohol and practically insoluble in chloroform and ether.

Chemical Properties

If a small quantity of the cyclobarbitone calcium is added to a mixture of vanillin in alcohol, sulphuric acid and water, shaken and allowed to stand for 5 minutes, a greenish-yellow colour is formed slowly. It becomes dark red when it is heated on a water bath for ten minutes.

Stability and Storage

It should be kept in an airtight container.

Uses

Sedative and hypnotic.

Official

Cyclobarbitone Calcium, B.P.

Brand Names

For cyclobarbitone : Sonaform, Hexemal, Cyclodorm, Phanodorm etc.

For cyclobarbitone calcium : Pronox, Hexemal calcium, Itridal, Cyclobarbital calcium.

4. PARALDEHYDE

Paraldehyde is a polymer of acetaldehyde. It is a trimer and consists of three molecules of acetaldehyde. When concentrated HCl or H_2SO_4 is added to acetaldehyde, polymerization of acetaldehyde to paraldehyde takes place.

Physical Properties

Paraldehyde is a transparant, colourless or pale yellow liquid with a strong and characteristic odour. It solidifies at low temperature to produce a crystalline mass. It should be liquefied before use. During storage it may be oxidized to acetic acid. So if the container of the drug has been kept open for 24 hours, it should not be used since oxidation occurs easily in opened containers. It is soluble in water but less soluble in boiling water. It is miscible with ethanol, ether, chloroform and volatile oils. Since it has solvent action on certain types of plastic, it should not be taken in a plastic syringe for injection. It boils at about 123°C to 126°C.

Chemical Properties

It can be decomposed by boiling with sulphuric acid. Acetaldehyde, which can be recognised by its odour, is produced. Since it is made up of 3 molecules of acetaldehyde, it gives the silver mirror test. If ammonical silver nitrate is added to a solution of paraldehyde and heated on a water bath, silver is deposited as a mirror on the side of the test tube.

171

Stability and Storage

Since it is easily oxidised to acetic acid, paraldehyde should be kept in a small, well-filled, airtight container, protected from light and stored at a low temperature (8 to 15°C). If the material in the container is found to have solidified, it must be fully liquefied before use.

Uses

Hypnotic. It is a powerful hypnotic with a short lasting action. Even though it has no analgesic or anticonvulsant action, it is able to control certain convulsions because of strong CNS depression.

Official

Paraldehyde, I.P., B.P.
Paraldehyde Injection, B.P.

Brand Names

Paraldehyde, Paracetaldehyde.

5. NITRAZEPAM

Nitrazepam is a benzodiazepine derivative. Benzodiazepine is formed by the fusion of one benzene ring and one diazepine ring which is a 7-membered ring containing two nitrogen atoms. It contains also one phenyl radical and a nitro group as substituents.

Physical Properties

Nitrazepam is a yellow, crystalline powder without odour. It melts at about 226°C with decomposition. It is practically insoluble in water, slightly soluble in ethanol and ether and sparingly soluble in chloroform.

172

Chemical Properties

If nitrazepam is dissolved in methanol and dilute sodium hydroxide solution is added, an intense yellow colour is produced. Since nitrazepam contains a nitro group on the benzene ring, it can be reduced to amino group and diazotised by adding hydrochloric acid and sodium nitrite. This, after adding sulphamic acid, can be coupled with N-(1-naphthyl) ethylenediamine hydrochloride to give a red colour

Stability and Storage

Since it is affected by light, store it in well-closed, light-resistant containers.

Uses

Hypnotic. It is a long-acting hypnotic with good sedation.

Official

Nitrazepam, I.P., B.P.
Nitrazepam Tablets, I.P., B.P.
Nitrazepam Capsules, B.P.
Nitrazepam Oral Suspension, B.P.

Brand Names

Sedamas, Hypnotex, Nirven etc.

6. METHYPRYLONE

Methyprylone is a derivative of 2,4-piperidinedione.

Properties

It is a white, crystalline powder. It has a bitter taste and a slight characteristic odour. It melts at about 76°-77°C. It is soluble in water. It is also soluble in alcohol, ether, benzene and chloroform. It is affected by light.

Stability and Storage

Store in well-closed containers, protected from light.

Uses

Hypnotic. It acts like glutethimide. It is not official in the latest I.P. or B.P.

Brand Names

Noludar, Noctan, Dimerin.

7. GLUTETHIMIDE

Glutethimide is also a derivative of 2,6-piperidinedione. It can also be considered to be a derivative of glutaric acid which is a dicarboxylic acid. Glutaric acid has the formula $HOOC(CH_2)_3COOH$. The acid combines with ammonia to form glutarimide.

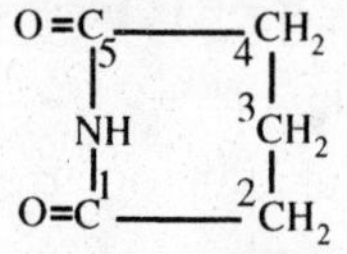

$$O=C\overset{5}{\underset{}{-}}\quad {}^{4}CH_2$$
$$NH \quad {}^{3}CH_2$$
$$O=\overset{1}{C}\overline{\quad\quad} {}^{2}CH_2$$

Numbering starts from a carboxylic group, that is from a -C=O now. One ethyl group and one phenyl group are substituted at the second carbon atom to give glutethimide which has the formula given below :

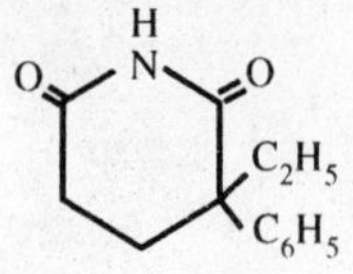

GLUTETHIMIDE

174

So glutethimide is *2-ethyl-2-phenylglutarimide*. If it is considered to be a derivative of piperidine, then the numbering will start from the nitrogen atom and the two keto groups are present at the 2 and 6 positions. The ethyl and phenyl groups are now considered to be at position 3. So glutethimide is *3-ethyl-3-phenyl-2, 6-piperidinedione*.

Physical Properties

Glutethimide occurs as a white or almost white powder or as colourless crystals. It melts at 86 to 89°C. It is practically insoluble in water, freely soluble in alcohol, soluble in ether and very soluble in dichloromethane. It is affected by light.

Chemical Properties

If the substance is dissolved in methanol and a cooled mixture of formalin and concentrated sulphuric acid is added and heated on a water bath, the solution becomes red and exhibits an intense blue fluorescence under ultraviolet light, that is at 365 nm.

Stability and Storage

Store in well-closed containers, protected from light.

Uses

Hypnotic. It was considered to be a safe non-barbiturate hypnotic. But later on it was found that it had all the disadvantages of barbiturates. So it is not very much used nowadays.

Official

Glutethimide, B.P.

Brand Names

Doriden, Elrodorm.

8. TRICLOFOS SODIUM

This is an ester of trichloroethanol and phosphoric acid and converted to the sodium salt. So triclofos sodium is *2,2,2-trichloroethanol sodium dihydrogen phosphate.*

Physical Properties

Triclofos sodium is a white or almost white powder. It is odourless or almost odourless and hygroscopic. It is freely soluble in water, slightly soluble in ethanol and practically insoluble in ether. In aqueous solution, which has a pH of 3 to 4.5, it slowly decomposes and releases chloride and phosphate ions.

Chemical Properties

If triclofos sodium is oxidised by heating with acidified permanganate on a water bath and the excess of permanganate is removed by adding oxalic acid and pyridine and sodium hydroxide solution are added and heated on a water bath, a pink colour is produced in the pyridine layer.

If triclofos sodium is dissolved in water, it decomposes liberating chloride ions. If silver nitrate solution is added, a white precipitate of silver chloride insoluble in ammonia and nitric acid is formed. If triclofos sodium is disintegrated by heating with sodium carbonate to dull redness it decomposes to liberate sodium phosphate and sodium chloride. The residue is extracted with water and filtered. The filterate answers the reactions of chlorides and phosphates.

Stability and Storage

It must be kept in a well-closed container.

Uses

Hypnotic. It is less irritating and stable but rarely used.

176

Official

Triclofos Sodium, B.P.
Triclofos Oral Solution, B.P.

Brand Names

Tricloryl, Triclos, Sodium trichlorofos.

Other hypnotics and sedatives clinically used are *secobarbitone, pentobarbitone, flurazepam, diazepam, flunitrazepam, temazepam, triazolam, midazolam, chloral hydrate and methaqualone.* The last two drugs are drugs of abuse, that is, drugs of addiction which should be avoided.

CHAPTER - 15

Central Nervous System Depressants
ANTICONVULSANTS
(Antiepileptic Drugs)

Epilepsy is a term which is applied to a disease caused by disorders of the central nervous system. In this disease convulsions or other abnormal body movements may occur. Consciousness also may be affected, that is, consciousness may be lost or disturbed. There are as many as seven types of epilepsy but the most important are grand mal, petit mal and psychomotor epilepsy. The anticonvulsant drugs are used to prevent the onset of convulsions. The majority of anticonvulsants are non-specific depressants of the central nervous system. It must also be borne in mind that all depressants of the central nervous system are not anticonvulsants.

CLASSIFICATION

I) **Hydantoins :**
   (1) Methoin
   (2) Phenytoin

II) **Barbiturates :**
   Phenobarbitone

III) **Succinimides :**
   Ethosuximide

IV) **Dibenzazepines :**
   Carbamazepine

V) **Oxazolidinediones :**
   Troxidone

178

1. PHENYTOIN

Hydantoins : Hydantoin is the 2,4-diketo derivative of imidazolidine, which is the completely saturated form of imidazole .

Phenytoin is *5,5-diphenylydantoin*, that is, two phenyl groups are substituted in the 5th position.

PHENYTOIN
5,5-Diphenylhydantoin

Physical Properties

Phenytoin is a white, crystalline powder which has no odour. It melts at 295-298°C. It is very slightly soluble in water, soluble in ethanol and slightly soluble in ether and chloroform. It is official as phenytoin sodium.

Phenytoin sodium is a white, odourless, crystalline powder which is slightly hygroscopic. It is soluble in water. The solution becomes turbid due to absorption of carbon dioxide from the atmosphere and liberation of phenytoin base. It is also soluble in ethanol and practically insoluble in ether and chloroform.

Chemical Properties

When phenytoin sodium is dissolved in water and acidified with dilute hydrochloric acid, it is decomposed and phenytoin is liberated as a white precipitate. If phenytoin sodium is dissolved in a 10% solution of pyridine, cupric sulphate with pyridine solution is added and it is allowed to stand for 10 minutes, a blue precipitate is produced.

179

Stability and Storage

Since it is slightly hygroscopic, store it in tightly-closed containers.

Uses

Anticonvulsant and antiarrhythmic. It is one of the most popular drugs for epilepsy. It is especially useful in the treatment of grand mal, status epilepticus (this is a condition in which major epileptic fits occur without recovery of consciousness in between) and trigeminal neuralgia (pain in the face due to unknown cause confined to branches of trigerminal nerve). It is also used in the treatment of cardiac arrhythmias (deviations from the normal rhythm of the heart).

Official

Phenytoin, B.P.
Phenytoin Sodium, I.P., B.P.
Phenytoin Capsules, B.P.
Phenytoin Sodium Injection, I.P.
(Phenytoin Injection, B.P.)
Phenytoin Sodium Tablets, I.P
(Phenytoin Tablets, B.P.)

Brand Names

Dilantin, Epileptin, Epsolin, Eptoin, Diphentoin, Solantoin etc.

2. METHOIN (MEPHENYTOIN)

Methoin is *5-ethyl-3-methyl-5-phenylhydantoin.*

Properties

It is a colourless, crystalline powder melting at 136-137°C. It is almost insoluble in water but soluble in organic solvents. It can be converted into methoin sodium which, when dissolved in water, has an alkaline reaction. It is not official in B.P. or I.P.

Stability and Storage

Store in a well-closed container.

Uses

Anticonvulsant. It has sedative property also. It may be used in cases which are resistant to phenytoin. However since it causes blood dyscrasias, it is rarely used now.

Brand Names

Methoin, Mesantoin, Phenantoin, Nesantoin etc.

3. PHENOBARBITONE

See the chapter on "Hypnotics and Sedatives"

4. ETHOSUXIMIDE

Succinimides : These are derived from succinic acid

$$CH_2-COOH$$
$$|$$
$$CH_2-COOH$$

which is a dicarboxylic acid.

When ethyl succinate is shaken with ammonia and heated, succinimide is formed.

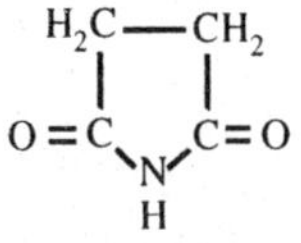

$$H_2C - CH_2$$
$$O=C \diagdown_N \diagup C=O$$
$$H$$

SUCCINIMIDE

181

Ethosuximide is α-*ethyl*-α-*methyl succinimide*, that is one ethyl and one methyl groups are substituted at the position marked as α.

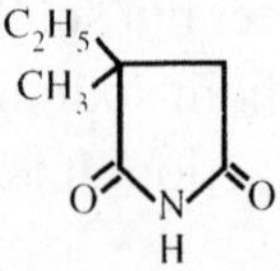

C_2H_5
CH_3

O   O
   N
   H

ETHOSUXIMIDE
α-*ethyl*-α-*methylsuccinimide.*

Physical Properties

It is a white or almost white powder or waxy solid. It melts at 45° to 50°C. It is freely soluble in water and very soluble in ethanol and ether. The sodium salt of ethosuximide has a bright green fluorescence.

Chemical Properties

When ethosuximide is dissolved in methanol and cobalt chloride, calcium chloride and sodium hydroxide solutions are added, a purple colour is produced. No precipitate is produced.

Stability and Storage

Since it is affected by light, store it in well-closed, light-resistant containers.

Uses

Anticonvulsant. It is effective in petit mal and is the drug of choice.

Official

Ethosuximide, I.P., B.P.
Ethosuximide Capsules, I.P., B.P.
Ethosuximide Oral Solution, B.P.
Ethosuximide Syrup, B.P.

Brand Names

Zarontin, Mesentol, Suximal, Ethymal etc.

5. CARBAMAZEPINE

Dibenzazepines : These are derivatives of dibenzazepine in which two benzene rings are fused with the azepine nucleus at the positions 2,3 and 6,7.

In carbamazepine the nitrogen atom carries a carbamoyl (-CONH₂) group as a substitutent.

Therefore carbamazepine is given the systematic name *1-carbamoyl-2, 3:6,7-dibenzazepine.*

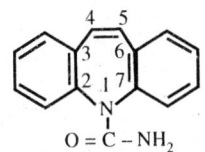

CARBAMAZEPINE
1-Carbamoyl-2,3: 6,7-dibenzazepine

Properties

It is a white or yellowish-white, crystalline powder which has no odour. It exhibits polymorphism. It melts at 189° to 193°C. An intense blue fluorescence is seen when it is exposed to ultra-violet light (365 nm). It is practically insoluble in water as well as in ether and soluble in ethanol and acetone.

Stability and Storage

It is stable in air. So store in well-closed containers only.

Uses

Anticonvulsant. Carbamazepine is an effective drug in epilepsy. It is highly useful in the treatment of psychomotor epilepsy, grand mal and cortical focal epilepsy. It is the drug of choice for trigeminal neuralgia.

Official

Carbamazepine, I.P., B.P.
Carbamazepine Tablets, I.P., B.P.

Brand Names

Tegretol, Carbatol, Mazetol, Tegretol retard etc.

6. TROXIDONE (TRIMETHADIONE)

This is a compound of oxazolidine which is the saturated form of oxazole. Actually it is an oxazolidinedione since it contains two keto groups at positions 2 and 4. It also contains three methyl groups (that is why it is named also as tri-methadione) at positions 3 (one) and 5 (two) so troxidone is 3,5,5-trimethyl-2,4-oxazolidinedione.

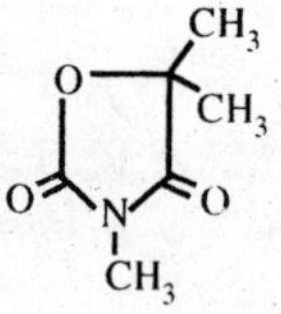

Physical Properties

It consists of almost colourless crystals with a camphoraceous odour melting between 45° and 47°C. It is soluble in water and very soluble in chloroform, ethanol and ether. It is affected by light.

Chemical Properties

If troxidone is dissolved in carbon dioxide-free water and barium hydroxide solution is added, a white precipitate is produced.

Stability and Storage

Since it is affected by light, store it in well-closed containers protected from light.

Uses

Anticonvulsant. It is specifically effective in the treatment of petit mal.

Official

Troxidone, I.P., B.P.
Troxidone Capsules, I.P.

Brand Names

Tridione, Absentol, Petidone etc.

Other anticonvulsants clinically used are *mephobarbitone, primidone, ethotoin, valproic acid, clonazepam, diazepam, phenacemide, vigabatrin etc.*

CHAPTER - 16

DRUGS USED TO TREAT MENTAL ILLNESS

A. ANTIPSYCHOTICS

Drugs used to treat mental illness and mental disorders are also known as psychotropic drugs and psycho-pharmacological agents. Mental disorders can be broadly divided into neuroses, psychoses and personality disorders. Of these, psychoses may be treated with antipsychotics. When the mental functioning of the individual is impaired enough to grossly interfere with the meeting of the ordinary demands of life by him, it is known as a *psychosis*.

When the disease is due to an organic disease (in the brain), it is known as *organic psychosis*. If it is due to some disturbance in the activity of the neurotrasmitters in the brain, it is known as *functional psychosis*. Functional psychoses can be further subdivided into *schizophrenia* and *affective disorders*. Schizophrenia is marked by behavioural abnormalities such as catatonia (state of generalized muscular silly behaviour), paranoia (feeling of persecution), oneirism (day dreaming), obsessions (unpleasant thoughts, feelings or actions which provoke anxiety but cannot be got rid of), delusions (irrational beliefs that cannot be corrected by rational argument) and hallucinations (imaginary sights and sounds etc.).

The schizophrenic patients are unable to cope with the external environment and their personality and behaviour get very much disorganised. The affective disorders are those in which the moods of the patients are affected and alterations in moods are the predominant symptoms.

The exact mechanism by which the antipsychotics act is not known. However they are supposed to have dopaminergic blocking action, that is binding to the receptors of dopamines such as noradrenaline in the brain limbic system and reducing their activity.

The antipsychotics do not cure the disease but provide the much needed relief. They also have antihistaminic, antiemetic, anticholinergic, local anaesthetic and secretory (gastric) actions also.

CLASSIFICATION OF ANTIPSYCHOTICS

1. **Phenothiazines**
   a) Chlorpromazine
   b) Prochlorperazine
   c) Trifluoperazine

2. **Ring Analog of Phenothiazine**
   Thiothixene

3. **Butyrophenones**
   a) Haloperidol
   b) Triperidol

1. CHLORPROMAZINE

Phenothiazines are derived from phenothiazine, a heterocyclic compound with three six membered rings. The central ring is a thiazine with sulphur and nitrogen. The other two rings are benzene rings.

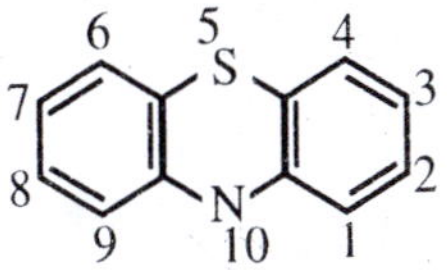

PHENOTHIAZINE

Chlorpromazine has a chlorine atom in the second position and a propyl group in the 10th position. The third carbon atom of the propyl radical carries a dimethylamino group ($-N(CH_3)_2$). Therefore chlorpromazine is *2-chloro-10-(3-dimethylaminopropyl) phenothiazine.* It is official as the hydrochloride.

CHLORPROMAZINE

Physical Properties

Chlorpromazine hydrochloride is a white or creamy-white, crystalline powder without odour and with a bitter taste. It melts between 194°C and 198°C. It is affected by air and light. It becomes yellow, then pink and finally violet on exposure to air and light. It is very soluble in water, freely soluble in ethanol, soluble in chloroform and practically insoluble in ether. It is acidic, a 10% solution in water has a pH of 4.

Chemical Properties

If a small quantity of the substance is dissolved in water, a cherry red colour is produced. It darkens slowly on standing. If this solution is divided into two parts and one portion is warmed, it changes to brown and then magenta. If decinormal potassium dichromate is added to the other portion, the colour changes to brownish red. In another test if ferric chloride solution is added to an aqueous solution of the substance, a stable red colour is produced.

Stability and Storage

Since it is affected by air and light, store it in a tightly-closed, light-resistant container.

Uses

Antipsychotic and antiemetic. It is also known as a **major tranquiliser.** It has effective antipsychotic action and is used in the treatment of schizophrenia to control hyperkinetic states and aggression. It is also an antiemetic and used in the treatment of nausea and vomiting and also intractable hiccup.

Official

Chlorpromazine Hydrochloride, I.P., B.P.
Chlorpromazine Hydrochloride Injection, I.P.
(Chlorpromazine Injection, B.P.)
Chlorpromazine Oral Solution, B.P.
Chlorpromazine Hydrochloride Tablets, I.P.
(Chlorpromazine Tablets, B.P.)

Brand Names

Chlorpromazine, Largactil, Chloractil, Torazine, Taroctyl etc.

2. PROCHLORPERAZINE

Prochlorperazine has almost the same structure as chlorpromazine. However the –N(CH$_3$)$_2$ group attached to the end carbon atom of the propyl group at the 10th postion is replaced by a methylpiperazino group. It is official as the maleate.

Physical Properties

Prochlorperazine maleate is a white or pale yellow, crystalline powder which is odourless It is very slightly soluble in water and ethanol and practically insoluble in ether and chloroform. It is affected by light. The mesylate and the edisylate are water soluble.

Chemical Properties

The maleic acid component of the prochlorperazine maleate can be tested by extracting the prochlorperazine base from an alkaline solution of the substance. For this purpose prochlorperazine maleate is triturated with water and sodium hydroxide solution and extracting with ether, thus removing the prochlorperazine in ether.

One portion of the aqueous layer containing the sodium salt of maleic acid is first treated with resorcinol and concentrated sulphuric acid and heated on a water bath. No colour is produced. However if another portion of the aqueous solution is first treated with bromine solution and heated on a water bath, the maleic acid is oxidised to dibromosuccinic acid. If this solution is treated with resorcinol and concentrated sulphuric acid and heated on a water bath, a dye is produced which is indicated by the solution turning blue. Compare this with the preparation of eosin (see "Fluorescein Sodium" in Chapter 33).

Stability and Storage

Since it is affected by light, store it in a well-closed container protected from light.

Uses

Antipsychotic and antiemetic. It has the same effects as chlorpromazine but at lower doses.

Official

Prochlorperazine Maleate, I.P., B.P.
Prochlorperazine Maleate Tablets, I.P.
(Prochlorperazine Tablets, B.P.)
Prochlorperazine Mesylate, I.P., B.P.
Prochlorperazine Mesylate Injection, I.P.
(Prochlorperazine Injection, B.P.)

Brand Names

Stemetil, Nipodal, Tementin etc.

3. TRIFLUOPERAZINE

Trifluoperazine has the same structure as prochlorperazine in the sense that it contains the same side chain at position 10. However it contains a trifluoromethyl group at position 2 in place of the chloro group in prochlorperazine. It is official as the hydrochloride.

Physical Properties

Trifluoperazine hydrochlordie is a white to pale yellow, crystalline powder. It is almost odourless and slightly hygroscopic. An aqueous solution of the substance is found to be intensely acidic. It is freely soluble in water, soluble in ethanol, slightly soluble in chloroform and insoluble in ether. It is affected by light.

Chemical Properties

If trifluoperazine hydrochloride is dissolved in concentrated sulphuric acid and allowed to stand for 5 minutes, an orange colour is produced. If, however, an aqueous solution of the substance is first treated with bromine solution and shaken and concentrated sulphuric acid is added and shaken vigorously, a red colour is produced. If an aqueous solution of the substance is treated with concentrated nitric acid, a dark red colour is produced. It finally becomes pale yellow.

Stability and Storage

Since it is slightly hygroscopic and is also sensitive to light, store it in a well-closed, light-resistant container.

Uses

Antipsychotic and antiemetic. It has the same actions and uses as chlorpromazine.

Official

Trifluoperazine Hydrochloride, I.P., B.P.
Trifluoperazine Hydrochloride Injection, I.P.
Trifluoperazine Hydrochloride Tablets, I.P.
(Trifluoperazine Tablets, B.P.)

Brand Names

Espazine, Trinicalm, Eskazine, Stelazine, Terfluzine etc.

4. THIOTHIXENE

Thiothixene is a ring analog of chloropromazine in that it is not derived from phenothiazine but from thioxanthene. It is used as the hydrochloride. It occurs in three forms :- cis, trans, and cis-trans mixture of which the cis isomer is preferred for pharmacological use.

Properties

Thiothixene hydrochloride is a white, crystalline powder with a slight odour. It is soluble in water, ethanol and chloroform and practically insoluble in ether and acetone. It is affected by light.

Stability and Storage

Since it is affected by light, store it in well-closed containers protected from light.

Uses

Antipsychotic. It has the same uses as chlorpromazine as an antipsychotic. It is very potent and its sedative action is less. It is effective in both types of schizophrenia, that is in both depressed and agitated schizophrenics.

Official

Thiothixene Hydrochloride Injection, U.S.P.

Brand Names

Tiotixene, Orbinamon and Navane.

5. HALOPERIDOL

Haloperidol is a butyrophenone, that is the keto group is present between the phenyl radical and a propyl group (which becomes the butyro group including the keto). The phenyl group carries a fluoro (-F) group in the para position whereas the end carbon atom of the butyro group carries a piperidino group which itselt has a hydroxyl and a p-chlorophenyl group in the 4th position.

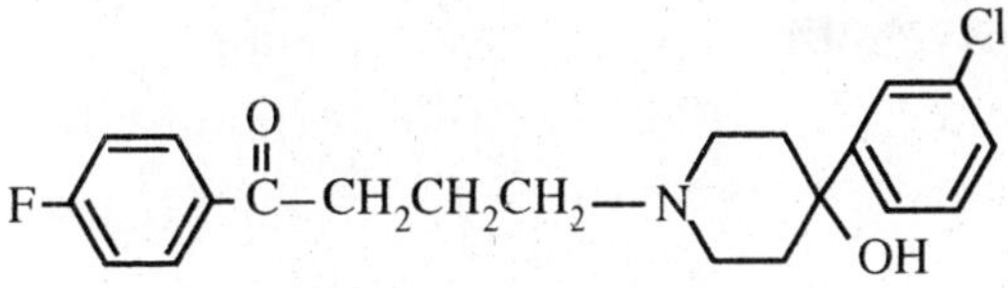

HALOPERIDOL

4-(4-Chlorophenyl)-4-hydroxypiperidino-4'-fluorobutyrophenone.

Physical Properties

Haloperidol is a white or slightly yellowish, amorphous or crystalline powder which is without odour. It melts at about 150°C. It is practically insoluble in water, soluble in chloroform, sparingly soluble in ethanol and slighly soluble in ether. It is affected by light.

Chemical Properties

If an alcoholic solution of haloperidol is treated with dinitrobenzene solution and 2M ethanolic potassium hydroxide, a violet colour is produced. It becomes brownish

193

red after 20 minutes. If an alcoholic solution of the substance is mixed with a mixture of alizarin red S solution and zirconyl nitrate solution, the red colour of the solution becomes yellow. The molecule of haloperidol can be disintegrated by acidifying with 0.5M sulphuric acid. The solution now answers the reactions of chlorides since the nuclear chlorine in the p-chlorophenyl group attached to the piperidine is now present in the inorganic state.

Stability and Storage

Since it is affected by light, store it in airtight containers protected from light.

Uses

Antipsychotic. It is a powerful antipsychotic. Its side effects are much less compared to the phenothiazines. It is used to treat acute schizophrenia and other diseases.

Official

Haloperidol, I.P., B.P.
Haloperidol Injection, I.P., B.P.
Haloperidol Oral Solution, I.P., B.P.
Strong Haloperidol Oral Solution, B.P.
Haloperidol Tablets, I.P., B.P.

Brand Names

Serenace, Hexidol, Hexidol Plus, Aloperidine, Brotopon, Halidol, Depidol etc.

Other antipsychotics in clinical use are *triflupromazine, thioridazine, fluphenazine, thioproperazine, triperidol, droperidol, chlorprothixene, flupenthixel, pimozide, reserpine, clozapine, molindone, sulpiride etc.*

B. ANTIANXIETY AGENTS (ANXIOLYTICS)

Anxiety is an unpleasant mental state characterised by mental discomfort, a feeling of uneasiness and a vague fear of some unknown threat or danger. The antianxiety drugs counteract these symptoms and produce a restful or peaceful state of mind without interfering with normal mental or physical functions. They resemble closely sedatives and hypnotics and also have anticonvulsant effect. They are also drugs of abuse and produce physical dependence.

CLASSIFICATION

a) **Benzodiazepines**
   1. Chlordiazepoxide
   2. Diazepam
   3. Lorazepam

b) **Miscellaneous**
   Meprobamate

Diazepines are unsaturated seven-membered rings with two nitrogen atoms in the rings. Depending on the positions of the nitrogen atoms, they are known as 1,2 or 1,3 or 1,4 diazepines. **Benzodiazepines** are formed by the fusion of one benzene ring and one diazepine ring.

1. CHLORDIAZEPOXIDE

Chlordiazepoxide is a 1,4-benzodiazepine derivative. It has totally 5 double bonds, three in the benzene ring and two in the diazepine nucleus. The substituents in the benzodiazepine ring are one methylamino group in the second position, a chlorine atom at position 7, a phenyl group at position 5 and an oxygen linked to the nitrogen at the 4th position through a coordinate covalent linkage (indicated by an arrow.)

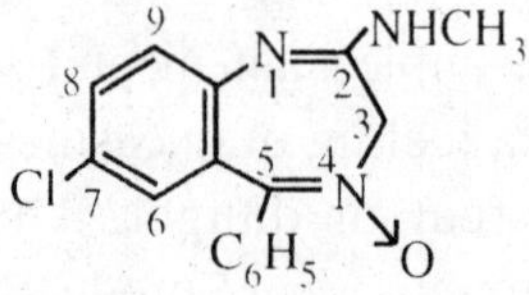

CHLORDIAZEPOXIDE

Physical Properties

Chlordiazepoxide is a white or light yellow, crystalline powder which is bitter and odourless. It is practically insoluble in water, sparingly soluble in ethanol and slightly soluble in ether. It is affected by light. It is used as the hydrochloride also which is very soluble in water.

Chemical Properties

The compound can be disintegrated by boiling with hydrochloric acid. The decomposition product answers the reaction of primary aromatic amines such as getting diazotised and coupled with α-naphthol or N-(1-naphthyl)ethylene diamine dihydrochloride to give a red or reddish violet azo dye.

Stability and Storage

Since it is affected by light, store it in a well-closed container protected from light.

Uses

Anxiolytic. It acts as a sedative and minor tranquilizer. It is slowly absorbed but its action is long lasting. In the body active metabolites are produced extending its duration of action. It is liable to be abused.

196

Official

Chlordiazepoxide. I.P., B.P.

Chlordiazepoxide Tablets, I.P., B.P.

Chlordiazepoxide Hydrochloride, B.P.

Chlordiazepoxide Capsules, B.P.

Chlordiazepoxide Hydrochloride Tablets, B.P.

Brand Names

Librium, Equilibrium, Mesricem, Mesural etc.

2. DIAZEPAM

Diazepam is also a 1,4-benzodiazepine derivative. It has totally 4 double bonds, three in the benzene ring and one in the diazepine nucleus. The substituents are a methyl group at the first position, a keto group at position 2, a phenyl group at position 5 and a chloro group in position 7 as in chlordiazepoxide.

DIAZEPAM

Physical Properties

Diazepam is a white to pale yellow, crystalline powder which is almost without odour. It is sparingly soluble in water but freely soluble in chloroform and soluble in ethanol. It melts between 131°C and 135°C. It is affected by light.

Chemical Properties

If diazepam is dissolved in sulphuric acid, the solution exhibits a greenish yellow fluorescence when examined under ultraviolet light. The compound can be disintegrated and the

197

organic chlorine is converted into sodium chloride by using the oxygen-flask combustion technique and using sodium hydroxide solution as the absorbing liquid. After this solution is acidified with dilute sulphuric acid and boiled, it is able to give the reactions of chloride.

Stability and Storage

Since it is affected by light, it may be stored in well closed, light-resistant containers.

Uses

Anxiolytic, sedative and anticonvulsant. It has anxiolytic, sedative, anticonvulsant, muscle relaxant and amnestic actions. It is quickly absorbed. Initially the action is strong and it is followed by a mild long-lasting effect due to production of active metabolites. It is used in the control of muscle spasm of tetanus.

Official

Diazepam, I.P., B.P.
Diazepam Capsules, I.P., B.P.
Diazepam Injection, I.P., B.P.
Diazepam Oral Solution, B.P.
Diazepam Tablets, I.P., B.P.

Brand Names

Valium, Calmpose, Levium, Tranquase etc.

3. LORAZEPAM

Lorazepam is also a 1,4-benzodiazepine derivative which has almost the same structure as diazepam but has no methyl group at position 1 but has a hydroxyl group at position 3.

Properties

Lorazepam is a white or almost white, crystalline powder without odour and melting at 166 to 168°C. It is practically insoluble in water, sparingly soluble in ethanol and slightly soluble in chloroform. It is affected by light.

Stability and Storage

It is slowly absorbed. It has, however, relatively short duration of action since no active metabolite is produced. It is a good sedative also apart from being a good antianxiety agent.

Official

Lorazepam, B.P.
Lorazepam Injection, B.P.
Lorazepam Tablets, B.P.

Brand Names

Larpose, Ativam, Calmese, Lorax etc.

4. MEPROBAMATE

Meprobamate is a relatively simple compound, being the biscarbamate of a diol. It is actually *2-methyl-2-n-propyl-1, 3-propanediol dicarbamate*. It was introduced in medicine in 1954.

Physical Properties

Meprobamate is a white or almost white, crystalline or amorphous powder. It is odourless and has a characteristic bitter taste. It melts at 104°C to 108°C. It is slightly soluble in water and ether and freely soluble in ethanol. Though it is an ester, it is stable in dilute acid and alkali.

Chemical Properties

Meprobamate answers a colour reaction in which it is dissolved in ethanolic potassium hydroxide and boiled. Then glacial acetic acid and a solution of cobalt (II) nitrate in absolute ethanol are added. A deep blue colour is produced.

Stability and Storage

Store it in airtight containers.

Uses

Anxiolytic. It is used as tablets and capsules in the treatment of anxiety and tension. However it is less effective than the benzodiazepines and more toxic. It also induces tolerance, both physical and psychological. It is rarely used now.

Official

Meprobamate, B.P.

Brand Names

Equanil, Miltown, Calmate, Equinil etc.

Other antianxiety agents in clinical use are *oxazepam, alprazolam, hydroxyzine, buspirone, flurazepam, medazepam and prazepam etc.*

C. ANTIDEPRESSANTS

Antidepressants are used for treating depressive illness which means they are used to overcome or counteract mental depression. Depression may arise in mentally ill patients such as after a schizophrenic attact or even in normal persons sometimes which may lead to suicidal tendencies also. Mental depression is believed to be caused due to disturbances in the levels of certain biogenic amines in the brain. The balance is restored by antidepressants through different mechanisms.

CLASSIFICATION

1. **Betaphenylethylamine and Related Derivatives**
   a) Phenelzine
   b) Tranylcypromine

2. **Tricyclic Compounds**
   a) Amitriptyline
   b) Nortriptyline
   c) Imipramine

1. PHENELZINE

Phenelzine and tranylcypromine are what are known as monoamine oxidase inhibitors. Monoamine oxidase is an enzyme which combines with and destroys biogenic amines such as noradrenaline etc. By inhibiting this enzyme the monoamine oxidase inhibitors (MAO_2) promote the accumulation of biogenic amines in the brain.

Phenelzine is *phenylethylhydrazine*. It is official as the sulphate.

Physical Properties

Phenelzine sulphate is a white powder or it may consist of pearly platelets. It has a pungent and peculiar odour. It melts at 164°C to 168°C. It is freely soluble in water and practically insoluble in ether, ethanol and chloroform. It is affected by light.

Chemical Properties

An aqueous solution of the substance made alkaline with sodium hydroxide solution and treated with cupric-tartrate solution gives a red precipitate.

201

Stability and Storage

Since it is affected by light, store it in well-closed containers and protected from light.

Uses

Antidepressant (monoamine oxidase inhibitor). It elevates the mood of depressed patients and is used in the treatment of severe mental depression.

Official

Phenelzine Sulphate, B.P.
Phenelzine Tablets, B.P.

Brand Names

Nardil, Stinerval etc.

2. TRANYLCYPROMINE

Tranylcypromine is a nonhydrazine compound and also a cyclopropane derivative. It is a primary amine. It is official as the sulphate.

Physical Properties

Tranylcypromine sulphate is a white or almost white, crystalline powder with a faint odour which is the same as that of cinnamaldehyde. It is soluble in water, very slightly soluble in ethanol and ether and insoluble in chloroform.

Chemical Properties

If ninhydrin is added to a suspension of the substance in ethanol, a purple colour is produced within fifteen minutes.

Stability and Storage

Store it in well-closed containers.

202

Uses

Antidepressant (monoamine oxidase inhibitor). Its actions and uses are similar to those of phenelzine.

Official

Tranylcypromine Sulphate, B.P.
Tranylcypromine Tablets, B.P.

Brand Names

Parnate, Tylciprine etc.

3. AMITRIPTYLINE

Amitriptyline is a derivative of dibenzcycloheptene in which two benzene rings are fused with a seven-membered unsaturated carbocyclic ring, that is, a cycloheptene. It is official as the embonate and the hydrochloride.

Physical Properties

Amitriptyline hydrochloride consists of colourless crystals or is a white or almost white powder which has no odour. It melts between 195°C and 199°C. It is freely soluble in water, ehtanol, chloroform and methanol and practically insoluble in ether.

Chemical Properties

If quinhydrone in methanol solution is added to an aqueous solution of the substance, no red colour is produced within 15 minutes. This is a distinction from nortriptyline which gives a red colour within fifteen minutes when similarly treated.

Stability and Storage

Store in well-closed containrs.

Uses

Antidepressant. This class of tricyclic antidepressants is believed to act by inhibiting the reuptake of biogenic amines such as noradrenaline and 5-HT. They have usually potent anticholinergic action also. Amitriptyline is used in the treatment of mental depression and nocturnal enuresis (bed wetting at night).

Official

Amitriptyline Embonate, B.P.
Amitriptyline Oral Suspension, B.P.
Amitriptyline Hydrochloride, I.P., B.P.
Amitriptyline Hydrochloride Tablets, I.P.
(Amitriptyline Tablets, B.P.)

Brand Names

Amilene, Quietal, Tryptanol, Sarotex etc.

4. NORTRIPTYLINE

Nortriptyline has also almost the same structure as amitriptyline. It is also a dibenzcycloheptene derivative. It is official as the hydrochloride.

Physical Properties

Nortriptyline hydrochloride is a white to off white powder with a slight, characteristic odour. It melts between 215°C and 220°C. It is sparingly soluble in water and methanol, freely soluble in ethanol and chloroform and practically insoluble in ether. It is affected by light.

Chemical Properties

It answers the quinhydrone reaction given under amitriptyline and gives a red colour within 15 minutes.

Stability and Storage

Since it is affected by light, store it in tightly closed, light-resistant containers.

Uses

Antidepressant. It has the same actions and uses of amitriptyline. It is less sedating.

Official

Nortriptyline Hydrochloride, I.P., B.P.
Nortriptyline Capsules, B.P.
Nortriptyline Hydrochloride Tablets, I.P.
(Nortriptyline Tablets, B.P.)

Brand Names

Sensival, Nortrilen, Norzepine. Vivedyl, Pamelor etc.

5. IMIPRAMINE

Imipramine is a dibenzazepine derivative, whereas amitriptyline and nortriptyline are derivatives of dibenzcycloheptene. The carbon atom at postion no.5 in dibenzcycloheptene is replaced by a nitrogen atom to give dibenzazepine. In the structure of imipramine there is a dimethylaminopropyl group attached to the nitrogen.

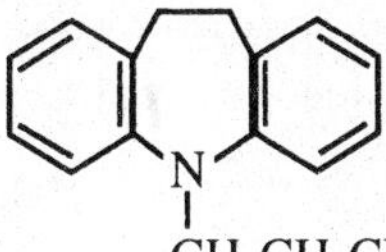

$$CH_2CH_2CH_2N(CH_3)_2$$

IMIPRAMINE

Physical Properties

Imipramine is official as imipramine hydrochloride which is a white or slightly yellow, crystalline powder without odour. It is affected by light and becomes yellow to red in colour. It melts between 170°C and 174°C. It is freely soluble in water, ethanol and chloroform and practically insoluble in ether.

Chemical Properties

If it is dissolved in nitric acid, it gives an intense blue colour. If quinhydrone test is applied to imipramine, it does not answer it like amitriptyline and no red colour is produced.

Stability and Storage

Since it is affected by light, it may be stored in well-closed, light-resistant containers.

Uses

Antidepressant. It has the same actions and uses as amitriptyline. It also is less sedating.

Official

Imipramine Hydrochloride, I.P., B.P.
Imipramine Hydrochloride Tablets, I.P.
(Imipramine Tablets, B.P.)

Brand Names

Tofranil, Depsonil, Imiprin, Iramil etc.

Other antidepressants in clinical use are *isocarboxacid, clorgiline, moclobemide, selegiline, doxepin, dothiepin, clomipramine, mianserin, amoxapine, maprotilene, trazodone, fluoxetine etc.*

CHAPTER - 17

NARCOTIC ANALGESICS

Narcotic Analgesics : Analgesics are drugs which give relief from pain without causing loss of consciousness. Narcotic analgesics are drugs which not only give relief from pain but also may cause *narcosis* (unconsciousness induced by narcotics) by depression of the central nervous system.

CLASSIFICATION

1) **Naturally Occuring Opium Alkaloids**
   a) Morphine
   b) Codeine

2) **Synthetic Morphine Substitutes**
   a) Pethidine
   b) Methadone
   c) Dextropropoxyphene
   d) Pentazocine

Naturally Occuring Opium Alkaloids

Opium is the dried latex obtained from the unripe capsules of opium poppy, *Papaver somniferum*. About twenty five alkaloids have been extracted from opium. The most important is morphine followed by codeine.

1. MORPHINE

Morphine is the principal alkaloidal constituent of opium. Good samples of opium contain about 10% of morphine. It is present in opium not in the free state but as sulphate and meconate.

Physical Properties

Morphine is a colourless, crystalline substance melting at 254°C with decomposition. It has novel solubility properties for an alkaloid. Just like any other alkaloid it is very sparingly soluble in water and slightly more soluble in ethanol. However unlike many other alkaloids which are soluble in organic solvents, morphine is only slightly soluble in organic solvents such as ether, chloroform, benzene and acetone. It is more soluble in amyl alcohol and much more soluble in benzyl alcohol. It is slightly soluble in ammonia. Since morphine is both phenolic and basic, it is freely soluble in solutions of fixed alkali and alkaline earth hydroxides and in mineral acids. So if to a solution of morphine sulphate in water, sodium hydroxide solution is added, morphine is not precipitated like any other alkaloid but dissolves in the alkali solution forming the sodium salt. It is intensely bitter. It is a monacid tertiary base forming salts with one equivalent of an acid. Morphine is official in the I.P. as morphine sulphate. *Morphine sulphate* consists of white, acicular crystals or cubical masses or occurs as a white, crystalline powder. It is soluble in cold water and freely soluble in hot water. It is slightly soluble in ethanol, more soluble in hot ethanol and practically insoluble in ether and chloroform. It is affected by light.

Chemical Properties

When any salt of morphine is dissolved in water and ammonia is added, morphine is precipitated but it dissolves on the addition of sodium hydroxide solution indicating its phenolic nature. The phenolic nature is further confirmed by the fact that a solution of a morphine salt gives with ferric chloride solution a blue colour. If potassium ferricyanide and ferric chloride solutions are added, it gives a bluish green colour. It changes rapidly to blue. These tests help to distinguish morphine from codeine which is non-phenolic.

Morphine liberates iodine from iodic acid. So when the aqueous solution of any morphine salt is added to a solution of potassium iodate acidified with dilute sulphuric acid and containing starch mucilage, a deep blue colour is produced. The liberated iodine gives the blue colour with starch.

When morphine is dissolved in concentrated sulphuric acid, heated on a water bath for about 15 minutes, the solution cooled and a few drops of dilute nitric acid are added, a blood red colour is produced. When a small quantity of morphine is dissolved in concentrated nitric acid, an orange red colour is produced.

When a dilute solution of morphine in dilute hydro chloric acid is added to a crystal of sodium nitrite and an excess of ammonia is added, a red colour is produced. If a few milligrams of a morphine salt are added to a mixture of concentrated sulphuric acid and formaldehyde solution, a purple colour is produced.

Stability and Storage

Since it is affected by light, store it in well-closed, light-resistant containers.

Uses

Narcotic analgesic. Morphine acts as a powerful analgesic to relieve severe pain and also as a sedative in the presence of pain. It is also used as preanaesthetic medication in some cases and also to produce constipation by reducing peristaltic movements in diarrhoea. It is a very good antitussive (a drug which suppresses cough) though codeine is preferred for this purpose. Its side effects include depression of respiratory centre leading to respiratory failure, depression of temperature regulating centre leading to hypothermia (reduced body temperature) and depression of vasomotor centre leading to vasodilatation (relaxation or increase in diameter of the blood vessels). It is a dangerous drug of addiction (habit-forming drug) since it produces euphoria (exaggerated sense of well-being called as pleasurable experience or *high* by addicts). Since it is a drug of abuse, the cultivation, collection, distribution and sale of opium and morphine and morphine derivatives such as heroin are regulated by the government.

Official

Morphine Hydrochloride, B.P.
Morphine Suppositories, B.P.
Morphine Sulphate, I.P., B.P.
Chloroform and Morphine Tincture, B.P.
Morphine Sulphate Injection, I.P., B.P.
Morphine Sulphate and Atropine Sulphate Injection, I.P.
(Morphine and Atropine Injection, B.P.)
Morphine Tablets, B.P.

Brand Names

Morphine sulphate, Morphia, Morphium, MST-1 continus.

2. CODEINE

Codeine is the methyl ether of morphine. In its structure the phenolic -OH group in morphine is methylated and converted to $-OCH_3$. It is present to the extent of 0.1 to 3% in opium. It is prepared either by extraction from opium or by synthesis by methylation of morphine. Codeine is official as codeine phosphate in I.P. and as codeine, codeine hydrochloride, codeine phosphate and codeine phosphate sesquihydrate in the B.P.

Physical Properties

Codeine consists of colourless crystals or occurs as a white, crystalline powder. It melts between 155° and 159°C. It contains one molecule of water of hydration and effloresces slowly in dry air. It is soluble in cold water (1 in 120), more soluble in ethanol (1 in 2) and in chloroform (1 in 5) and in toluene. Its aqueous solution has an alkaline pH (more than 9). It is a monacid tertiary base which dissolves freely in dilute acids. But since it does not contain a phenolic -OH like morphine, it is insoluble in solutions of alkali hydroxides. It is affected by light.

Codeine phosphate occurs as a white, crystalline powder or as colourless crystals. It is freely soluble in water, slightly soluble in ethanol, sparingly soluble in chloroform and practically insoluble in ether. Codeine phosphate contains ½ molecule of water of hydration and codeine phosphate sesquihydrate contains 1½ molecules of water of hydration.

Chemical Properties

Since codeine does not contain a phenolic -OH group like morphine, it does not give blue colour with ferric chloride nor does it give a bluish-green colour with potassium ferricyanide and ferric chloride. It does not also give yellow colour with nitrous acid and ammonia. On warming a small amount of codeine with concentrated sulphuric acid and ferric chloride solution, a blue colour is produced. It changes to red on the addition of dilute nitric acid. Being a typical alkaloid it answers the reactions of alkaloids. For example it gives an orange or orange red colour when it is acidified with dilute hydrochloric acid and Dragendorff's reagent (potassium bismuth iodide) is added.

211

Stability and Storage

Since it is affected by light, codeine and its salts should be kept in well-closed containers protected from light.

Uses

Narcotic analgesic, antidiarrhoeal and cough suppressant. It is less potent than morphine as an analgesic. It has only $1/6$ to $1/10$ the activity of morphine. Even though it is only $1/3$ as potent as morphine as a cough suppressant, it is still preferred to morphine as an antitussive, since its liability as a drug of abuse is low. It is also used as an antidiarrhoeal to control diarrhoea. Constipation is the most common side effect when it is used as an analgesic or antitussive.

Official

Codeine, B.P.

Codeine Hydrochloride, B.P.

Codeine Phosphate, I.P., B.P.

Codeine Phosphate Syrup, I.P.

Co-cadamol Tablets, B.P.

(Codeine phosphate and paracetamol tablets)

Co-cadaprin Tablets, B.P.

(Codeine and aspirin tablets)

Dispersible Co-cadaprin Tablets, B.P.

Codeine Linctus, B.P.

Paediatric Codeine Linctus, B.P.

Codeine Phosphate Oral Solution, B.P.

Codeine Phosphate Tablets, B.P.

Brand Names

Codicept, Methylmorphine.

212

3. PETHIDINE

Pethidine is, structurally, an ester and a tertiary base. It is derived from piperidine. Pethidine is *ethyl-1-methyl-4-phenylpiperidine-4-carboxylate.*

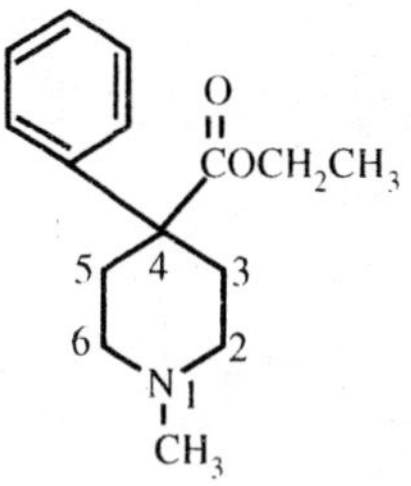

PETHIDINE
(Ethyl-1-methyl-4-phenylpiperidine-4-carboxylate)

Physical Properties

Pethidine is a strong, tertiary base and also an ester. It is official as the hydrochloride. Pethidine hydrochloride is a white, crystalline powder melting at 187° to 189°C. It is very soluble in water, freely soluble in chloroform and ethanol and practically insoluble in ether. When an alkali solution is added to an aqueous solution of pethidine hydrochloride, the base is liberated as an oil solidifying at 30°C. It is affected by light.

Chemical Properties

A cream-coloured precipitate is formed when an aqueous solution of pethidine hydrochloride is treated with potassium mercuri-iodidie solution. An orange-red colour is produced when formaldehyde solution and concentrated sulphuric acid are added to an aqueou solution of pethidine hydrochloride.

Stability and Storage

Since it is affected by light, store it in well-closed, light-resistant containers.

213

Uses

Narcotic analgesic. It is a good synthetic morphine substitute for analgesic action. It has equal sedative action and causes equal euphoria compared to morphine. It is used for preanaesthetic medication but not for treating diarrhoea or cough. Like morphine, it is also an addiction-causing drug.

Official

Pethidine Hydrochloride, I.P., B.P.
Pethidine Hydrochloride Injection, I.P.
(Pethidine Injection, B.P.)
Pethidine Hydrochloride Tablets, I.P.
(Pethidine Tablets, B.P.)

Brand Names

Dolantin, Demerol, Dolvanol, Meperidine etc.

4. METHADONE

Methadone is a ketone and it is a derivative of the hydrocarbon heptane. It is an aliphatic compound. It is official as the hydrochloride.

Physical Properties

Methadone hydrochloride is a white, odourless, crystalline powder with a bitter taste. It melts between 233° and 236°C. It is soluble in water, freely soluble in ethanol and chloroform and practically insoluble in ether. It is affected by light.

Chemical Properties

If methadone hydrochloride is dissolved in water and dilute hydrochloric acid and ammonium thiocyanate solution are added, a white, amorphous precipitate is produced. It becomes crystalline on stirring for a few minutes. After it is dried at 105°C, its melting point may be found out. Its melting range is between 143° and 148°C.

Stability and Storage

Since it is affected by light, store it in well-closed containers protected from light.

Uses

Narcotic analgesic. It is somewhat more potent than morphine. It has analgesic, antitussive, respiratory depressant, emetic and contipating actions like morphine. It produces less sedation and narcosis than morphine.

Official

Methadone Hydrochloride, I.P., B.P.
Methadone Hydrochloride Injection, I.P.
(Methadone Injection, B.P.)
Methadone Linctus, B.P.
Methadone Hydrochloride Tablets, I.P.
(Methadone Tablets, B.P.)

Brand Names

Physeptone, Dolophine, Depridol etc.

5. DEXTROPROPOXYPHENE

Dextropropoxyphene is also a tertiary base and an ester like pethidine. It is official as the hydrochloride.

Properties

Dextropropoxyphene hydrochloride is a white or almost white, crystalline powder. It melts at about 165°C. It is very soluble in water, freely soluble in ethanol and practically insoluble in ether. It is affected by light.

Stability and Storage

Since it is affected by light, it should be kept in a well-closed container and protected from light.

Uses

Narcotic analgesic. It is used as a mild analgesic given orally usually in combination with aspirin and paracetamol. Its abuse potential is low.

Official

Dextropropoxyphene Hydrochloride, B.P.
Co-praxamol Tablets, B.P.
(Dextropropoxyphene hydrochloride and paracetamol
tablets)
Dextropropoxyphene Napsylate, B.P.
Dextropropoxyphene Capsules, B.P.

Brand Names

Proxyvon (dextropropoxyphene + paracetamol), Parvon, Walagesic and Sudhinol (dextropropoxyphene + paracetamol + diazepam).

6. PENTAZOCINE

Pentazocine has a complex structure.

Physical Properties

It is a white or pale cream powder. It is practically insoluble in water, freely soluble in chloroform, soluble in ethanol and sparingly soluble in ether. It melts between 150° and 155°C. It is affected by light.

Chemical Properties

If pentazocine is treated with concentrated sulphuric acid containing ammonium molybdate, an intense blue colour is produced. It changes to bluish green, then to green and finally to yellow on standing. If pentazocine is dissolved in concentrated sulphuric acid and ferric chloride solution is added, a yellow colour is produced. It deepens slightly on warming. The yellow colour is unchanged when nitric acid is added.

Stability and Storage

Store in well-closed containers protected from light.

Uses

Narcotic analgesic. Its actions and uses are similar to those of morphine.

Official

Pentazocine, I.P., B.P.
Pentazocine Injection, B.P.
Pentazocine Hydrochloride, I.P., B.P.
Pentazocine Hydrochloride Tablets, I.P.
(Pentazocine Tablets, B.P.)
Pentazocine Lactate, I.P.
Pentazocine Lactate Injection, I.P.

Brand Names

Fortwin, Meriwyn, Sosegon, Liticon etc.

Other narcotic analgesies clinically used are *ethylmorphine, fentanyl, ethoheptazine, levorphanol, levallorphan, dipipanone, dextromoramide etc.*

217

CHAPTER - 18

ANTIPYRETIC ANALGESICS AND NONSTEROIDAL ANTIINFLAMMATORY AGENTS

Unlike narcotic analgesics, the nonnarcotic analgesics not only relieve pain but also reduce elevated body temperature. They are also antiinflammatory agents which reduce inflammation and relieve the pain due to inflammation. Inflammation due to arthritis, rheumatism, ankylosing spondylytis, lupus erythematosus etc. is relieved. The analgesic action is used for the relief of pain due to toothache, headache, arthralgias, myalgias, neuralgias and dysmenorrhea. Some of them have uricosuric properties also.

CLASSIFICATION

1) **Salicylate**
   Aspirin

2) **Para-aminophenol derivate**
   Paracetamol

3) **Pyrazole derivatives**
   1. Analgin
   2. Phenylbutazone
   3. Oxyphenbutazone

4) **Arylpropionic acid derivative**
   Ibuprofen

5) **Substituted indole derivative**
   Indomethacin

1. ASPIRIN

Aspirin is the acetyl derivative of salicylic acid. In this the -OH group of salicylic acid has been esterified with acetic acid. Aspirin is also known as *acetylsalicylic acid.*

ASPIRIN
(Acetylsalicylic acid)

Physical Properties

Aspirin consists of colourless needle-like crystals or occurs as a white, almost odourless, crystalline powder which melts at 142°C. It has a slightly acid taste. It is stable in dry air but in moist air and in contact with moisture it is gradually hydrolysed to acetic and salicylic acids. It is slightly soluble in water, freely soluble in ethanol and soluble in ether and chloroform.

Chemical Properties

Aspirin may be hydrolysed to salicylic acid by boiling with sodium hydroxide solution and adding dilute sulphuric acid. The salicylic acid may be collected, dissolved in water and ferric chloride test solution added. A deep violet colour is produced. The filtrate in this test containing acetic acid may be warmed with ethanol and concentrated sulphuric acid. The characteristic odour of ethyl acetate may be noticed.

Stability and Storage

Since it is affected by exposure to moist air, it must be stored in tightly closed containers in a cool, dry place.

Uses

Antipyretic analgesic, antirheumatic and antithrombotic. As an antirheumatic it is used to treat acute rheumatic fever, rheumatoid arthritis and osteoarthritis. As an antithrombotic it reduces platelet aggregation and lowers the incidence of reinfarction. Since it irritates the gastric mucosa, it should not be taken on empty stomach.

Official

Aspirin, I.P., B.P.
Dispersible Aspirin Tablets, B.P.
Effervescent Soluble Aspirin Tablets, B.P.
Soluble Aspirin Tablets, I.P.
Aspirin and Caffeine Tablets, I.P., B.P.
Co-codaprin Tablets, B.P.
(Aspirin and Codeine Tablets)
Dispersible Co-codaprin Tablets, B.P.

Brand Names

Aspirin, Disprin, Asabuf, Micropyrin, Aspro, Biospirin etc.

2. PARACETAMOL

Paracetamol is *p-acetamido (paraacetylamino) phenol.* In this the p-amino group in p-aminophenol is acetylated.

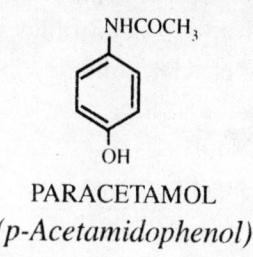

PARACETAMOL
(p-Acetamidophenol)

Physical Properties

Paracetamol is a white, odourless, crystalline powder with a slightly bitter taste. It melts between 168° and 172°C. It is sparingly soluble in water, freely soluble in ethanol and acetone and very slightly soluble in ether, chloroform, benzene and petroleum ether. It is affected by light.

Chemical Properties

When it is boiled with concentrated hydrochloric acid, water added and cooled, no precipitate is produced. If potassium dichromate is added, a violet colour develops. It does not turn red.

Stability and Storage

Since it is affected by light, store it in well-closed, light-resistant containers.

Uses

Antipyretic analgesic. Paracetamol is a safe antipyretic and analgesic. It does not cause any gastric irritation, ulceration and bleeding and can be given to ulcer patients safely. It does not have any significant antiinflammatory action.

Official

Paracetamol, I.P., B.P.
Co-cadamol Tablets, B.P.
(Codeine phosphate and paracetamol tablets)
Co-dydramol Tablets, B.P.
(Dihydrocodeine and paracetamol tablets)
Co-praxamol Tablets, B.P.
(Dextropropoxyphene hydrochloride and paracetamol tablets)
Paediatric Paracetamol Oral solution, B.P.
Paracetamol Oral Suspension, B.P.
Paracetamol Syrup, I.P.
Paracetamol Tablets, I.P., B.P.

Brand Names

Crocin, Metacin, Tylenol, Amadil, Dymadon etc.

3. ANALGIN

Analgin is a pyrazoline derivative. Pyrazoline is a partially saturated form of pyrazole and one double bond is present. The other name of analgin is metamizole.

Physical Properties

Analgin is a white or almost white, odourless, crystalline powder with a scarcely preceptible yellowish tinge and with a bitter taste. It is freely soluble in water, slightly soluble in ethanol and practically insoluble in chloroform and ether. It is slightly hygroscopic.

Chemical Properties

If, to a mixture of analgin in water, ethanol and dilute hydrochloric acid, potassium iodate solution is added, a crimson colour is produced. When more potassium iodate solution is added, the colour deepens. If analgin is heated with dilute hydrochloric acid, it is decomposed and the odour of sulphur dioxide and formaldehyde may be noticed in that order.

Stability and Storage

Since it may be slightly hygroscopic, store it tightly-closed containers.

Uses

Analgesic and antipyretic. It is a powerful and speedily acting analgesic and antipyretic but is a poor antiinflammatory agent. It irritates the gastric mucosa and is also toxic with chances of agranulocytosis being induced on continuous use. Therefore its use as a routine antipyretic and analgesic is not advisable.

Official

Analgin. I.P.

Analgin Tablets. I.P.

Brand Names

Analgin, Novalgin, Metamizol, Benalsin etc.

4. PHENYLBUTAZONE

Phenylbutazone is a derivative of pyrazolidine which is the completely saturated form of pyrazole and no double bond is present. Phenylbutazone has two phenyl groups at positions 1 and 2, one butyl group at position 4 and two keto groups at postions 3 and 5. Therefore it is *1,2-diphenyl-4-butylpyrazolidine-3, 5-dione.*

$$CH_3(CH_2)_3 \quad \overset{O}{\diagup}$$
$$O \diagup \underset{\underset{C_6H_5}{|}}{N} \diagdown {}^{N-C_6H_5}$$

PHENYLBUTAZONE

Physical Properties

Phenylbutazone is a white or almost white, odourless, crystalline powder. It is practically insoluble in water, freely soluble in chloroform and acetone, soluble in ether and sparingly soluble in ethanol. It melts between 104° and 107°C.

Chemical Properties

By heating phenylbutazone under reflux for 30 minutes with glacial acetic acid and concentrated hydrochloric acid, it is decomposed and the resulting compound with a primary amino group may be treated with sodium nitrite, when a yellow colour is produced. It can then be coupled with 2-naphthol in sodium carbonate solution when a reddish-brown to reddish violet precipitate is produced.

Stability and Storage

Since it is stable in air, it is enough if it is stored in well-closed containers.

Uses

Non-steroidal antiinflammatory and analgesic. It is a potent non-corticosteroid antiinflammatory agent. Comparatively its analgesic and antipyretic action is rather poor and slow in onset. It is more toxic than aspirin. Adverse effects include nausea, vomiting, epigastric distress, peptic ulceration, diarrhoea, bone marrow depression, agranulocytosis, oedema etc. It is used to treat rheumatoid arthritis, spondylitis, rheumatic fever, osteoarthritis and acute gout.

Official

Phenylbutazone, I.P., B.P.
Phenylbutazone Tablets, I.P.

Brand Names

Zolandin, Butazolidin, Zolapen etc.

5. OXYPHENBUTAZONE

Oxyphenbutazone has almost the same structure as phenylbutazone. The difference is that it has a p-hydroxyphenyl group in the first position instead of just a phenyl group present in phenylbutazone. So oxyphenbutazone is *1-p-hydroxyphenyl-2-phenyl-4-butylpyrazolidine-3, 5-dione.*

Physical Properties

Oxyphenbutazone is a white to yellowish white, almost odourless crystalline powder. It melts at 96°C. It is practically insoluble in water, freely soluble in ethanol and soluble in acetone, chloroform and ether. It dissolves in dilute solutions of alkali hydroxides.

Chemical Properties

If a solution of 2,6-dichloroquinone-4-chlorimide in ethanol and sodium carbonate solution are added to a solution of oxyphenbutazone in ethanol, an intense green colour is produced. As in the case of phenylbutazone, the oxyphenbutazone is also hydrolysed by boiling with glacial acetic acid and hydrochloric acid and diazotised by adding sodium nitrite and coupled with 2-naphthol in sodium carbonate solution. An orange-red precipitate is produced.

Stability and Storage

Since it is affected by exposure to light, store it in tightly-closed, light-resistant containers.

Uses

Non-steroidal antiinflammatory and analgesic. It has the same actions and adverse effects of phenylbutazone. The use of these two drugs is banned in some countries.

Official

Oxyphenbutazone, I.P., B.P.
Oxyphenbutazone Tablets, I.P.
Oxyphenbutazone Eye Ointment, B.P.

Brand Names

Suganril, Inflavan, Reparil, Tanderil etc.

6. IBUPROFEN

Ibuprofen is an arylpropionic acid derivative. The aryl part is a 4-isobutylphenyl group attached to the α-carbon atom of the propionic acid.

Physical Properties

Ibuprofen is a white or almost white, crystalline powder with a slight odour. It melts at 75° to 77°C. It is practically insoluble in water and freely soluble in acetone, chloroform, ethanol and ether. Being an acid, it dissolves in dilute solutions of alkali hydroxides and carbonates.

Stability and Storage

Since it is stable in air, store it in well-closed containers.

Uses

Non-steroidal antiinflammatory and analgesic. It is popularly used for treating rheumatoid arthritis, osteoarthritis and other similar diseases. It is also used to reduce swelling and inflammation in tooth extraction, vasectomy, fractures, tissue injuries etc. It has some analgesic and antipyretic action equal to the low dose of aspirin. Its side effects include gastric discomfort, nausea and vomiting, dizziness, blurring of vision, fluid retention etc., but they are less severe than with other drugs.

Official

Ibuprofen, I.P., B.P.
Ibuprofen Tablets, I.P., B.P.

Brand Names

Brufen, Ibugesic, Ibusynth, Ibuprocin etc.

7. INDOMETHACIN

Indomethacin is an indoleacetic acid derivative unlike ibuprofen which is a propionic acid derivative. In indomethacin the acetic acid is in the 3rd postion of the indole nucleus. The first has a 4-chlorobenzoyl group attached. In the 2nd position there is a methyl group and in the 5th position there is a methoxy group. So indomethacin is *1-(4-chlorobenzoyl)-5-methoxy-2-methylindole-3-acetic acid.*

CO—⟨ ⟩—Cl

N—CH₃

CH₃O   CH₂COOH

INDOMETHACIN

Physcial Properties

Indomethacin is a white to pale yellow, odourless, crystalline powder. It melts between 158°C and 162°C. It exists in two different crystalline forms (polymorphs) which melt at 155°C and 162°C. It is decomposed by exposure to sun light and also by strong alkali. It is practically insoluble in water, soluble in chloroform and sparingly soluble in ethanol and ether.

Chemical Properties

A violet pink colour is produced when a freshly prepared mixture of hydroxylamine hydrochloride and sodium hydroxide solutions followed by dilute hydrochloric acid and ferric chloride solution is added to a solution of indomethacin in alcohol and heated, if necessary.

Stability and Storage

Since it is affected by light, store it in well-closed, light-resistant containers.

Uses

Non-steroidal antiinflammatory and analgesic. It is a powerful antiinflammatory drug but a lot of gastrointestinal and CNS effects are produced. It is particularly useful in ankylosing spondylitis and acute gout.

Official

Indomethacin, I.P., B.P.
Indomethacin Capsules, I.P., B.P.
Indomethacin Suppositories, I.P., B.P.

Brand Names

Indocid, Idicin, Indocap, Indocin, Mezolin etc.

Other non-steroidal antiinflammatory analgesic antipyretics clinically used are *salicylamide, benorylate, diflunisal, propiphenazone, sulindac, naproxen, ketoprofen, fenoprofen, flurbiprofen, mephenamic acid, enphenamic acid, diclofenac sodium, piroxicam, ketorolac, nefopam etc.*

CHAPTER - 19

ADRENERGIC DRUGS
(Sympathomimetic Amines)

The adrenergic drugs are drugs whose pharmacological actions are very much like the effect obtained by stimulation of adrenergic or sympathetic nerves. Many of these substances have an intact or substituted amino group and for this reason they are also known as sympathomimetic amines. Chemically they are known as phenylethylamine derivatives.

They mainly give three types of actions :-

1) *Pressor* (blood pressure raising effect), due to direct stimulation of the heart and constriction of the smaller arterioles, *(2) Bronchodilator*, due to relaxation of the bronchial smooth muscle, and *(3) Central stimulant* actions.

In view of the above actions naturally they are used in the treatment of hypotension and heart block and to give relief in asthma and nasal congestion. Some of them like amphetamine are used for their central stimulant action and for inducing anorexia (loss of appetite) in obese (fat) persons.

CLASSIFICATION
They are divided into two groups :-

I. Catecholamines
  a) Adrenaline
  b) Noradrenaline
  c) Isoprenaline

II. Noncatecholamines

   a) Phenylephrine
   b) Salbutamol
   c) Terbutaline
   d) Ephedrine
   e) Pseudoephedrine

1. ADRENALINE

Adrenaline is secreted by the medula of the adrenal glands. It is secreted in good quantity to meet conditions of stress.

Structurally adrenaline is *1-(3,4-dihydroxyphenyl)-2-methylaminoethanol.*

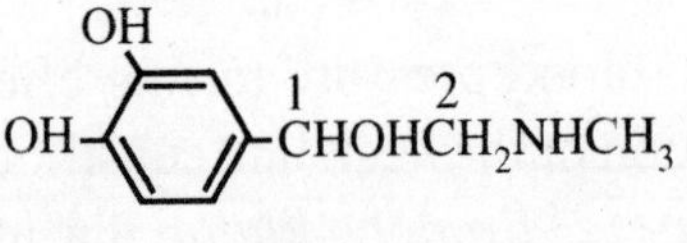

To the first carbon atom of the ethanol (marked as 1) is attached the 3,4-dihydroxyphenyl group (which is nothing but catechol, that is orthohydroxyphenol). To the second carbon atom (marked as 2) is attached the methylamino group ($-NHCH_3$). Therefore adrenaline is *1-(3,4-dihydroxyphenyl)-2-methylaminoethanol.*

Physical Properties

Adrenaline is a white or creamy white, microcrystalline powder or occurs as small granules. It slowly darkens on exposure to air and light and becomes brown. This is due to the oxidation of the catechol nucleus and adrenochrome is formed. Adrenochrome is ineffective as adrenergic agent but is of value in stopping bleeding associated with haemorragic disseage or postoperative seepage when given orally or intramuscularly. The decompostion is faster at higher temperatures and in the presence of moisture. It is sparingly soluble in water and insoluble in ethanol and ether. However it is soluble in solutions of mineral acids and in solutions of alkali hydroxides. It is not soluble in aqueous ammonia and solutions of alkali carbonates. It is unstable in alkali or neutral solution becoming red when exposed to air. It is stable in slightly acid solution. Solutions are stabilised by the inclusion of a reducing agent like sodium metabisulphite in a concentration of 0.1% and are buffered to pH 4.2.

Chemical Properties

Since adrenaline contains a catechol nucleus in its structure, an emerald green colour is formed when ferric chloride solution is added to a slightly acid solution of adrenaline. If sodium bicarbonate solution is added gradually, the emerald green colour first changes to blue and then to red. This test is answered by all sympathomimetic amines containing a catechol nucleus such as noradrenaline and isoprenaline.

Stability and Storage

Considering what is stated under Physical Properties, adrenaline should be kept in tightly-closed, light-resistant, dry containers which are preferably filled with nitrogen.

Uses

Sympathomimetic. Adrenaline is used locally to stop haemorrhage and to enhance the activity of local anaesthetics by local vasocontriction. It is also used to relax the bronchioles in asthma and in anaphylactic collapse. It is used in the form of injections, aqueous or oily solutions and also in the form of ointments or suppositories. Adrenaline is always used in the form of its salts such as adrenaline malate and adrenaline bitartrate in injections and aqueous solutions.

Official

Adrenaline, I.P., B.P.

Adrenaline Bitartrate, I.P.

(Adrenaline Acid Tartrate, B.P.)

Adrenaline Bitartrate Injection, I.P.

(Adrenaline Injection, B.P.)

Adrenaline Eye Drops, B.P.

Adrenaline Solution, B.P.

Bupivacaine and Adrenaline Injection, B.P.

Lignocaine and Adrenaline Injection, B.P.

(Lignocaine Hydrochloride and Adrenaline Bitartrate Injection, I.P.)

Brand Names

Adrenaline, Epinephrine, Suprarenin, Levorenin etc. and Brovon inhalant (0.5% solution).

2. NORADRENALINE

Noradrenaline is the transmitter at most postganglionic sympathetic nerve endings and also in certain parts of the brain. It is also secreted by the adrenal medulla. Structurally noradrenaline is the lower homologue of adrenaline. It has the same structure as adrenaline except for the fact that it contains a primary amino group ($-NH_2$) instead of the methylamino group ($-NHCH_3$) present in adrenaline. Therefore noradrenaline is *1-(3,4-dihydroxyphenyl)-2-aminoethanol.*

Noradrenaline is used as the bitartrate.

232

Physical Properties

Noradrenaline bitartrate is a white or almost white, crystalline powder which has no odour. It has a bitter taste. Since it also contains a catechol nucleus, it darkens gradually on exposure to air and light due to oxidation. It is freely soluble in water, slightly soluble in ethanol and practically insoluble in chloroform and ether. Aqueous solutions of noradrenaline are slowly oxidized when exposed to air and light.

Chemical Properties

Since noradrenaline also contains a catechol nucleus like adrenaline, it also answers the ferric chloride test like adrenaline. Therefore it gives an intense green colour when treated with ferric chloride solution and it changes first to blue and then to red on the addition of sodium bicarbonate solution.

Stability and Storage

It should be stored in tightly-closed, light-resistant containers or it may be kept preferably in sealed containers which are filled with an inert gas like nitrogen.

Uses

Sympathomimetic. It is used to maintain blood pressure in acute hypotensive conditions like trauma, central vasomotor depression and haemorrhage. It is administered by infusion in isotonic saline, glucose, plasma or blood intravenously.

Official

Noradrenaline Bitartrate, I.P.
(Noradrenaline Acid Tartrate, B.P.)
Noradrenaline Bitartrate Injection, I.P.
Noradrenaline Hydrochloride, B.P.

Brand Names

Noradrenaline, Nordrin, Norepinephrine, Levarterenol.

3. ISOPRENALINE

Isoprenaline is the isopropyl homologue of adrenaline and it is prepared by synthesis. It has the same structure as adrenaline, the only difference being that it contains the isopropyl group ($-CH(CH_3)_2$) attached to the amino group in place of the methyl group present in adrenaline. So isoprenaline is *1-(3,4-dihydroxyphenyl)-2-isopropylaminoethanol.*

$$OH-\langle\,\rangle-CHOHCH_2NH(CH_3)_2$$

Isoprenaline is official as the hydrochloride and the sulphate.

Physical Properties

Isoprenaline sulphate is a white or almost white, crystalline powder. It is odourless. Since it also contains the catechol nucleus, it also darkens gradually when exposed to air and light. It is freely soluble in water and practically insoluble in ethanol, ether and chloroform. Aqueous solution of isoprenaline becomes pink on standing.

Chemical Properties

Since isoprenaline is also a catecholamine derivative, it answers the test with ferric chloride in the same way like adrenaline and noradrenaline by giving an emerald green colour which turns blue first and then red on adding a solution of sodium bicarbonate. When to an aqueous solution of insoprenaline sulphate, silver nitrate solution is added, a greyish precipitate is produced on standing for ten minutes and the supernatant liquid becomes pink.

Stability and Storage

Since it is affected by air and light, store it in tightly-closed, light-resistant containers.

Uses

Sympathomimetic (beta-adrenoceptor agonist). Isoprenaline can be administered orally unlike adrenaline and noradrenaline. It is used in the symptomatic treatment of mild as well as moderately severe asthma. It should not be given parenterally because of its intense stimulation of the heart muscle. It produces peripheral vasodilation and a consequent fall in blood pressure. It may be given by infusion to treat bradycardia and as a stimulant in heart attack.

Official

Isoprenaline Hydrochloride, I.P.
Isoprenaline Hydrochloride Injection, I.P.
(Isoprenaline Injection, B.P.)
Isoprenaline Sulphate, I.P., B.P.
Isoprenaline Sulphate Tablets, I.P.

Brand Names

Neoepinine (sublingual tablets), Isoprin (injection), Autohaler (inhaler), Isoproterenol, Novadrin etc.

4. PHENYLEPHRINE

Phenylphrine is a noncatecholamine which means that it is not a catechol derivative. It contains only one hydroxyl group on the benzene ring in the third position. Otherwise it has the same structure as adrenaline. So phenylephrine is *1-(3-hydroxyphenyl-2-methylaminoethanol*. It is used as the hydrochloride.

235

Physical Properties

Phenylephrine hydrochloride is a white or almost white, bitter, crystalline powder which is without odour. It is freely soluble in water and ethanol and practically insoluble in chloroform. It melts at 140-145°C. The aqueous solution has a specific rotation between -43° and -47°.

Chemical Properties

Phenylephrine hydrochloride can be decomposed by adding dilute ammonia to its aqueous solution and scratching the side of the test tube with a glass rod. Phenylephrine crystals, which are precipitated, may be washed with iced water and dried at 105°C for two hours. The melting range of the dried crystals is between 171° and 176°C. Phenylephrine also answers a colour reaction in which the aqueous solution of the hydrochloride is treated with copper sulphate solution and sodium hydroxide solution. A violet colour is produced. This colour is not extracted by ether. This can be found by adding ether and shaking. The ether layer remains colourless.

Stability and Storage

Since it is affected by light, store it in well-closed, light-resistant containers.

Uses

Sympathomimetic. It is used in the treatment of hypotension. Since it is a vasoconstrictor, it prolongs the action of local anaesthetics. It is also used as a mydriatic.

Official

Phenylephrine Hydrochloride, I.P.
Phenylephrine Hydrochloride Injection, I.P.
(Phenylephrine Injection, B.P.)

Brand Names

Drosyn, Pupiletto, Dristan, Fenox, Decangin, Sinustin etc.

5. SALBUTAMOL

Sulbutamol is also a noncatecholamine. Like phenylephrine it also contains only one hydroxyl group on the benzene ring. It also contains a -CH$_2$OH group ortho to the phenolic -OH. The side chain contains a tertiary amino group.

Physical Properties

Salbutamol is a white or almost white, crystalline powder with no odour. It is sparingly soluble in water, soluble in ethanol and slightly soluble in ether. Salbutamol sulphate is a white or almost white, crystalline powder. It is freely soluble in water and slightly soluble in ethanol and ether.

Chemical Properties

When treated with borax solution, aminophenazone solution, potassium ferricyanide solution and chloroform and shaken, salbutamol gives an orange-red colour in the chloroform layer.

Stability and Storage

Since it is affected by light, keep it in well-closed, light-resistant containers.

Uses

Sympathomimetic (beta-adrenoceptor agonist). It is mainly used as a bronchodilator in bronchial asthma and in premature labour. It is administered orally, intramuscularly and by inhalation.

Official

Salbutamol. I.P., B.P.
Salbutamol Inhaler, I.P.
(Salbutamol Pressurised Inhalation, B.P.)
Salbutamol Sulphate, I.P., B.P.
Sulbutamol Sulphate Injection, I.P.
(Salbutamol Injection, B.P.)
Salbutamol Sulphate Syrup, I.P.
Salbutamol Sulphate Tablets, I.P.
(Salbutamol Tablets, B.P.)

Brand Names

Asthalin, Croysal, Albuterol etc.

6. TERBUTALINE

Terbutaline has almost the same structure as adrenaline. The only difference is that it is not a catechol derivative but an orcinol derivative. Orcinol is a dihydric phenol with the two hydroxyl groups meta to each other. Secondly terbutaline has a t-butylamino group in place of the methylamino group present in adrenaline.

Properties

Terbutaline is used as the sulphate. Terbutaline sulphate is a white or almost white, crystalline powder. It has no odour. It is freely soluble in water, slightly soluble in ethanol and practically insoluble in chloroform and ether.

Stability and Storage

Since it is affected by light, keep it in well-closed, light-resistant containers.

Uses

Sympathomimetic (beta-adrenoceptor agonist). It is used in the same way as salbutamol.

Official

Terbutaline Sulphate, I.P., B.P.
Terbutaline Sulphate Inhaler, I.P.
Terbutaline Sulphate Injection, I.P.
Terbutaline Sulphate Tablets, I.P.
(Terbutaline Tablets, B.P.)

Brand Names

Terbutaline, Bricarex, Bricanyl Misthaler, Terbasmin etc

7. EPHEDRINE

Ephedrine is an alkaloid obtained from the stems of Ephedra or *Ma Huang* such as *E.vulgaris, E.sinica and E.equisetina*. It was known to the Chinese as early as 2800 B.C. It has the following structure :-

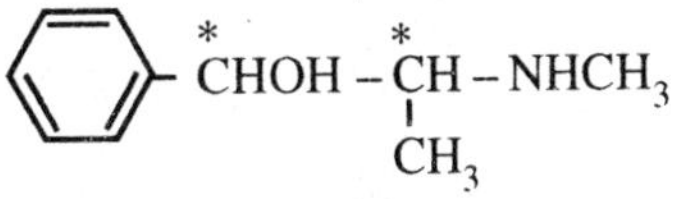

$$\text{C}_6\text{H}_5 - \overset{*}{\text{C}}\text{HOH} - \overset{*}{\text{C}}\text{H} - \text{NHCH}_3$$
$$|$$
$$\text{CH}_3$$

In this structure, ephedrine differs from adrenaline in having no phenolic -OH group and also in the side chain extended to three carbon atoms, that is it is not an ethanol but a propanol. So it is *1-phenyl-2-methylaminopropanol*. It has two asymmetric carbon atoms at carbon atoms 1 and 2 marked with *. So there are four optical isomers, that is, D- and L - ephedrine and D- and L - pseudoephedrine. D- and L- ephedrine have the erythro configuration. The biologically active form is

239

the D-(-)- ephedrine. It can be obtained by extraction from the stems of Ephedra or by synthesis starting from benzaldehyde and a sugar like D-glucose using yeast.

Physical Properties

Ephedrine occurs as a waxy solid or colourless crystalls or granules or as a white, crystalline powder. It has a characteristic and pronounced odour. It gradually decomposes on exposure to light and darkens. It contains ½ molecule of water of hydration and melts at 40° to 43°C. The anhydrous substance melts at about 36°C. It is soluble in water and chloroform, very soluble in ethanol and freely soluble in ether. If the hydrated material is dissolved in chloroform, the water of hydration separates and the solution appears turbid. It has unique solubility in water in that it is soluble to the extent of 5% (1 in 20). This solubility is even more than that of caffeine which is soluble in water only to the extent of 1 in 60. The free alkaloid is a strong base and the aqueous solution of ephedrine has a pH above 10. It decomposes chloroform in the cold giving rise to chloride ions. It combines readily with acids to form salts such as ephedrine hydrochloride and ephedrine sulphate.

Chemical Properties

As a already stated under Physical Properties, ephedrine decomposes chloroform in the cold. If ephedrine is dissolved in choloroform and set aside for 12 hours and the chloroform evaporated slowly, crystals of ephedrine hydrochloride separate. They can be washed with chloroform and dried at 100°C. The crystals have a melting range between 217° and 220°C and also give the reactions of chlorides.

Ephedrine also gives a colour reaction. When it is dissolved in dilute hydrochloric acid and copper sulphate solution and sodium hydroxide solution are added, a violet colour is produced. If ether is added and shaken, the ether layer becomes purple and the aqueous layer is blue.

Stability and Storage

Keep it in well-closed, light-resistant containers, since it is affected by light.

Uses

Sympathomimetic (bronchodilator). Ephedrine has a similar action to adrenaline. However its pressor and local vasoconstrictor effects are more long lasting than adrenaline. It may be given orally or by injection. It can be used to produce rise in blood pressure and to cause vaso-constriction of small capillaries on mucous membranes in sinusitis, asthma, hay fever etc. However its present day use is restricted to giving relief in mild chronic bronchial asthma. Sometimes it is also used to treat postural hypotension and urinary incontinence.

Official

Ephedrine, I.P., B.P.
Anhydrous Ephedrine, B.P.
Ephedrine Hydrochloride, I.P., B.P.
Ephedrine Hydrochloride Oral Solution, I.P.
Ephedrine Elixir, B.P.
Ephedrine Nasal Drops, B.P.
Ephedrine Hydrochloride Tablets, I.P., B.P.

Brand Names

Ephedrine (Tablets & injection)
Endrine (Nasal drops)
Efedrina

8. PSEUDOEPHEDRINE

Pseudoephedrine is one of the optical isomers of ephedrine. It is also obtained from Ephedra species.

Properties

Pseudoephedrine hydrochloride is a white, crystalline powder which is very soluble in water, freely soluble in chloroform, soluble in ethanol and slightly soluble in ether. It has a faint, characteristic odour and melts at 181-182°C.

Stability and Storage

Keep in well-closed containers, protected from light.

Uses

Sympathomimetic. It is not a good branchodilator like ephedrine. It is only used as a decongestant of nose.

Official

Pseudoephedrine Hydrochloride, I.P., B.P.

Pseudoephedrine Hydrochloride Syrup, I.P.

Pseudoephedrine Hydrochloride Tablets, I.P.

(Pseudoephedrine Tablets, B.P.)

Brand Names

Pseudoephedrine, Sudafed.

Other adrenergic drugs in clinical use are *dopamine, methoxamine, metaraminol, mephentermine, prenalterol, dobutamine, orciprenaline, xylometazoline, oxymetazoline, naphazoline, amphetamine, dexamphetamine, methamphetamine, fenfluramine, diethylpropion, mazindol, isoxsuprine, nylidrine etc.*

242

CHAPTER - 20

ADRENERGIC BLOCKING AGENTS

The adrenergic blocking agents are drugs which antagonise the actions of adrenergic drugs. These drugs block either alpha or beta adrenergic receptors. They prevent the response of the effector organs to adrenaline and noradrenaline, both internally produced and externally administered.

Many of these sympathetic depressants and adrenolytic agents also interfere with the transmission of postganglionic sympathetic impulses by preventing the release of noradrenaline. This may be due to depletion of the nonadrenaline store or interference with its synthesis in nerves and various body tissues or just preventing the release of stored noradrenaline.

CLASSIFICATION

I. **Alpha Receptor Blockers**
   Tolazoline
II. **Beta Receptor Blockers**
   1. Propranolol
   2. Practalol

1. TOLAZOLINE

Tolazoline is a synthetic drug and is *2-benzyl-2-imidazoline*. Imidazoline is a partially saturated form of imidazole. Tolazoline has a benzyl group in the second position of the imidazoline. It is used in the form of its hydrochloride.

Physical Properties

Tolazoline hydrochloride is a white or creamy-white, odourless, crystalline powder with a bitter taste. It melts between 172° and 176°C. It is freely soluble in water, ethanol and chloroform. Aqueous solution is slightly acidic to litmus. It is affected by light.

Chemical Properties

Tolazoline answers some colour reactions. When ammonium reineckate solution is added to an aqueous solution of the substance, a pink precipitate with a pearly lustre is produced. When tolazoline hydrochloride is dissolved in methanol, solutions of sodium nitroprusside and sodium hydroxide are added and after about 10 minutes sodium bicarbonate solution is added, a rose violet colour is produced.

Stability and Storage

Since it is affected by light, store it in a well-closed container, protected from light.

Uses

Adrenergic blocking drug. It is used as a peripheral vasodilator in the treatment of peripheral vascular disorders.

Official

Tolazoline Hydrochloride, B.P. '88
Tolazoline Tablets, B.P. '88

Brand Names

Priscol, Priscoline, Lambril, Kasimid etc.

2. PROPRANOLOL

See **Antiarrythmic Agents** under **Cardiovascular Agents** (Chapter 24.)

3. PRACTOLOL

Practolol has a comparatively simpler structure to propranolol. It is a crystalline substance melting at 135° to 136°C and soluble in hot isopropanol.

Uses

Adrenergic blocking drug. Like propranol it is a β-adrenoceptor antagonist and has the same uses.

Other adrenergic blocking drugs in clinical use are *phenoxybenzamine, dibenamine, ergotamine, ergotoxine, dihydroergotamine, dihydroergotoxine, phentolamine, chlorpromazine, prazosin, trimazosin, indoramine, urapidil, yohimbine etc.*

CHAPTER - 21

CHOLINERGIC DRUGS AND ANTICHOLINESTERASE AGENTS

Acetylcholine is a chemical substance which is the acetyl ester of the quarternary ammonium alcohol choline. It acts as the neurohumoral tranmitter in the body, that is, it is a chemical which carries the message from one nerve ending to another nerve ending or muscle or gland. Acetylcholine is the neurohumoral transmitter mainly at both the sympathetic and parasympathetic ganglia and at postganglionic parasympathetic neuromuscular junction. The action of acetylcholine can be divided into two parts :-

(1) muscarinic (2) nicotinic.

The *muscarinic* action is so named because it resembles the action of an alkaloid known as muscarine. Because of the muscarinic action, the heart will slow down, the pupil of the eye is contracted, the secretions of the salivary and other glands are increased, there is vasodilatation of the peripheral blood vessels; peristatic movements of the intestine are increased and the smooth muscle of the urinary bladder is contracted. The muscarinic action of acetycholine is blocked by atropine. The other part of the action of acetylcholine is the *nicotinic* which involves mainly stimulation of skeletal muscles. The stimulation of parasympathetic nerves gives actions which are similar to the actions of acetylcholine, confirming that acetylcholine is the neurohumoral transmitter.

Acetylcholine, as soon as its function is over, is hydrolysed and destroyed in the body by an enzyme acetylcholinesterase. There are some compounds which are structurally similar to acetylcholine and give the same actions. However

246

they take a longer time to be destroyed by the acetylcholinesterase and so give the actions of acetylcholine for a longer time. They are known as cholinergic agents. However there are other substances which fix the acetylcholinesterase by combining with it. Because of this the enzyme is said to be inhibited. Such compounds are known as anticholinesterases or anticholinesterase agents. These allow the acetylcholine to accumulate at the receptor site and prolong its action.

The cholinergic agents and anticholinesterases are used to stimulate intestinal peristalsis in post-operative atony, to induce micturition (passing of urine) in atony of the bladder, to bring down the intraocular pressure in the eye disease glaucoma and in certain cardiac arrythmias. They may also be used to relieve the muscular weakness in myasthenia gravis.

CLASSIFICATION

I. Cholinergic (cholinomimetic) drug

Pilocarpine

II. Anticholinesterases

1. Neostigmine
2. Pyridostigmine
3. Physostigmine

III. Antidote for Cholinesterase Inhibition

Pralidoxime chloride

1. PILOCARPINE

Pilocarpine is an alkaloid extracted from the dried leaflets of *Pilocarpus jaborandi or Pilocarpus microphyllus*. It directly acts on the cholinergic smooth muscles and glands and stimulates them. It is clinically used as the hydrochloride and the nitrate. It has a relatively simple structure being a compound of imidazole linked to a furan drivative.

Physical Properties

Pilocarpine hydrochloride melts at 204° to 205°C and occurs in the form of colourless crystals or as a white or almost white, hygroscopic, crystalline powder. It is very soluble in water and ethanol, slightly soluble in chloroform and practically insoluble in ether. It is affected by light.

Chemical Properties

When pilocarpine hydrochloride is dissolved in carbon dioxide free water and potassium dichromate solution, hydrogen peroxide solution and chloroform are added and shaken, a violet colour is produced in the chloroform layer.

Stability and Storage

Since the substance is hygroscopic and is also affected by light, store it in an airtight container and protected from light.

Uses

Cholinergic drug. It is mainly used as a miotic, that is, for constricting the pupil of the eye to reduce intraocular tension in the eye disease glaucoma.

Official

Pilocarpine Hydrochloride, B.P.
Pilocarpine Eye Drops, B.P.
Pilocarpine Nitrate, I.P., B.P.

Brand Names

Pilocar, Carpo-miotic, Almocarpin, Pilomiotin etc.

2. NEOSTIGMINE

Neostigmine is a synthetic compound and it is used as neostigmine bromide and neostigmine methyl sulphate. Neostigmine is an anticholinesterase and enhances the action of acetylcholine.

$$(CH_3)_2NCO.O-\!\!\!\!\bigcirc\!\!\!\!-\overset{+}{N}(CH_3)_3Br^-$$

NEOSTIGMINE BROMIDE

Dimethycarbamic ester of 3-hydroxy-N,N.N-trimethylanilinium bromide.

Carbamic acid is H_2NCOOH. Dimethylcarbamic acid is $(CH_3)_2NCOOH$. It has esterified 3-hydroxyaniline. The amino part of the aniline is converted into a quarternary ammonium compound by methylation with methyl bromide, CH_3Br. Therefore neostigmine is *dimethylcarbamic ester of 3-hydroxy-N,N,N-trimethylanilinium bromide.*

Physical Properties

Neostigmine bromide occurs as colourless crystals or as a white, very hygroscopic, crystalline bitter powder. It is odourless. It melts at 171° to 176°C with decomposition. It is very soluble in water, freely soluble in chloroform and ethanol and practically insoluble in ether. It is affected by light.

Chemical Properties

Whem neostigmine is disintegrated by boiling with dilute sodium hydroxide solution, dimethylamine is produced and the smell of dimethylamine can be noticed. When neostigmine is treated with potassium hydroxide and ethanol, warmed on a water bath replacing the ethanol from time to time, cooled and dilute diazobenzene sulphonic acid solution is added, an orange red colour is produced.

Stability and Storage

Since it is hygroscopic and is also affected by light, keep it in a well-closed container protected from light.

Uses

Anticholinesterase. It is useful in the treatment of paralytic ileus (intestinal obstruction due to paralysis of the muscles of peristalsis), postoperative urinary retention and myasthenia gravis (disorder characterized by abnormal fatigue of striated muscle).

Official

Neostigmine Bromide, I.P., B.P.
Neostigmine Bromide Tablets, I.P.
(Neostigmine Tablets, B.P.)
Neostigmine Methylsulphate, I.P., B.P.
Neostigmine Methylsulphate Injection, I.P.
(Neostigmine Injection, B.P.)

Brand Names

Prostigmin, Neostigmin, Proserine, Syntigmin etc.

3. PYRIDOSTIGMINE

This has almost the same structure as neostigmine except for the fact that the aniline is substituted by a heterocyclic ring pyridine. So it is the *dimethylcarbamic ester of 3-hydroxy-1-methylpyridinium bromide.*

Properties

Pyridostigmine bromide is a white, crystalline powder with an agreeble, characteristic odour. It melts at 152° to 154°C. It is deliquescent and is freely soluble in water, alcohol and chloroform and practically insoluble in acetone, benzene and ether. It is affected by light.

Stability and Storage

Since it is deliquescent and is also affected by light, store it in an airtight, light-resistant container.

Uses

Anticholinesterase. It is mainly used in myasthenia gravis. It is less potent and longer acting than neostigmine.

Official

Pyridostigmine Bromide, B.P. '88
Pyridostigmine Injection, B.P. '88
Pyridostigmine Tablets, B.P. '88

Brand Names

Kalymin, Regonol, Mestinon bromide.

4. PHYSOSTIGMINE

Physostigmine has a complex structure and is an indole-pyrrole derivative. It is also a methylcarbamic ester. It is an alkaloid obtained by extraction from the calabar beans, seeds of *Physostigma venenosum*. It is used in the form of its salicylate and sulphate.

Physical Properties

Physostigmine salicylate consists of colourless crystals melting at about 182°C with decomposition. The substance and its aqueous solution turn gradually red on exposure to air and light and also in contact with traces of metals. This change is brought about more rapidly when the substance is also exposed to moisture. This is because of oxidative changes in the substance and this can be prevented by adding a reducing agent like sodium sulphite. The aqueous solution is most stable at pH 6 and should not be sterilized by heat.

It is sparingly soluble in water, soluble in chloroform and ethanol and very slightly soluble in ether. It is affected by light.

251

Chemical Properties

When an aqueous solution of physostigmine salicylate is treated with dilute sodium hydroxide solution, a white precipitate is produced. It turns pink. The precipitate dissolves when excess of dilute sodium hydroxide solution is added, producing a red solution.

Another colour reaction involves the heating of physostigmine salicylate with a few drops of dilute ammonia and evaporating it. The residue has an orange colour and is soluble in ethanol producing a blue solution. When glacial acetic acid is added, the colour becomes violet. When it is diluted with water, an intense red fluorescence is seen.

Stability and Storage

Since it is affected by light and also turns red on exposure to air, light and moisture, store it in an airtight container and protected from light.

Uses

Anticholinesterase. It is used as a miotic in the form of eye drops in glaucoma.

Official

Physostigmine Salicylate, I.P., B.P.
Physostigmine Salicylate Injection, I.P.
Physostigmine Sulphate, B.P.
Physostigmine Eye Drops, B.P.

Brand Names

Eserine, Physostol, Bi-miotic (with pilocarpine)

Other cholinergic drugs in clinical use are *methacholine, carbachol, bethanechol etc.* Other anticholinesterases in clinical use are *ambenonium, edrophonium, demecarium, echothiophate etc.*

252

5. PRALIDOXIME CHLORIDE

Pralidoxime is the aldoxime (aldehyde oxime) of N-methylpyridinium chloride. This means that there is an aldehydic group (-CHO) present at the 2nd position of the pyridine nucleus and that it is also converted to its oxime (-CH=NOH).

Properties

Pralidoxime chloride is a white to pale yellow, odourless, crystalline powder. It melts between 215° and 225°C with decomposition. It is freely soluble in water and sparingly soluble in ethanol. If ferric chloride solution is added to an aqueous solution of pralidoxime chloride, an amber-brown colour is produced.

Stability and Storage

Store it in well-closed containers.

Uses

Antidote for cholinesterase inhibitors. Pralidoxime is also known as 2-PAM. It is a quarternary ammonium compound and also is an oxime. If the cholinesterase enzyme is poisoned by organophosphorus compounds (irreversible inhibition), it is released by pralidoxime forming the oxime-phosphonate. Thus cholinesterase is reactivated. Pralidoxime is used to restore neuromuscular transmission in the case of cholinesterase inhibition by organophosphate poisioning or by neostigmine, pyridostigmine etc.

Official

Pralidoxime Chloride, I.P.
Pralidoxime Chloride Injection, I.P.

Brand Names

2-PAM chloride, Protopam chloride.

CHAPTER - 22

CHOLINERGIC BLOCKING AGENTS

Anticnolinergic drugs block the action of acetylcholine in the parasympathetic part of the ANS and also in the CNS. They mainly block the muscarinic action of acetylcholine at the postganglionic parasympathetic nerve endings and also at the autonomic ganglia (both sympathetic and parasympathetic - these are known as ganglion blockers) and at the neuromusecular junction (neuromuscular blockers).

Because of this, antispasmodic, antiulcer, antisecretory, antiparkinsonism, mydriatic and cycloplegic actions are exhibited by anticholinergic drugs. These are competitive antagonists.

Therefore anticholinergic drugs have the following three uses :-

a) *antispasmodic* - they reduce the tone and motility by the gastrointestinal tract providing relief from spasm of bowel.

b) *antisecretory* - they reduce the secretion of salivary and sweat glands and also acid secretion in the stomach. So they are useful in ulcers.

c) *mydriatic and cycloplegic* - they dilate the pupil of the eye and also paralyse the ciliary structure of the eye.

CLASSIFICATION

I. Solonaceous Alkaloids and Related Compounds

1. Atropine
2. Hyoscine
3. Homatropine

254

II. Synthetic Compounds

1. Propantheline
2. Benztropine
3. Tropicamide
4. Biperiden

1. ATROPINE

The solanaceous alkaloids are obtained from various plants belonging to the family *Solanaceae*. These alkaloids are mainly hyoscyamine and hyoscine. Various species of *Atropa, Datura, Duboisia, Hyoscyamus, Mandragora and Scopolia* contain these alkaloids in varying quantities. It is doubtful if atropine is present in the plants. It is formed by racemisation of (-) hyoscyamine during extraction. It can also be made from (-) hyoscyamine by adding alcoholic alkali.

These alkaloids are tertiary bases as well as esters of aminoalcohols with acids. (-)-hyoscyamine and atropine are esters of the aminoalcohol tropine with tropic acid, the only difference being that (-) - hyoscyamine is laevorotatory and atropine is optically inactive because it is a racemic mixture of (+) and (-)-hyoscyamine.

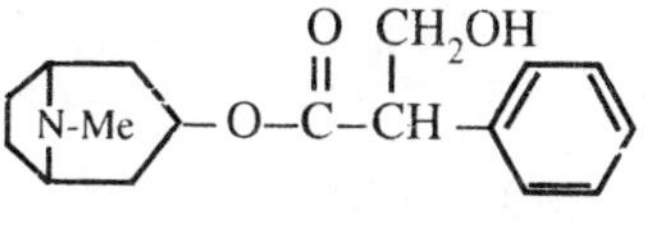

ATROPINE

(Tropyltropine)

Homatropine is also an ester of the aminoalcohol tropine but with mandelic acid which is a lower homologue of tropic acid.

255

$$\text{N-Me} - \text{O} - \overset{\overset{\text{O}}{\|}}{\text{C}} - \overset{\overset{\text{OH}}{|}}{\text{CH}} - \text{(benzene ring)}$$

HOMATROPINE
(Mandelytropine)

Atropine is official as the methyl bromide, methonitrate and sulphate. Other atropine salts in clinical use are the hydrochloride and the hydrobromide.

Physical Properties

Atropine occurs in colourless crystals or as a crystalline powder, When pure, it melts at 115°-115.5°C. The melting point is lowerred if it contains small quantities of hyoscyamine as impurity. It is slightly soluble in water (1 in 460), readily soluble in alcohol (1 in 2) and in chloroform (1 in 1) and soluble in ether (1 in 25). It is optically inactive. It is a monacid tertiary base and forms salts with one equivalent of acids. The saturated aqueous solution of atropine is alkaline to phenolphthalein. It has a pKa of 10 which is rather strong for an alkaloid.

Atropine sulphate is a white, crystalline powder or occurs as colourless crystals. It is very soluble in water, freely soluble in ethanol and glycerin and practically insoluble in chloroform and ether. It is efflorescent in dry air and should be protected from light. Aqueous solutions of atropine sulphate are unstable and should be freshly prepared. They should be preferably in acid solution at pH 6 to be stable.

Chemical Properties

Atropine answers **Vitali's test**. To a small amount of the substance fuming nitric acid is added and evaporated to dryness on a water bath. The residue is cooled and acetone and potassium hydroxide in methanol solution are added. A violet colour is produced. When an aqueous solution of the substance is treated with dilute hydrochloric acid and Dragendorff's reagent, an orange or orange red precipitate is formed immediately. Atropine in dilute hydrochloric acid gives a lemon yellow precipitate with gold chloride solution. This precipitate melts at 137° to 139°C. It also gives a yellow amorphous precipitate with a saturated solution of bromine in hydrobromic acid (Wormley's reagent). Atropine forms atropine picrate with picric acid solution in rectangular plates which melt at 197°-200°C.

A delicate biological test for atropine is for its power of producing mydriasis in the eye. A 1 in 40,000 solution of atropine is found to be sufficient for dilating the pupil of a cat within an hour.

Stability and Storage

Since atropine sulphate is efflorescent and is also affected by light, store it in well-closed, light-resistant containers.

Uses

Anticholinergic drug and antidote to cholinesterase inhibitors. Atropine and its salts are useful in the treatment of ulcers, parkinsonism, coryza (the common cold), hay fever (allergic rhinitis) and rhinitis (inflammation of the nose) and for the relief of biliary and renal colics. It is also used for dilating the pupil of the eye. Atropine methonitrate is used in the treatment of pyloric stenosis (contraction or narrowing of pylorus which is the region of the junction between the stomach and the duodenum). The extract and tincture of belladonna are both used as antispasmodics for the relief of spasm in the bowels.

Official

Atropine Methobromide, B.P.

Atropine Methonitrate, I.P., B.P.

Atropine Sulphate, I.P., B.P.

Atropine Eye Drops, B.P.

Atropine Sulphate Eye Ointment, I.P.

(Atropine Eye Ointment, B.P.)

Atropine Sulphate Injection, I.P.

(Atropine Injection, B.P.)

Atropine Sulphate Tablets, I.P.

(Atropine Tablets, B.P.)

Morphine and Atropine Injection, B.P.

Brand Names

DL-Hyoscyamine, Atropine sulphate. Tropine tropate.

2. HYOSCINE

Hyoscine or scopolamine is obtained from the mother liquor after hyoscyamine has been crystallised out. It is got by extraction from solanaceous plants such as *Daturc metel, Duboisia myoperoides, Scopolia carniolica and Hyoscyamus niger*. It can be called as epoxyhyoscyamine since it is obtained by the combination of the aminoalcohol scopine (which is tropine with an epoxy ring) and tropic acid. It is clinically used in the form of its hydrobromide and butylbromide.

Physical Properties

Hyoscine hydrobromide consists of colourless crystals or occurs as a white, crystalline powder without odour. It is efflorescent. After drying over phosphorus pentoxide for 24 hours and then at 100° to 105°C for two hours, it melts at about 197°C with decomposition. It is freely soluble in water, soluble in ethanol and practically insoluble in chloroform and ether.

Chemical Properties

Hyoscine answers the Vitali's test (see atropine). Wormley's reagent (bromine in hydrobromic acid) gives with hyoscine initially an amorphous precipitate which soon becomes crystalline. It does not give a crystalline precipitate with iodine in potassium iodide solution as readily as atropine. Hyoscine is more sensitive in the gold chloride test giving crystals from a 1 in 1000 solution also. Hyoscine pictrate melts at 188° to 193°C.

Stability and Storage

Since hyoscine hydrobromide is efflorescent and is also affected by light, it must be stored in a well-filled, air-tight, small container which is protected from light and stored at a temperature not exceeding 15°C. To avoid repeated exposure to the atmosphere, a well-filled, small container must be used.

Uses

Parasympatholytic (anticholinergic). It is used as an **antiemetic, mydriatic and cycloplegic.** Hyoscine butylbromide is used mainly as an antispasmodic. Hyoscine is also used in the treatment of nausea, parkinsonism, acute mania and delirium (extravagant talking and raving, generally due to high fever). Along with morphine or pethidine, it produces partial amnesia (partial loss of memory) leading to 'twilight sleep'.

Official

Hyoscine Butylbromide, I.P., B.P.
Hyoscine Butylbromide Injection, I.P., B.P.
Hyoscine Butylbromide Tablets, I.P., B.P.
Hyoscine Hydrobromide, I.P., B.P.
Hyoscine Eye Drops, B.P.
Hyoscine Hydrobromide Injection, I.P.
(Hyoscine Injection, B.P.)
Hyoscine Hydrobromide Tablets, I.P.
(Hyoscine Tablets, B.P.)

Brand Names

Scopolamine, Transderm-V, Scopine tropate.

3. HOMATROPINE

Homatropine is the lower homologue of atropine. It is produced by the combination of the aminoalcohol tropine with mandelic acid. In atropine, tropine is combined with tropic acid. So homatropine is mandelyltropine. See atropine for the structure of homatropine. Homatropine is official as homatropine hydrobromide and homotropine methylbromide. While the hydrobromide is mainly used as a mydriatic and cycloplegic, the methylbromide is used as a general anticholinergic.

Physical Properties

Homatropine is a synthetic alkaloid melting at 99° - 100°C. Just like any alkaloid, it is sparingly soluble in water but soluble in organic solvents such as alcohol, ether, benzene, chloroform, acetone etc.

Homatropine hydrobromide consists of colourless crystals or is a white, crystalline powder without odour. It is freely soluble in water, sparingly soluble in ethanol and slightly soluble in ether. It is affected by light.

Chemical Properties

Homatropine does not answer Vitali's test (see atropine). So any contamination or deliberate adulteration of homatropine with atropine or hyoscyamine can be easily detected by subjecting it to Vitali's test which is answered by the natural solanaceous alkaloids. Homatropine can be extracted by chloroform from the aqueous solution of the hydrobromide by adding dilute ammonia. The chloroform extract may be evaporated to dryness and the residue (homatropine) is treated with alcoholic mercuric chloride solution. A yellow colour is produced. On warming it becomes red. Homatropine picrate melts at 182° to 186°C.

Stability and Storage

Since homatropine hydrobromide is affected by light, store it in well-closed, light-resistant containers.

Uses

Mydriatic and cycloplegic. The methyl bromide is used as an anticholinergic. Mydriatic action is shorter and more rapid than atropine. It is about 10 times less potent than atropine and is the most commonly used mydriatic in adults.

Official

Homatropine Hydrobromide, I.P., B.P.
Homatropine Hydrobromide Eye Drops, I.P.
(Homatropine Eye Drops, B.P.)
Homatropine Methyl Bromide, B.P.

Brand Names

Homarin, Mandelyltropine, Tropine mandelate.

4. BENZTROPINE

Benztropine is not an ester like atropine or homatropine but is an ether. It is produced by the combination of the aminoalcohol tropine with benzhydryl alcohol. It is official as the mesylate (methane sulphonate).

Physical Properties

Benztropine mesylate is a white crystalline powder, almost without odour melting at 142° to 144°C. It is slightly hygroscopic. It is very soluble in water, freely soluble in ethanol and practically insoluble in ether.

Chemical Properties

When fuming nitric acid is added to the substance, a reddish colour is produced. It is evaporated to dryness. A brownish yellow, oily residue is obtained. It becomes yellow on the addition of acetone. When potassium hydroxide in methanol solution is added, a brownish red precipitate is produced.

In the second test, the substance may be dissolved in conc.sulphuric acid. An orange solution is produced. Divide it into two parts. To one part add dilute potassium dichromate solution, warm and allow to stand. The colour slowly changes to brown. To the other part add water. A colourless, opalescent solution is produced. Benztropine picrate melts at 185°C.

Stability and Storage

Since it is slightly hygroscopic, store it in a well-closed container.

Uses

Central anticholinergic. It is mainly used in the treatment of parkinsonism (a disorder of the middle aged and elderly people characterised by tremor, rigidity and lack of spontaneous movements. It is a disease affecting the basal ganglia of the brain). It has antihistaminic and local anaesthetic action also along with the anticholinergic action.

Official

Benztropine Mesylate, B.P.
Benztropine Injection, B.P.
Benztropine Tablets, B.P.

Brand Names

Cobrentin, Cogentin, Cogentinol.

262

5. PROPANTHELINE

Propantheline is a choline-homologue ester of 9-xanthencarboxylic acid. Xanthen is a dibenzpyran. In the 9th position of xanthen there is a substitution of a carboxylic acid group. Propantheline is the ester of 9-xanthencarboxylic acid and a quarternary alcohol known as methyldiisopropylaminoethyl alcohol. It is official as the quarternary bromide.

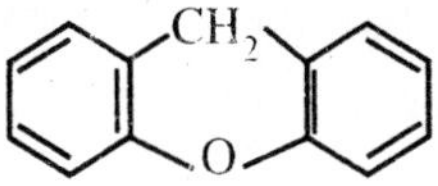

XANTHEN

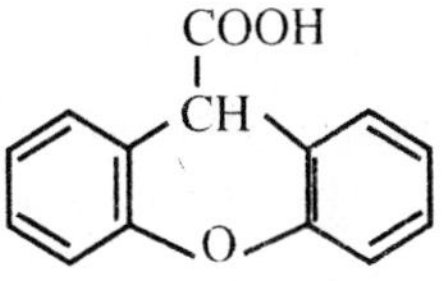

9-XANTHEN CARBOXYLIC ACID

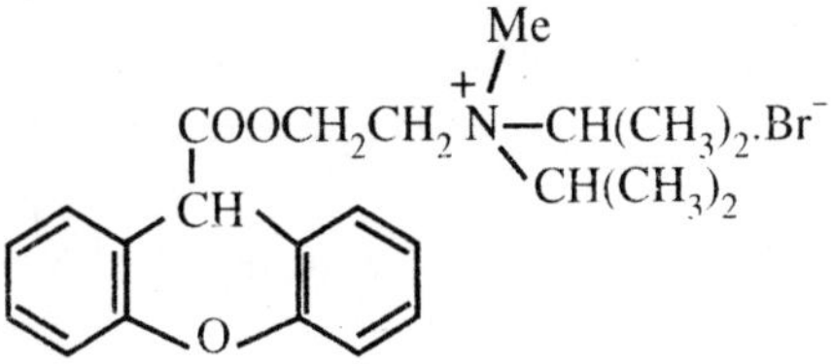

PROPANTHELINE BROMIDE

Physical Properties

Propantheline bromide is a white to yellowish white, crystalline powder. It has no odour and is slightly hygroscopic. It melts at 159° to 161°C. It is very soluble in water, ethanol and chloroform and practically insoluble in ether.

Chemical Properties

When an aqueous solution of the substance is boiled with sodium hydroxide solution, dilute hydrochloric acid added, cooled and filtered and the residue treated with concentrated sulphuric acid, an intense yellow colour is produced and it fluoresces strongly in ultraviolet light.

Stability and Storage

Since propantheline bromide is slightly hygroscopic, store it in well-closed containers.

Uses

Antispasmodic and parasympatholytic. It is the most popular drug used for providing relief in peptic ulcer. It is reported to reduce gastric secretion. Only weak side effects are produced. It is also used in gastritis, acute pancreatitis, enuresis (absence of voluntary control over the passing of urine) and spasm of the g.i.t. and biliary and urinary tracts.

Official

Propantheline Bromide, I.P., B.P.
Propantheline Bromide Tablets, I.P.
(Propantheline Tablets, B.P.)

Brand Names

Probanthine, Ketaman, Pantheline, Ercotina.

6. TROPICAMIDE

Tropicamide is an amide of tropic acid. Actually it is *N-ethyl-N-(4-pyridylmethyl) tropamide*.

Physical Properties

Tropicamide is a white or almost white, odourless, crystalline powder melting at 95° to 98°C. It is slightly soluble in water but freely soluble in ethanol, chloroform and in solutions of strong acids. It is affected by light.

Chemical Properties

If the substance is dissolved in a mixture of acetic anhydride, acetic acid and citric acid and heated on a water bath for 5 to 10 minutes, a reddish yellow colour is produced.

Stability and Storage

Since it is affected by light, store it in well-closed, light-resistant containers.

Uses

Mydriatic and cycloplegic. It is powerful and is speedy and brief in mydriatic action. It produces complete cycloplegia in children.

Official

Tropicamide, I.P., B.P.
Tropicamide Eye Drops, I.P., B.P.

Brand Names

Mydriacyl, Bistropamide.

7. BIPERIDEN

Biperiden is a piperidinopropanol. It is clinically used as the hydrochloride.

Properties

Biperiden hydrochloride is a white, crystalline powder without odour and melting at 275°C (dec). It is optically inactive. It is slightly soluble in water but freely soluble in chloroform. It is sparingly soluble in methanol. It is affected by light.

Stability and Storage

Since it is affected by light, store it in well-closed, light-resistant containers.

Uses

Antiparkinsonism drug. Even though it has anticholinergic action (mainly muscarinic), it is primarily used to treat all types of parkinsonism.

Official

Biperiden Hydrochloride Tablets, U.S.P.

Biperiden Lactate Injection, U.S.P.

Brand Names

Akinophyl, Kineton.

Other anticholinergic drugs in clinical use are *ipratropium bromide, cyclopentolate, oxyphenonium, clidinium, penthienate, pipenzolate, mepenzolate, isopropamide, glycopyrrolate, dicyclomine, pirenzepine, trihexyphenidyl, procyclidine, cycrimine, ethopropazine etc.*

CHAPTER - 23

HISTAMINE AND ANTIHISTAMINIC AGENTS

HISTAMINE

Histamine is an amine found in many tissues and also synthesized by intestinal bacteria. Chemically it is *4-(2-aminoethyl) imidazole.* It is released, along with other substances, during allergic and anaphylactic reactions in the body which are caused by sensitising substances known as antigens. The antigens may be derived from food or the immediate environment or even a drug.

Histamine is supposed to act on two type of receptors, H_1 and H_2. The following are the effects due to action on H_1 receptors :-

(a) Dilation and increased permeability of capilaries giving rise to flare reaction on the skin and leading to oedema and fall of blood pressure.

(b) Strong stimulation of bronchial smooth muscle leading to bronchiolar constriction.

(c) Stimulation of the secretion of acid in the stomach and also nasal and lacrimal secretions.

(d) Stimulation of the heart producing cardiac acceleration.

ANTIHISTAMINES

Antihistamines are drugs which abolish or reduce the H_1 receptor action of histamine. Therefore they are used in allergic diseases like urticaria, hay fever, asthma, rhinitis etc. Some of them also show other types of activity such as local anaesthetic action, antispasmodic effects, sedation, antiemetic and antipruritic effects. So they are useful in motion sickness, vomiting such as post-operative vomiting and vomiting due to pregnancy and also for anaesthetic premedication.

HISTAMINE

As already stated, it is β-*imidazolylethylamine*. It is found to be present in ergot and some other plants and also in mast cells in the body. Skin, gastric and intestinal mucosa, lungs, liver and placenta are rich in histamine. It is also present in blood and many body secretions. It is synthesized in the body from the aminoacid histidine which is decarboxylated to histamine. It is official as the phosphate and dihydrochloride.

Physical Properties

Histamine phosphate consists of colourless, long prismatic, odourless crystals. It is freely soluble in water and slightly soluble in ethanol. It is affected by light.

Chemical Properties

When an aqueous solution of histamine phosphate is treated with sodium hydroxide and diazotised sulphanilic acid, a deep red colour is produced.

Stability and Storage

Keep it in well-closed, light-resistant containers.

Uses

Diagnostic acid (gastric secretion indicator). It is injected subcutaneously to find out the capacity of the stomach to secrete acid.

Official

Histamine Phosphate, I.P., B.P.
Histamine Phosphate Injection, I.P.
Histamine Dihydrochloride, B.P.

Brand Names

Ergamine, Peremine, Amin-Glaukosan etc.

CLASSIFICATION OF ANTIHISTAMINICS

H_1 RECEPTOR ANTAGONISTS

(a) Aminoalkyl ethers
   Diphenhydramine

(b) Ethylenediamines
   Mepyramine

(c) Alkylamines
   1. Pheniramine
   2. Chlorpheniramine

(d) Phenothiazines
   Promethazine

(e) Miscellaneous
   Cyproheptadine

1. DIPHENHYDRAMINE

Ethers have the structure R-O-R′. R and R′ are alkyl groups which may be the same or different, When the alkyl groups carry amino groups attached to them, they are known as aminoalkyl ethers.

In diphenyhydramine the two alkyl groups on either side of the ether oxygen are methyl and ethyl groups. The first carbon atom of the ethyl group carries a dimethylamino [$-N(CH_3)_2$] group. Now it is known as dimethylethylamine. The methyl radical on the other side carries two phenyl groups. Including the ether oxygen this part is known a diphenylmethoxy [$(C_6H_5)_2CHO-$] group. Therefore the systematic name of diphenhydramine is *2-diphenylmethoxy-N, N-dimethylethylamine* and its formula is given below :-

DIPHENYDRAMINE
(2-Diphenylmethoxy-N,N-dimethylethylamine)

Diphenhydramine is official as the hydrochloride.

Physical Properties

Diphenhydramine hydrochloride is a white or almost white, odourless, crystalline powder. It melts between 168° and 172°C. It is very soluble in water. pH of the aqueous solution is between 4 and 6. It is freely soluble in chloroform and ethanol and practically insoluble in ether. It slowly darkens on exposure to light.

Chemical Properties

If the aqueous solution of the substance is treated with concentrated hydrochloric acid, an intense yellow colour is produced. When concentrated nitric acid is added, the yellow colour changes to red. When it is cooled, mixed with water, chloroform added and shaken, an intense violet colour is produced in the chloroform layer.

Stability and Storage

Since it darkens on exposure to light, keep it in well-closed, light-resistant containers.

Uses

Antihistaminic (histamine H_1-receptor antagonist). It is also used in cough mixtures and as an antiemetic. It is also used to treat symptoms of parkinsonism and to treat hay fever, urticaria, bronchial asthma and vasomotor rhinitis. The side effects are sedation and drowsiness. Dimenhydrinate (salt with theoclic acid) is used in the control of motion sickness).

Official

Diphenhydramine Hydrochloride, I.P., B.P.
Diphenhydramine Hydrochloride Capsules, I.P.
Diphenhydramine Oral Solution, B.P.

Brand Names

Benadryl, Dramamine, Diatrinate, Gravel etc.

2. MEPYRAMINE

Ethylenediamine has the structure $H_2NCH_2CH_2NH_2$. In mepyramine the amino group on one side carries two methyl groups and the amino group on the other side has 4-methoxybenzyl (CH_3O-C_6H_4-CH_2-) and 2-pyridyl (pyridine connected in the 2nd position) groups. Mepyramine is official as the maleate.

Properties

Mepyramine maleate is a white or slightly yellow, odourless, crystalline powder. It melts between 99° and 103°C. It is very soluble in water, freely soluble in ethanol and chloroform and very slightly soluble in ether.

Stability and Storage

Since it is affected by light, keep it in well-closed, light-resistant containers.

Uses

Antihistaminic (histamine H_1 -receptor antagonist). It is used for treating allergic conditions, insect bites and stings etc. It has also got somewhat good local anaesthetic effect. It is also used as an antiemetic.

Official

Mepyramine Maleate, I.P., B.P.
Mepyramine Maleate Tablets, I.P.
(Mepyramine Tablets, B.P.)

Brand Names

Mepyramine, Anthisan, Paraminyl, Mepiren etc.

3. PHENIRAMINE

It is the derivative of an alkylamine. The alkylamine reffered to here is a tertiary amine carrying three alkyl groups. In pheniramine, the three alkyl groups are one propyl and two methyl groups. The third atom of the propyl radical carries two substituents, a 2-pyridyl group and a phenyl group. Therefore pheniramine is *3-phenyl-3-(-2 pyridyl)propyl dimethylamine*. It is official as the maleate.

PHENIRAMINE MALEATE
[3-Phenyl-3-(2-pyridyl)propyldimethylamine]

Properties

Pheniramine maleate is a white or almost white, crystalline powder having no odour. It melting point is between 106° and 109°C. It is freely soluble in water, chloroform and ethanol and very slightly soluble in ether. It is affected by light.

Stability and Storage

Since it is affected by light, keep it in tightly-closed, light-resistant containers.

Uses

Antihistaminic (histamine H_1 -receptor antagonist). It has less potency compared to other antihistaminics.

Official

Pheniramine Maleate, I.P., B.P.
Pheniramine Maleate Injection, I.P.
Pheniramine Maleate Tablets, I.P.

Brand Names

Avil, Daneral, Inhiston, Trimeton.

4. CHLORPHENIRAMINE

Chlorpheniramine has almost the same structure as pheniramine but for the fact that it has a chloro group extra in the para postion of the phenyl group attached to the third postion of the propyl radical of the tertiary amine. Therefore it is *3-(4-chlorophenyl)-3-(2-pyridyl)propyldimethylamine*. It is official as the maleate.

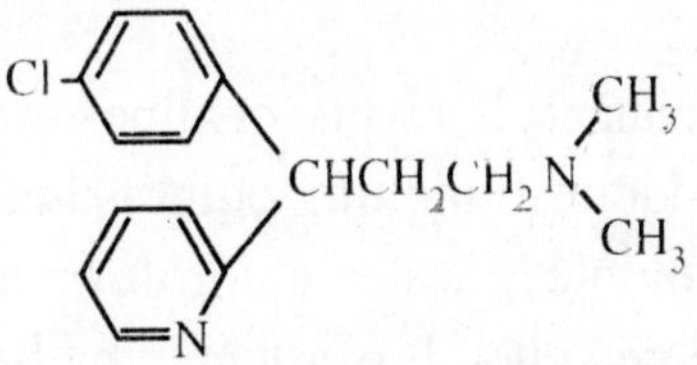

CHLORPHENIRAMINE

Properties

Chlorpheniramine maleate is an odourless, white, crystalline powder. It melts between 132° and 135°C. It is freely soluble in water, soluble in ethanol and slightly soluble in ether. It is affected by light.

Stability and Storage

Since it is affected by light, keep it in tightly-closed, light-resistant containers.

Uses

Antihistaminic (histamine H_1-receptor antagonist). It is one of the most potent antihistaminics unlike pheniramine. The activity is increased 20 times because of the presence of the para chloro group in the benzene ring. Its advantage is also that it is only mildly sedative and also has low anticholinergic activity.

Official

Chlorpheniramine Maleate, I.P., B.P.
Chlorpheniramine Maleate Injection, I.P., B.P.
Chlorpheniramine Oral Solution, B.P.
Chlorpheniramine Maleate Tablets, I.P.
(Chlorpheniramine Tablets, B.P.)

274

Brand Names

Piriton, Zeet, Alumex, Histalen etc.

5. PROMETHAZINE

Promethazine is a phenothiazine derivative. In its structure it carries at the 10th position a 2-dimethylaminopropyl group. Therefore promethazine is *10-(2-dimethylaminopropyl) phenothiazine*. It is official as the hydrochloride.

Physical Properties

Promethazine hydrochloride is a white or faintly yellow, crystalline powder. It is very soluble in water, freely soluble in chloroform and ethanol and practically insoluble in ether. It is oxidized to a blue compound on prolonged exposure to light. It melts at about 222°C with decomposition.

Chemical Properties

When concentrated nitric acid is added to an aqueous solution of promethazine hydrochloride, a precipitate is produced. It dissolves rapidly to give a red solution. The colour changes first to orange and finally to yellow. If the solution is heated to boiling, the colour again becomes orange and finally an orange-red precipitate is produced.

Stability and Storage

Since it is affected by light, keep it in well-closed, light-resistant containers.

Uses

Antihistaminic (histamine H_1 -receptor antagonist). Also sedative, antiemetic and tranquiliser. It has anticholinergic and some local anaesthetic actions also. It is included in many cough mixtures and syrups. It is used also topically in various skin conditions due to allergy. Promethazine theoclate is used in the control of motion sickness.

275

Official

Promethazine Hydrochloride, I.P., B.P.
Promethazine Hydrochloride Injection, I.P.
(Promethazine Injection, B.P.)
Promethazine Oral Solution, B.P.
Promethazine Hydrochloride Syrup, I.P.
Promethazine Hydrochloride Tablets, I.P., B.P.
Promethazine Theoclate, I.P., B.P.
Promethazine Theoclate Tablets, I.P., B.P.

Brand Names

Phenergan, Atosil, Remsed, Protazine etc.

6. CYPROHEPTADINE

Cyproheptadine is a dibenzcycloheptene derivative. It is official as the hydrochloride.

Properties

Cyproheptadine hydrochlordie is a white or slightly yellow, odourless, crystalline powder. It is slightly soluble in water, freely soluble in methanol, soluble in water, freely soluble in methanol, soluble in chloroform, sparingly soluble in ethanol and practically insoluble in ether. It melts between 252° and 254°C with decomposition.

Stability and Storage

Since it is affected by light, store it in well-closed, light-resistant containers.

Uses

Antihistaminic (histamine H_1-receptor antagonist). It has moderately sedative and high anticholinergic actions also. It is also used in the treatment of migraine and vascular headaches and also in itching and Cushings's disease.

Official

Cyproheptadine Hydrochloride, I.P., B.P.
Cyproheptadine Hydrochloride Syrup, I.P.
Cyproheptadine Hydrochloride Tablets, I.P.
(Cyproheptadine Tablets, B.P.)

Brand Names

Periactin, Peritol, Anarexol, Cipractin etc.

Other antihistaminics clinically used are *hydroxyzine (atarax), antazoline (antistine), trimeprazine (vellergan), meclizine (ancolan), buclizine (longifene), methdilazine (dilosyn), dimethindene (foristal), triprolidine (actidil), mebhydroline (incidal), cyclizine (marezine), clemastine (tavist)), terfenadine (trexyl), astemizole (stemizole), loratadine, cetirizine and cinnarizine (stugeron).*

CHAPTER - 24

CARDIOVASCULAR AGENTS

Cardiovascular agents are drugs which are able to alter cardiovascular function. They affect either the heart or the circulation. Five categories of cardiovascular drugs, namely cardiac glycosides, antiarrhythmic drugs, antihypertensive agents, vasodilators and lipid lowering agents will be considered in this chapter. Diuretics and anticoagulants are also useful in treating some of the cardiovascular diseases.

A. CARDIAC GLYCOSIDES

Cardiac glycosides are found widely in nature from both plant and animal sources. The plant sources are digitalis *(Digitalis lanata and Digitalis purpurea)*, strophanthus *(S.gratus and S.kombe)*, squill *(Scilla maritima)* and lily of the valley *(Convallaria majalis)*. The animal source is the poison of toad *(Bufo)*.

Cardiac glycosides improve the function of the heart by increasing the force and efficiency of the heart muscle without a corresponding increase in oxygen consumption, when administered in congestive heart failure. Because of this there is increased cardiac output. The heart rate comes down. Because of the improved blood pressure due to better cardiac output, the kidney functions more efficiently and diuresis is the result. There is also improved ventilation in the lungs. Cardiac glycosides also slow the heart rate in atrial fibrillation and other arrhythmias.

Chemically cardiac glycosides are composed of two portions, a sugar and a steroid nucleus. The sugar component may be made up of one or more sugars. The steroid part is known as the aglycone. This aglycone is responsible for the cardiotonic activity of the glycoside. However the sugar component provides water solubility.

In fact the plants contain glycosides which have sugar residues upto four. During the extraction process some of these sugars may be shed due to hydrolysis and new glycosides with less number of sugars are formed. For example the official digitalis glycosides digitoxin and digoxin are got by the hydrolysis of the original glycosides lanatosides A and C.

In the case of the plant glycosides there is a five membered α,β, -unsaturated lactone ring at position 17 in the steroid or aglycone moiety. The aglycones are also referred to as genins. The aglycones of the digitals glycosides have the structures given below :

DIGOXIGENIN   R = -OH

DIGITOXIGENIN   R = -H

The C_{17} side chain above is an α,β-unsaturated 5-membered lactone ring. The compounds having this side chain are known as **cardenolides** and they occur mostly in plants. In the toad poison the side chain is a 6-membered lactone ring and these are the **bufadienolides.** The bufadienolides occur in plants belonging to the Liliaceae and Ranunculaceae and in the toad poison. The sugars are linked with the hydroxyl group in the 3rd position of the genin.

The following are the crude drugs and cardiac glycosides official in the I.P. or B.P. or both :-

1. DIGITALIS LEAF

Digitalis consists of the leaves of *Digitalis purpurea Linn* which were dried in the dark at a temperature below 60°C soon after collection from the plant. It contains not less than 0.3% of cardenolic glycosides, calculated as digitoxin. It has a faint and characteristic odour and a bitter taste. It has the macroscopical and microscopical characters prescribed in the B.P. It is affected by light and moisture. It responds to the usual colour tests for digitalis glycosides. For example an extract of the digitalis leaf powder containing the glycosides may be evaporated to dryness on a water bath and to the residue, 3:5-dinitrobenzoic acid and sodium hydroxide solution are added. A reddish violet colour develops. In another test xanthydrol solution is added to the residue of glycosides and heated for 3 minutes on a water bath. A red colour is produced.

Stability and Storage

It should be kept in a well-closed container which is protected from moisture and light.

Uses

Cardiotonic glycoside. See the introduction to this chapter for details of pharmacological action.

Official

Digitalis Leaf, B.P.
Powdered Digitalis Leaf, B.P.

Note

Powdered Digitalis Leaf is Digitalis Leaf reduced to moderately coarse powder. It is required to contain not less than 0.3% of cardenolic glycosides, calculated as digitoxin. It is a green to greyish green powder.

2. DIGITOXIN

The glycoside lanatoside A contains in its structure the aglycone digitoxigenin attached to which there are two molecules of digitoxose, one molecule of acetyldigitoxose and one molecule of β-D-glucose.

If the glycose residue is shed and the acetyl group in the acetyldigitoxose is also removed through enzymatic hydrolysis and mild alkaline hydrolysis, digitoxin is obtained. Digitoxin is actually not present in the plant as such but is formed during the extraction process and extracted as such. It contains the aglycone digitoxigenin and three molecules of digitoxose (sugar). The structure of digitoxin is already given in the introduction in the chapter.

Physical Properties

It is a white or almost white powder melting at 256-257°C. It is affected by light, moisture and temperature exceeding 15°C. It is practically insoluble in water, freely soluble in a mixture of equal volumes of chloroform and methanol, sparingly soluble in chloroform and slightly soluble in ethanol and methanol.

Chemical Properties

It also answers the 3,5-dinitrobenzoic acid test. When it is suspended in 60% alcohol and 3,5-dinitrobenzoic acid and sodium hydroxide solutions are added, a violet colour is produced. This is known as Kedde's reaction and it is due to the aglycone part of the molecule. It also answers the Keller Killiani reaction. In this digitoxin is dissolved in glacial acetic acid, allowed to cool and ferric chloride test solution is added (even a trace of ferric chloride is enough). Then concentrated sulphuric acid is added without mixing. A brown ring is produced at the interface and a green colour which changes to blue is found in the upper layer. Other reactions answered by it include the Baljet's reaction in which it gives an orange-red colour with alkaline picrate solution and the Raymond's test in which it gives a blue colour with m-dinitrobenzene in strongly alkaline solution). These reactions are answered by all digitals glycosides.

Stability and Storage

It should be kept in a well-closed container, protected from light and stored at a temperature below 15°C.

Uses

Cardiac glycoside. It is useful in the treatment of congestive heart failure and cardiac arrhythmias such as atrial fibrillation, atrial flutter etc.

Official

Digitoxin, I.P., B.P.
Digitoxin Tablets, I.P., B.P.

Brand Names

Digitalin, Griefon, Digilong, Digimerck etc.

3. DIGOXIN

Digoxin is also obtained in the same way like digitoxin from lanatoside C. It contains in its structure the aglycone digoxigenin and 3 molecules of digitoxose. It is also formed during the process of isolation and extraction of glycosides.

Physical Properties

It consists of colourless crystals or occurs as an odourless, microcrystalline powder. It melts at 230°-235°C with decomposition. It is practically insoluble in water, freely soluble in a mixture of equal volumes of chloroform and methanol and slightly soluble in ethanol and chloroform. It is affected by light.

Chemical Properties

It answers both Kedde's reaction and the Keller-Killiani reaction in the same way as digitoxin.

Stability and Storage

It should be kept in a well-closed, light-resistant containr.

Uses

Cardiac glycoside. It has the same uses as digitoxin. It is often given by intravenous injection for rapid digitalization.

Official

Digoxin, I.P., B.P.
Digoxin Injection, I.P., B.P.
Paediatric Digoxin Injection, B.P.
Digoxin Paediatric Solution, I.P.
(Paediatric Digoxin Oral Solution, B.P.)
Digoxin Tablets, I.P., B.P.

Brand Names

Digoxin, Lanoxin, Cardioxin, Davoxin, Lenoxin etc.

4. DESLANOSIDE

This is desacetylanatoside C which means that it is obtained from lanatoside C by removal of the acetyl group in acetyldigitoxose by mild alkaline hydrolysis. It contains in its structure digoxigenin linked to three digitoxose and one β-D-glucose molecules.

Physical Properties

It consists of white crystals or occurs as a fine white, hygroscopic, crystalline powder. It melts between 265° and 268°C with decomposition. It loses water even in an atmosphere of low humidity. It is practically insoluble in water, chloroform and ether and very slightly soluble in ethanol and methanol.

Chemical Properties

It also answers both Kedde's reaction and the Keller-Killiani reaction in the same way as digitoxin and digoxin.

Stability and Storage

Since it is hygroscopic, store in tightly-closed, light-resistant containers in a cool place.

Uses

Cardiac glycoside. It is a quick-acting, cardiotonic agent which is useful in emergencies.

Official

Deslanoside, I.P., B.P.

Deslanoside Injection, I.P.

Brand Names

Deslanoside, Deacetyldigilanide C, Purpurea glycoside C, Deacetyllanatoside C, Cedilamid D etc.

5. LANATOSIDE C

This is the original glycoside present in the plant along with lanatosides A and B. It is also known as digilanide C. It contains in its structure digoxigenin, two molecules of digitoxose, one molecule of acetyldigitoxose and one molecule of β-D-glucose.

Physical Properties

It is a white or slightly yellow finely crystalline powder. It is hygroscopic and also loses water in an atmosphere of low relative humidity. It melts at 248° to 250°C with decomposition. It is practically insoluble in water, chloroform and ether. It is soluble in methanol.

Chemical Properties

It answers the Kedde's reaction and the Keller-Killiani reaction in the same way as other glycosides.

Stability and Storage

It should be kept in an airtight, well-filled glass container, protected from light and stored at a temperature below 10°C.

Uses

Cardiac glycoside. The actions and uses of this cardiotonic glycoside are the same as those of digoxin.

Official

Lanatoside C, I.P., B.P.
Lanatoside C Tablets, I.P.

Brand Names

Cedilanid, Lanimerck, Digilanide C etc.

Other cardiac glycosides clinically used are *strophanthin -K, ouabain, acetyldigoxin, gitoxin, acetyldigitoxin etc.*

B. ANTIARRHYTHMIC AGENTS

Antiarrhythmic drugs are compounds which are used to correct cardiac arrhythmias in which the heart beats without any rhythm. They act by directly depressing the heart muscle and also by increasing the refractory period between contractions.

They may be classified as below :

(a) Drugs that depress the heart muscle.

1. Quinidine
2. Procainamide
3. Lignocaine
4. Phenytoin

(b) Drugs that act through the autonomic nervous system.

Sympatholytics (B-adrenergic blockers)

Propranolol

1. QUINIDINE

Quinidine is the stereoisomer of quinine, the antimalarial. So it has the same structure as quinine. Quinidine is dextrorotatory and quinine is laevorotatory. In its structure quinidine consists of a quinoline ring linked to a quinuclidine ring through a -CHOH group.

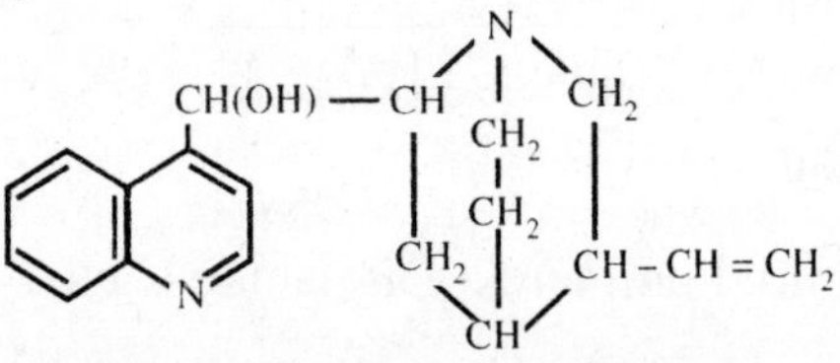

QUINOLINE   QUINUCLIDINE

QUINIDINE

Quinidine is extracted from the barks of the *Cinchona* species.

Physical Properties

Quinidine, when anhydrous, melts at 171.5°C. It is slightly soluble in water and more soluble in 80% ethanol and ether. It is dextrorotatory in alcohol-chloroform solution. It is official as the sulphate.

Quinidine sulphate is an almost white, crystalline powder or may consist of needle-like crystals. It has no odour. It is sparingly soluble in water, soluble in ethanol and chloroform and practically insoluble in ether.

Chemical Properties

Quinidine has almost the same chemical properties as quinine. It exhibits a strong blue fluorescence in dilute sulphuric acid like quinine and also answers the Thalleioquin test (see the Chemical Properties of Quinine in the chapter on "Antimalarials"). In another test silver nitrate solution is added to a solution of quinidine sulphate and stirred with a glass rod. After a small interval a white precipitate is produced. It is soluble in nitric acid (distinction from quinine and many other alkaloids).

Stability and Storage

Since it is affected by light, store it in well-closed, light-resistant containers.

Uses

Antiarrhythmic. Quinidine is a myocardial depressant. It depresses the excitability of the myocardium (heart muscle) and increases conduction time and refractory period. It is used in the treatment of atrial tachycardia (increased rate of the auricle), atrial flutter (rapid regular contraction of the atrial muscle of the heart) and fibrillation (uncoordinated contraction of the heart muscle).

Official

Quinidine Bisulphate, B.P.
Quinidine Sulphate, I.P., B.P.
Quinidine Sulphate Tablets, I.P., B.P.

Brand Names

Pitayine, Quiniduran, Kinichron etc.

2. PROCAINAMIDE

Its structure is given below :

$$
\underset{\substack{| \\ NH_2}}{C_6H_4} - \overset{\overset{O}{\|}}{C} - NH - CH_2 - CH_2 - N \overset{CH_2CH_3}{\underset{CH_2CH_3}{<}}
$$

PROCAINAMIDE

[p-Amino-N-(2-diethylaminoethyl) benzamide]

Procainamide is structurally related to procaine, the local anaesthetic. Whereas procaine is an ester, procainamide is an amide. Its systematic name is *p-amino-(N-2-diethylaminoethyl) benzamide*. It is derived from p-aminobenzamide, p-H_2N-C_6H_4-$CONH_2$ by replacement of a hydrogen in the amide nitrogen by the 2-diethylaminoethyl (-$CH_2CH_2NE_2$) group. It is official as the hydrochloride.

Physical Properties

Procainamide hydrochloride is a white or slightly yellow, odourless, hygroscopic, crystalline powder. It melts between 166° and 170°C. It is very soluble in water, freely soluble in ethanol, slightly soluble in acetone and chloroform and practically insoluble in ether.

Chemical Properties

Since it contains a primary aromatic amino group, it can be diazotised by treatment with sodium nitrite and hydrochloric acid and coupled with 2-naphthol to give an orange-red azo dye.

Stability and Storage

Since it is hygroscopic and also is affected by light, store it in tightly-closed, light-resistant containers.

288

Uses

Antiarrhythmic. Procainamide as a myocardial depressant like quinidine is dose to dose less potent. It causes less fall in B.P.

Official

Procainamide Hydrochloride, I.P., B.P.
Procainamide Hydrochloride Injection, I.P.
(Procainamide Injection, B.P.)
Procainamide Hydrochloride Tablets, I.P.
(Procainamide Tablets)

Brand Names

Pronestyl, Amidoprocain, Procamide, Proamide, Supicaine amide hydrochloride etc.

3. LIGNOCAINE

Since this is also a local anaesthetic, see the chapter on **LOCAL ANAESTHETICS.**

4. PHENYTOIN

Since this is also an anticonvulsant, see the chapter on **ANTICONVULSANTS.**

5. PROPRANOLOL

Propranolol is a beta-adrenergic blocking drug which is a naphthalene derivative. This prevents arrhythmia and also decreases the chance of angina pectoris, all through beta-adrenergic blockade of the sympathetic nerve to the heart.

It has a 2-hydroxy-3-isopropylaminopropoxy. $(CH_3)_2CHNHCH_2CH(OH)CH_2O$-, group in the naphthalene nucleus. It can be considered as an ether of 1-naphthol. It is official as the hydrochloride.

$$\underset{1}{OCH_2}\underset{2}{CH(OH)}\underset{3}{CH_2}NHCH\begin{smallmatrix}CH_3\\CH_3\end{smallmatrix}$$

PROPRANOLOL

Porperties

Propranolol hydrochloride is a white or creamy-white powder without odour. It melts between 163° and 166°C. It is soluble in water and ethanol. In aqueous solution propranolol is decomposed and the isopropylamine side chain is oxidised. The solution becomes discoloured and the pH drops to a low level. It is slightly soluble in chloroform and practically insoluble in ether.

Stability and Storage

Store in well-closed containers.

Uses

Antiarrhythmic, antianginal and antihypertensive agent (beta-adrenoceptor antagonist). It is very effective in the treatment of sympathetically mediated arrhythmias associated with pheochromocytoma (a small vascular tumour of the medulla of the adrenal gland) and chronic ventricular arrhythmias. It is also a mild antihypertensive.

Official

Propranolol Hydrochloride, I.P., B.P.
Propranolol Hydrochloride Injection, I.P.
(Propranolol Injection, B.P.)
Propranolol Hydrochloride Tablets, I.P.
(Propranolol Tablets, B.P.)

Brand Names

Inderal, Deralin, Inderex, Caridorol etc.

Other antiarrhythmic agents clinically used are *disopyramide, moricizine, mexiletine, tocainide, flecainide, encainide, propafenone, atenolol, sotalol, amiodarone, bretylium, verapamil, diltiazem, etc.*

C. ANTIHYPERTENSIVES

Hypertension is high blood pressure. It may be of two types : *(1) primary or essential hypertension*, where no definite cause is known for the rise in blood pressure and *(2) secondary hypertension*, caused as a secondary effect of renal, endocrine or vascular disease. If hypertension is left untreated, it may lead to heart, cerebrovascular and renal complications and premature death.

The drugs used to lower hypertension act through different mechanisms. Most of them reduce sympathetic vasomotor tone.

CLASSIFICATION

1. Calcium Channel Blocker
   Nifedipine
2. β-Adrenergic Blocker
   Propranolol
3. Direct Vasodilator
   Hydralazine
4. Central Sympatholytic
   a) Clonidine
   b) Methyldopa

5. Adrenergic Neurone Blocker

   a) Reserpine
   b) Guanethidine

6. Ganglion Blocker

   Pentolinium

1. NIFEDIPINE

Nifedipine is a pyridine derivative which is also a double ester. It contains an aromatic nitro group.

Physical Properties

Nifedipine is a yellow, crystalline powder. It melts between 171° and 175°C. When it is exposed to daylight and also when it is exposed to artificial light of some wavelengths, it is decomposed and is converted to a nitrosophenylpyridine derivative. It is practically insoluble in water, freely soluble in acetone and sparingly soluble in absolute alcohol.

Chemical Properties

When the substance is dissolved in ethanol and hydrochloric acid and granulated zinc are added, nascent hydrogen which is produced by the reaction between the acid and zinc reduces the aromatic nitro group to an aromatic amino group which can be diazotised by adding sodium nitrite and coupled with N-(1-naphthyl) ethylenediamine dihydrochloride. An intense red colour is produced. It remains for at least 5 minutes.

Stability and Storage

Since it is affected by exposure to light, nifedipine should be stored in a well-closed container protected from light.

Uses

Calcium channel blocker, antianginal and coronary vasodilator. This is the most popular and front line anti-hypertensive. It is preferred to most other earlier drugs because of the absence of many disadvantages associated with them.

Official

Nifedipine, I.P., B.P.
Nifedipine Capsules, I.P.
Nifedipine Tablets, I.P.

Brand Names

Cardipin, Cardules, Cardules Retard, Cardules Flus (Nifedipine+atenolol), Depicor, Depicor SR, Depin, Depin Retard, Nacten, Nicardia retard etc.

2. PROPRANOLOL

See earlier in this chapter under "ANTIARRHYTHMIC AGENTS".

3. HYDRALAZINE

Hydralazine is *1-hydrazinophthalazine*. Phthalazine is a heterocyclic compound in which two nitrogen atoms are present in the adjacent positions in naphthalene. The hydrazino group ($-NHNH_2$) is present at the first position. It is official as the hydrochloride.

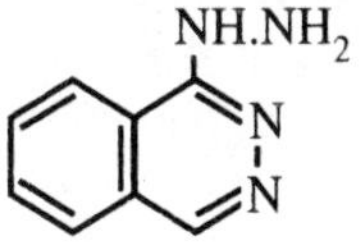

HYDRALAZINE

Physical Properties

Hydralazine hydrochloride is a white or almost white, crystalline powder melting at 273°C with decomposition. It has no odour. It is soluble in water, slightly soluble in methanol and ethanol and practically insoluble in chloroform and ether.

Chemical Properties

If hydralazine hydrochloride is dissolved in water and a solution of 2-nitrobenzaldehyde in ethanol (95%) is added, an orange precipitate is produced. When hydralazine hydrochloride is dissolved in very dilute hydrochloric acid, sodium nitrite solution added and allowed to stand for 10 minutes, a precipitate is produced. The precipitate may be washed with water and dried. It melts at 209° to 212°C.

Stability and Storage

Keep in well-closed containers.

Uses

Vasodilator and antihypertensive. Hydralazine directly acts as an arteriolar vasodilator. It is used to treat moderate to severe hypertension which is not responding to front line drugs. It is usually added in small doses to the drugs already being administered.

Official

Hydralazine Hydrochloride, I.P., B.P.
Hydralazine Hydrochloride Injection, I.P.
(Hydralazine Injection, B.P.)
Hydralazine Tablets, B.P.

Brand Names

Nepresol, Zinepress, Apresoline, Lopress etc.

4. CLONIDINE

Clonidine is an imidazolidine derivative. It is official as the hydrochloride.

Properties

Clonidine hydrochloride is a white or almost white, crystalline powder. It is freely soluble in water and ethanol, slightly soluble in chloroform and practically insoluble in ether.

Stability and Storage

It should be kept in a well-closed container.

Uses

Antihypertensive. Clonidine is an effective and cheap drug which is useful in reducing moderate hypertension. However a lot of side effects has limited its use.

Official

Clonidine Hydrochloride, I.P., B.P.
Clonidine Hydrochloride Injection, I.P.
(Clonidine Injection, B.P.)
Clonidine Hydrochloride Tablets, I.P.
(Clonidine Tablets, B.P.)

Brand Names

Catapres, Arkamin (tablets and injection), Clonidine - TTS (transdermal therapeutic delivery).

5. RESERPINE

Reserpine is one of the alkaloids extracted from the dried roots and bark of *Rauwolfia serpentina* and some other Rauwolfia species.

Physical Properties

Reserpine consists of small, white or slightly yellow crystals or occurs as a crystalline powder. It darkens slowly on exposure to light. It melts at 264-265°C with decomposition. It is odourless and tasteless. It is practically insoluble in water, freely soluble in chloroform, very slightly soluble in ethanol and practically insoluble in ether. On standing most of the solutions become yellow in colour and on exposure to light or by adding acid, fluorescence is seen to be present. It is also oxidised in solution and the green colour of the solution becomes orange.

Chemical Properties

Reserpine undergoes many colour reactions. If a solution of sodium molybdate in sulphuric acid is added to reserpine, a yellow colour is produced. It changes to blue within 2 minutes. If a solution of vanillin in acetic acid or hydrochloric acid is added to reserpine, a pink colour is produced within 2 minutes. If reserpine is mixed with 4-dimethylaminobenzaldehyde, glacial acetic acid and sulphuric acid, a green colour is produced. When more glacial acetic acid is added, the colour changes to red.

Stability and Storage

Since it is affected by light, it should be kept in a well-closed container protected from light.

Uses

Antihypertensive. Reserpine gradually depletes catecholamines and 5-HT. It acts through a combination of central sedation and central and peripheral depletion of pressor substances. Reserpine is seldom used now as an antihypertensive and also as an antipsychotic.

Official

Reserpine, I.P., B.P.

Reserpine Injection, I.P.

Reserpine Tablets, I.P.

Brand Names

Serpasil, Reserpex, Sandril, Serpasol etc.

6. GUANETHIDINE

Guanethidine has the structure given below :

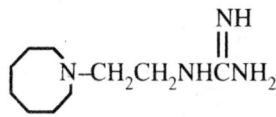

GUANETHIDINE

The eight-membered heterocyclic ring in this structure is known as octahydroazocine. A 2-guanidoethyl group is attached to the nitrogen of the heterocycle. So it can be called as 1-(2-guanidoethyl) octahydroazocine. It is official as the monosulphate.

Physical Properties

Guanethidine monosulphate is a colourless, odourless, crystalline powder melting at about 250°C with decomposition. It is freely soluble in water and practically insoluble in chloroform, ethanol and ether. It is affected by light.

Chemical Properties

Guanethidine monosulphate may be dissolved in water and sodium hydroxide solution, 1-naphthol solution and drop by drop with shaking sodium hypochlorite solution are added. A bright pink precipitate is produced. It becomes violet-red on standing. Guanethidine picrate may be prepared by dissolving the monosulphate in water and adding picric acid solution. The precipitate of guanethidine picrate may be washed and dried at 100° to 105°C. Its melting point is about 154°C.

Stability and Storage

It should be kept in a well-closed container protected from light.

Uses

Antihypertensive (adrenergic neurone blocking agent). It acts by preventing the release of noradrenaline at sympathetic nerve endings. Noradrenaline stores at sympathetic nerve endings and tissue noradrenaline are depleted (emptied). Guanethidine has almost gone out of use now.

Official

Guanethidine Monosulphate, B.P.
Guanethidine Tablets, B.P.

Brand Names

Iporal, Guethine, Ismelin, Isobarin.

7. PENTOLINIUM

Pentolinium tartrate is a quarternary ammonium compound which is a ganglion-blocking agent. In the structure of this two pyrrolidine rings are linked through their nitrogens by a pentamethylene bridge.

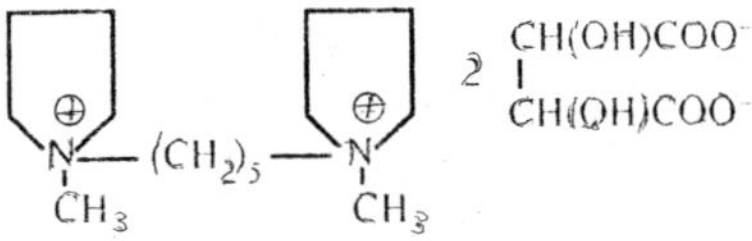

PENTOLINIUM TARTRATE

Properties

Pentolinium tartrate is an almost white powder which is very soluble in water, sparingly soluble in ethanol and practically insoluble in chloroform and ether. It is used as injection only.

Stability and Storage

It should be stored in a well-closed container.

Uses

Antihypertensive (ganglion blocking agent). It interferes with the nerve transmission of impulses at the ganglions. Sympathetic ganglions are blocked and it leads to peripheral vasodilatation and consequent reduction in blood pressure. It is rarely used now because of the serious side effects due to simulataneous parasympathetic blockade.

Official

Pentolinium Tartrate, B.P. '88

Pentolinium Injection, B.P. '88

8. METHYLDOPA

Methyldopa is the methyl derivative of the precursor of noradrenaline. It has the structure given below :

$$\text{OH} \quad \overset{\displaystyle OH}{\underset{}{\bigcirc}} - CH_2 - \overset{\displaystyle NH_2}{\underset{\displaystyle |}{C(CH_3)}} - COOH$$

METHYLDOPA

(-)-β-(3,4-dihydroxyphenyl)-α-methylalanine

Without the methyl group on the alpha carbon atom, it becomes the structure of DOPA (dihydroxyphenylalanine) from which noradrenaline is obtained. Structurally methyldopa is *(-)-β-3,4,-dihydroxyphenyl-α-methylalanine.*

Physical Properties

Methyldopa is a white to yellowish-white, fine powder. It may contain some lumps which are easily friable. It is slightly soluble in water, very slightly soluble in ethanol and practically insoluble in ether and chloroform. It dissolves easily in dilute hydrochloric acid.

Chemical Properties

When a solution of ninhydrin in sulphuric acid is added to methyldopa, a dark purple colour is produced within 5 to 10 minutes. If water is added, the colour changes to pale brownish-yellow.

Stability and Storage

Since it is affected by light, keep it in well-closed, light-resistant containers.

Uses

Antihypertensive. It is metabolized to α-methylnoradrenaline, a weak transmitter which replaces in the central nervous system noradrenaline, a strong transmitter. Bradycardia is the result. There is reduction in sympathetic tone also and consequent fall in blood pressure. It is used for treating mild to moderate hypertension. However its use is coming down because better drugs are now available.

Official

Methyldopa, I.P.
Methyldopa Tablets, I.P.

Brand Names

Aldomet, Emdopa, Medomet, Medopa, Presinol etc.

Other antihypertensives clinically used are *felodipine, nicardipine, diltiazem, verapamil, captopril, enalapril, lisinopril, perindopril, thiazides, furosemide, spironolactone, indapamide, metoprolol, atenolol, labetalol, prazosin, phentolamine, phenoxybenzamine, minoxidil, diazoxide, sodium nitroprusside, bethanidine, trimetaphan, ketanserin etc.*

D. CORONARY VASODILATORS

Angina pectoris or the so called heart attack takes place when the heart muscle or myocardium is starved of oxygen due to blockage of coronary arteries (atherosclerosis or narrowing of blood vessels due to fat depostits). When there is increased energy demand as during exercise, emotion or coitus (sexual intercourse), attacks are induced. Coronary vasodilators are drugs which dilate the coronary vessels giving an increased blood supply to the heart muscle. They are also called as antianginal drugs.

CLASSIFICATION

Nitrates

1. Ethyl nitrite
2. Glyceryl trinitrate

301

1. ETHYL NITRITE, $C_2H_5NO_2$

Ethyl nitrite is a very volatile liquid with a boiling point of 17°C. It is colourless or slightly yellowish, clear and inflammable. It has a burning, sweet taste and a characteristic, pleasant, ethereal odour. It is decomposed easily when exposed to air, light and moisture. During storage it slowly decomposes forming oxides of nitrogen. It is slightly soluble in water which hydrolyses it and more soluble in alcohol and ether. Previously it was used in the form of spirit of nitrous ether which is a solution of ethyl nitrite in alcohol. It has long since gone out of use.

Uses

Diaphoretic and coronary vasodilator.

2. GLYCERYL TRINITRATE (NITROGLYCERIN)

Glyceryl trinitrate is formed by the reaction of glycerol with nitric acid and has the following structure :-

$$
\begin{array}{l}
CH_2ONO_2 \\
| \\
CHONO_2 \\
| \\
CH_2ONO_2
\end{array}
$$

GLYCERYL TRINITRATE

It is official as concentrated glyceryl trinitrate solution and as the tablets.

Physical Properties

Glyceryl trinitrate is a pale yellow, heavy, inflammable oil. It has a sweet, burning taste. It explodes when struck with a hammer or on heating. It is slightly soluble in water and soluble in organic solvents such as ether and chloroform.

302

Concentrated glyceryl trinitrate solution is a clear, colourless to pale yellow solution which is miscible with acetone and ether.

Chemical Properties

When concentrated glyceryl trinitrate solution is mixed with ether and a small portion of the resulting solution evaporated to dryness and the residue dissolved in sulphuric acid containing a trace of diphenylamine, an intense blue colour is produced.

Stability and Storage

Concentrated glyceryl trinitrate solution should be kept in a well-closed container protected from light and stored at 8°C to 15°C.

Uses

Coronary vasodilator. It is used as sublingual tablets. The tablet may also be crushed and spread over the buccal mucosa from where it is absorbed into the circulation within 1 to 2 minutes terminating an attack.

Official

Concentrated Glyceryl Trinitrate Solution, I.P., B.P.
Glyceryl Trinitrate Tablets, I.P., B.P.

Brand Names

Angised, Nitromack retard, Angispan-TR, Angispan-SR, Myovin, Nitromack, Milliorol etc.

CHAPTER - 25

COAGULANTS AND ANTICOAGULANTS

A simplified outline of the coagulation or clotting of blood is given below :-

tissue damage ──→thromboplastin

    prothrombin ──↘→ thrombin

        fibrinogen ──↘→fibrin (clot)

        flibrinolysin ──↘→polypeptides.

Actually the process is very complicated and involves a dozen or more blood and tissue factors, a series of enzymes and their activators and calcium ions.

Coagulants are drugs which are used to promote clotting of blood and are usually employed in the treatment of severe haemorrhage and threatened haemorrhages.

Coagulants are classified as given below :-

I. COAGULANTS

a) Local Coagulant

Thrombin

b) Systemic Coagulant

Menadione

1. THROMBIN

Thrombin is an enzyme present in blood in the form of a precursor prothrombin. The prothrombin is isolated by the fractionation of plasma. By the addition of thromboplastin and calcium ions, it is converted into thrombin. After filtration the thrombin solution is freeze-dried in final containers containing 50, 250 and 500 units per ampoule. Thrombin is applied locally to control blood oozing out from puncture sites or due to surgery. So thrombin is a **local haemostatic.**

2. MENADIONE

Menadione is a synthetic substitute of vitamin K which is required for the synthesis of prothrombin and several other factors. Menadione is actually known as vitamin K_3. It has a simple structure and is a derivative of 1,4-napthoquinone. Actually it is *2-methyl-1, 4-naphthoquinone.*

MENADIONE

Physical Properties

Menadione is a pale yellow, crystalline powder with a faint, characteristic odour. It is affected by light and decomposes which is indicated by the substance darkening and becoming brown. It melts between 105° and 108°C. It is practically insoluble in water, freely soluble in chloroform and toluene, soluble in ether and sparingly soluble in ethanol and methanol.

Chemical Properties

If, to an alcoholic solution of menadione, dilute ammonia solution and ethyl cyanoacetate are added, an intense bluish violet colour is produced. It disappears on the addition of concentrated hydrochloric acid.

305

Stability and Storage

Since it is affected by light, store it in well-closed, light-resistant containers.

Uses

Synthetic vitamin K substitute. It promotes normal coagulation of blood by acting as a cofactor in the synthesis by liver of prothrombin and several other factors necessary for clotting.

Official

Menadiol Sodium Phosphate, B.P.
Menadiol Phosphate Injection, B.P.
Menadiol Phosphate Tablets, B.P.
Menadiol, I.P., B.P.

Brand Names

Gynae CVP, Kanone, Aquinone, Synkay etc.

Other coagulants are *vitamins K_1 and K_2, acetomena-phthone, human fibrinogen, adrenochrome monosemicarbazone, rutin etc.*

II. ANTICOAGULANTS

Anticoagulants are drugs which are used to prolong the clotting time and also to prevent clotting. They are useful in disseases such as venous thrombosis (coagulation of blood in the veins), pulmonary embolism (obstruction of blood vessels in the lung by clots) and myocardial infarction (small localized area of dead tissue produced in the heart muscle following coronary thrombosis). They are also used in the preservation and storage of blood. They are also used to prevent the development of clots during and after surgical operations.

CLASSIFICATION

a) Natural
Heparin

b) Synthetic
Coumarin derivatives :-
1. Bishydroxycoumarin
2. Warfarin sodium

1. HEPARIN

Heparin is a mucopolysaccharide obtained from ox lung or intestinal mucosa of pig, ox or sheep. It has the property of prolonging the clotting time of blood in man and other animals. It is thermolabile and is used as the calcium or sodium salt.

Physical Properties

Heparin sodium is a white or greyish-white, odourless, moderately hygroscopic powder. It is soluble in water and in saline solution forming a clear or straw-coloured solution.

Chemical Properties

Heparin sodium may be heated with sodium metal to bright red heat and the tube and the contents may be plunged into water. Then it is filtered and the filtrate may be boiled with ferrous sulphate. It is cooled, acidified with hydrochloric acid and ferric chloride test solution may be added. A blue colour is produced.

Stability and Storage

Since it is affected by microorganisms and is also hygroscopic, store it in tightly-closed and sealed containers in a dry place.

Uses

Anticoagulant. It is used to prevent thrombosis in cardiovascular surgery. It is also used in the treatment of arterial and venous thrombosis and in pulmonary embolism. It is not effective when given orally. It may be given by intravenous infusion or injection.

Official

Heparin Sodium, I.P., B.P.
Heparin Sodium Injection, I.P.
Heparin Calcium, B.P.
Heparin Injection, B.P.

Brand Names

Heparin sod, Beparine, Hepsal, Liquemin etc. - all heparin sodium brands. Calciparine - Heparin calcium.

2. BISHYDROXYCOUMARIN (DICOUMAROL)

Bishydroxycoumarin and warfarin are coumarin derivatives which act as anticoagulants. Bishydroxycoumarin is a creamy-white powder with a faint pleasant odour. It is practically insoluble in water, alcohol and ether and slightly soluble in chloroform. However it is soluble in solutions of alkali hydroxides.

Uses

Anticoagulant. It is given orally as tablets and capsules. Its action is slow but lasting.

Brand Names

Dicoumarol, Dicoumarin, Melitoxin etc.

3. WARFARIN SODIUM

Physical Properties

Warfarin sodium is a white, hygroscopic powder. Warfarin has an acidic enolic -OH group which enables it to form the sodium salt which is soluble in water. Warfarin base melts at 159° to 163°C. Warfarin sodium is very soluble in water and alcohol, soluble in acetone and very slightly soluble in ether and dichloromethane.

Chemical Properties

Since warfarin is a ketone, it forms an oxime on treatment with hydroxylamine and also a dinitrophenyl-hydrazone.

Stability and Storage

Since it is affected by light and also is hygroscopic, keep it in tightly-closed, light-resistant containers.

Uses

Anticoagulant. Heparin may be given with warfarin sodium for rapid anticoagulant effect.

Official

Warfarin Sodium, I.P., B.P.
Warfarin Sodium Tablets, I.P.
(Warfarin Tablets, B.P.)
Warfarin Sodium Clathrate, B.P.

Brand Names

Uniwarfin, Coumadin Sodium, Athrombin-K etc.

Other anticoagulants in clinical use are *acenocoumarin, ethyl biscoumacetate, nicoumalone, phenindione etc.*

CHAPTER - 26

DIURETICS

Diuretics are agents which increase the rate of urine flow. They are useful in diseases where fluid accumulation in the body takes place leading to increased weight and a condition known as dropsy or oedema. Dropsy is produced because of sodium and water retention. This condition is caused in diseases such as congestive heart failure or in hepatic, renal or pulmonary disease. In such cases, diuretics increase the excretion of sodium and water and eliminate dropsy.

Diuretics may also be used to counteract sodium and water retention promoted by other drugs. They may also be used to eliminte poisons and drugs taken in excess through the kidney. They are also used as adjuncts to drugs administered for reducing the blood pressure.

CLASSIFICATION

I. Sulphonamides
  1. Frusemide
  2. Chlorothiazide
  3. Hydrochlorothiazide
  4. Benzthiazide

II. Miscellaneous
  1. Urea
  2. Mannitol
  3. Ethacrynic acid

1. FRUSEMIDE (FUROSEMIDE)

The four compounds mentioned under sulphonamides in the classification contain the sulphonamido ($-SO_2NH_2$) group in their structure. Frusemide has the following structure:-

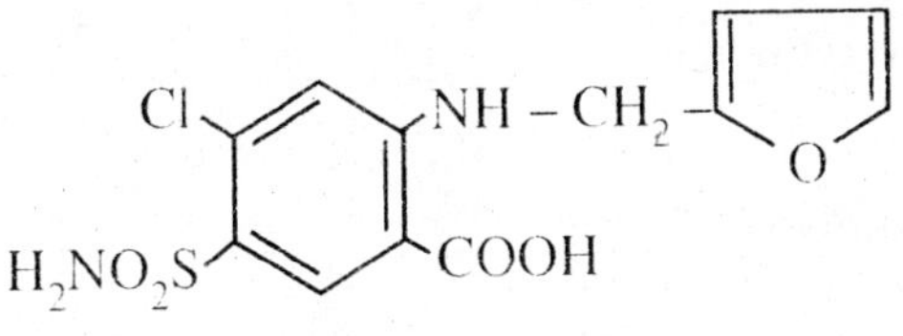

This is a sulphonamide derivative of anthranilic acid which has the structure given below:-

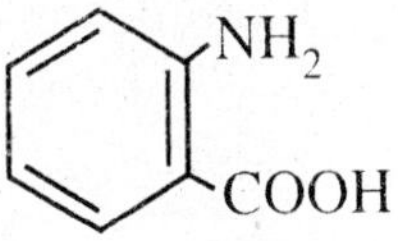

So in the structure of frusemide, counting from - COOH as no.1, there is one chloro group in the 4th position, a sulphonamido group in the 5th position and a furanylmethyl (or furfuryl) group attached to the nitrogen of the amino group in the 2nd position. So frusemide is *4-chloro-N-furfuryl-5-sulphamoylanthranilic acid*. It is prepared by synthesis.

Physical Properties

Frusemide is a white or almost white, odourless, crystalline powder. It is practically insoluble in water, sparingly soluble in ethanol, soluble in acetone and slightly soluble in ether. It dissolves in dilute aqueous solutions of alkali hydroxides. It melts at 210°C with decomposition. It is affected by light. Aqueous solution deteriorates spontaneously on exposure to light.

Chemical Properties

Frusemide can be hydrolysed by boiling with dilute hydrochloric acid and free anthranilic acid is released. The primary aromatic amino group in anthranilic acid is diazotised with sodium nitrite and coupled with N-(1-naphthyl) ethylene-diamine dihydrochloride to give a red-violet colour.

Stability and Storage

Since it is affected by light, keep it in well-closed, light-resistant containers.

Uses

Diuretic. It is a highly efficient diuretic which has only weak carbonic anhydrase inhibitory action, The onset of action is quick but duration is short. It promoters excretion of sodium and water.

Official

Frusemide, I.P., B.P.
Frusemide Injection, I.P., B.P.
Frusemide Tablets, I.P., B.P.

Brand Name

Lasix, Salinex, Diural, Urosemide etc.

2. CHLOROTHIAZIDE

Chlorothiazide, hydrochlorothiazide and benzthiazide can also be classified as benzothiadiazine derivatives in addition to their being classified as sulphonamides. Benzothiadiazine is a heterocyclic in which a benzene ring is fused with a thiadiazine ring which has sulphur in the first and two nitrogen atoms in the second and fourth positions in the ring. Chlorothiazide is so named because it has a chlorine atom as a substituent in the benzene part of the benzothiadiazine.

Physical Properties

Chlorothiazide is a white or almost white, odourless, crystalline powder. It is very slightly soluble in water, slightly soluble in ethanol and sparingly soluble in acetone. It dissolves in dilute solutions of alkali hydroxides.

312

Chemical Properties

Chlorothiazide can be disintegrated by boiling with sodium hydroxide. Ammonia, which turns red litmus blue, is evolved. The residue may be dissolved in dilute hydrochloric acid. Hydrogen sulphide is evolved and it turns lead acetate paper black.

Stability and Storage

Store in well-closed containers.

Uses

Diuretic. It is also used as an antihypertensive in the treatment of oedema and hypertension. It has quick onset of action and duration is 6 to 12 hours. All thiazides inhibit carbonic anhydrase and reduce the reabsorption of electrolytes and promote the excretion of sodium, bicarbonate and chloride ions.

Official

Chlorothiazide, B.P.
Chlorothiazide Tablets, B.P.

Brand Names

Diuresal, Diuril, Urinex, Minzil, Rochlorozide etc.

3. HYDROCHLOROTHIAZIDE

Hydrochlorothiazide has almost the same structure as chlorothiazide except for one difference. The double bond in the 3-4 position in the thiadiazine part of the nucleus is saturated and is not present in the case of hydrochlorothiazide. The structure of hydrochlorothiazide is given below :

Physical Properties

It is a white or almost white, crystalline, odourless powder. It is very slightly soluble in water, sparingly soluble in ethanol and soluble in acetone. It dissolves in dilute solutions of alkali hydroxides.

Chemical Properties

When hydrochlorothiazide is heated gently with a freshly prepared solution of chromotropic acid sodium salt in a cooled mixture of water and concentrated sulphuric acid, a violet colour is produced.

Stability and Storage

Keep in well-closed containers.

Uses

Diuretic. It is about 10 times more potent than chlorothiazide with reduced toxicity. Reduction of the 3,4 double bond has increased the potency. Otherwise it has the same action as chlorothiazide.

Official

Hydrochlorothiazide, I.P., B.P.
Co-amilozide Oral Solution, B.P.
Co-amilozide Tablets, B.P.
Hydrochlorothiazide Tablets, I.P., B.P.

Note

Co-amilozide is a mixture of amiloride and hydrochlorothiazide. Amiloride is also a diuretic.

Brand Names

Esidrex, Esidrix, Ro-hydrazide, Dichlorosal etc.

4. BENZTHIAZIDE

Benzthiazide also has almost the same structure as other benzothiadiazines with some minor modifications in structure. It is not official in I.P. or B.P.

Properties

It is a white, crystalline powder with characteristic odour and melting at 238°-239°C. It is practically insoluble in water and chloroform and slightly soluble in ethanol and acetone. It is freely soluble in dilute solutions of alkali hydroxides.

Stability and Storage

Keep in well-closed containers.

Uses

Diuretic. It is used in the same way as other benzothiadiazine compounds, that is, as a diuretic and antihypertensive.

Brand Names

Benzothiazide, Dihydrex, Edemex, Urese etc.

5. UREA

Structurally urea is NH_2-CO-NH_2. It is a normal constituesnt of urine and is a product of protein metabolism.

Physical Properties

Urea is a white, crystalline powder or occurs as transparent crystals. It is almost odourless but it may develop gradually a slight odour of ammonia upon standing for a long time. It is slightly hygroscopic. It melts at 132° - 133°C. It has a cooling, saline taste. Aqueous solutions are neutral to litmus.

Chemical Properties

Aqueous solution of urea, on heating, is decomposed and gives off some ammonia. Urea is easily oxidized by sodium hypochlorite in the cold and is converted to nitrogen and carbondioxide. Since it is weakly basic, it combines with acids like nitric acid and oxalic acid and gives white precipitates of urea nitrate and urea oxalate respectively. Urea forms biuret on heating. To the residue sodium hydroxide and copper sulphate solutions may be added. A reddish violet colour is produced.

Stability and Storage

Since it may be decomposed to ammonia on long standing, keep it in well-closed containers.

Uses

Osmotic diuretic. Urea is an excellent diuretic. It is not absorbed by the renal tubules and so is excreted with water. It can be administred orally as well as by intravenous infusion. It is used for reducing intraocular pressure in acute glaucoma. Since it is also an antiseptic, it can be used to treat wounds and promote healing. It is also a keratolytic.

It is used as a fertilizer, in animal feeds and in the preparation of plastics, resins and barbituric acid. It is also used in the preparation of certain dentifrices.

316

Official

Urea, I.P., B.P.
Urea Cream, I.P., B.P.

Brand Names

Carbamide, Aquacare, Basodexan, Ureaphil etc.

6. MANNITOL

Mannitol is a polyhydroxy alcohol with the structure $HOCH_2-(CHOH)_4-CH_2OH$. When it is injected intravenously, it is not metabolised and is excreted rapidly. Since it is non-reabsorbable, it carries with it a lot of sodium and water causing diuresis.

Physical Properties

Mannitol is a white, crystalline powder or it consists of free-flowing granules. It is odourless. It melts between 165° and 170°C. It is freely soluble in water, very slightly soluble in ethanol and insoluble in chloroform and ether. It is slightly soluble in pyridine.

Chemical Properties

If, to a saturated solution of mannitol, ferric chloride test solution and sodium hydroxide solution are added and shaken well, a clear solution is obtained. It remains clear when sodium hydroxide solution is further added.

If, to a solution of mannitol in carbon dioxide-free wate, a cooled mixture of concentrated sulphuric acid and catechol is added cooling in ice and heated gently over a naked flame, a pink colour is produced.

Stability and Storage

Store in well-closed containers.

Uses

Osmotic diuretic.

Official

Mannitol, I.P., B.P.

Mannitol Injection, I.P.

(Mannitol Intravenous Infusion, B.P.)

Brand Names

Mannitol, Mannite, Dismal, Osmitral.

7. ETHACRYNIC ACID

Ethacrynic acid is an unsaturated derivative of dichlorophenoxyacetic acid.

Physical Properties

It is a white or almost white, crystalline powder. It melts between 120 and 121°C. It is very slightly soluble in water and freely soluble in ethanol, chloroform and ether. It dissolves in ammonia and dilute aqueous solutions of alkali hydroxides and alkali carbonates.

Chemical Properties

If ethacrynic acid which contains two chloride atoms in its structure is disintegrated by subjecting it to the oxygen flask method using dilute sodium hydroxide solution as the absorbing liquid, acidified with dilute sulphuric acid and boiled, the solution gives the reactions of chlorides.

If, to ethacrynic acid, sodium hydroxide solution is added, cooled and concentrated sulphuric acid and chromotropic acid sodium salt are added and cautiously a further quantity of concentrated sulphuric acid is added, a deep violet colour is produced.

Stability and Storage

Keep it in well-closed containers.

Uses

Diuretic. Since it is rather toxic, it is not very popular.

Brand Names

Edecriin, Endecril, Hydromedin, Reomax etc.

Other diureties in clinical use are *mersalyl, bumetanide, piretanide, polythiazide, cyclopenthiazide, hydroflumethiazide, bendroflumethiazide, chlorthalidone, metolazone, xipamide, indapamide, acetazolamide, ethoxzolamide, spironolactone, triamterene, amiloride, theophylline, isosorbide, ammonium chloride, potassium citrate and potassium acetate.*

CHAPTER - 27

HYPOGLYCAEMIC AGENTS

Diabetes melitus is a disease caused by deficient secretion of insulin from the Islets of Langerhans in the pancreas. In this disease carbohydrate is not properly metabolised. There is accumulation of glucose in the blood (hyperglycaemia) and glucose also appears in the urine (glycosuria). Ketone bodies are also excreted in the urine. Administration of insulin or oral antidiabetic agents lowers the blood sugar by promoting its metabolism and remedies the situation.

CLASSIFICATION

I. Insulin and Insulin preparations

II. Oral antidiabetic agents

a) Sulphonylureas

1. Chlorpropamide
2. Tolbutamide
3. Glibenclamide

b) Biguanides

1. Phenformin
2. Metformin

I. INSULIN

Human insulin is a polypeptide made up of 51 amino acids. It contains two chains A and B containing 21 and 30 amino acids respectively. The two chains are joined at two places through two disulphide bridges. It is amphoteric forming salts with both weak acids and weak alkalis. It is not active orally as it is destroyed by the proteolytic enzymes. Therefore it is given parenterally, usually by the subcutaneous route.

Insulin is the antidiabetic hormone naturally obtained from the pancreas of the ox or the pig (bovine or porcine respectively). This is the raw material for preparing insulin injection.

Properties

It is a white or almost white powder. It is practically insoluble in water, ethanol, chloroform and ether. However since it is amphoteric, it dissolves in dilute mineral acids and also in dilute solutions of alkali hydroxides with decomposition. It is affected by light.

Stability and Storage

Insulin should be kept in tightly-closed, light-resistant containers below -20°C until it is released by the manufacturer. After it is thawed, it should be stored at 2° to 8°C and converted into insulin preparations within a short period of time.

Uses

Hypoglycaemic. It is used for the manufacture of insulin preparations like insulin injection.

Deficiency of insulin leads to diabetes mellitus with symptoms like hyperglycaemia (high amount of glucose in the blood), glycosuria (appearance of glucose in the urine), hyper-lipemia (high concentration of fats in the blood), negative nitrogen balance and sometimes ketonaemia (ketone bodies in the blood). Complications like atherosclerosis (narrowing of blood vessels due to deposition of cholesterol etc), retinopathy (disorder of the retina resulting in loss of vision), neuropathy (disease of the peripheral nerves causing weakness and numbness) and peripheral vascular insufficiency etc. may ensue. Administration of insulin reverses and relieves most of these complications.

There are various insulin preparations clinically used and a list is given below :-

1. **Insulin Injection :** This is insulin dissolved in water for injection and adjusted to a pH of 2.5 to 3.5 by adding hydrochloric acid. It contains 1.45 to 1.75% v/v of glycerol and 0.1 to 0.25% of phenol or any other bactericide. It is a clear solution which is sterilised by the filtration method and distributed into final sterile multiple dose containers (vials) which are then sealed. It is stored at a temperature between 2° and 8°C. It should not be allowed to freeze. It has a strength of 40 units or 80 units per ml. Its onset of action is from ½ to one hour which reaches its peak in 2 to 4 hours and the total duration of action is from 6 to 8 hours.

2. **Biphasic Insulin Injection :** This is sterile buffered solution of bovine (cattle) insulin in a solution of porcine (pig) insulin. It is a white suspension. It is adjusted to a pH of 6.6 to 7.2. It is both quick acting and long acting. It starts acting in 30 minutes and lasts upto 18 to 22 hours.

3. **Isophane Insulin Injection :** This is a sterile buffered solution of insulin with a suitable protamine and zinc. It has a pH of 6.9 to 7.5. It is a white suspension which on standing deposits a white sediment which can be redistributed by shaking. It starts acting in one to two hours and lasts upto 24 hours.

4. **Biphasic Isophane Insulin Injection :** This is either a sterile buffered suspension of pork insulin, complexed with protamine in a solution of pork insulin or a sterile

buffered suspension of human insulin complexed with protamine in a solution of human insulin. It is a white suspension which on standing deposits a white sediment which can be redistributed by gentle shaking. It has a pH of 6.9 to 7.5.

5. **Insulin Zinc Suspensions :** These are zinc compounds of insulin without a protein like protamine. They are in amorphous or crystalline form suitably buffered. pH 6.9 to 7.5 and strength 40 or 80 units per ml. The Insulin Zinc Suspension (Amorphous) is short acting and lasts about 12 to 16 hours. The Insulin Zinc Suspension (Crystalline) lasts for about 30 to 36 hours. Both may be combined in suitable proportions according to individual needs to give Insulin Zinc Suspension and administered. I.P. suggests that 3 volumes of Insulin Zinc Suspension (Amorphous) may mixed with 7 volumes of Insulin Zinc Suspension (Crystalline).

6. **Protamine Zinc Insulin Injection :** This is a sterile buffered suspension of insulin in the form of a complex with a suitable protamine and zinc. It contains sodium phosphate as buffering agent, glycerol to render it isotonic and a suitable bactericide. The usual strength is about 40 units per ml. pH is between 6.9 and 7.5. It starts acting in 4 to 6 hours and lasts upto 24-36 hours.

7. **Human Insulin :** This is also called as biosynthetic human insulin or semisynthetic human insulin. It is prepared by recombinant DNA technology of the bacterium *Escherichia coli* or a type of yeast. It is also prepared by the enzymatic modification of porcine insulin. More than 75% of patients in developed countries use human insulin. It is more water soluble and lipophilic than the other insulins. It is absorbed more easily from the site of injection and has a slightly shorter duration of action.

Official

Insulin, I.P.
Insulin Injection, I.P., B.P.
Biphasic Insulin Injection, B.P.
Biphasic Isophane Insulin Injection, B.P.
Insulin Zinc Suspension, I.P., B.P.
Insulin Zinc Suspension (Amorphous), I.P., B.P.
Insulin Zinc Suspension (Crystalline), I.P., B.P.
Isophane Insulin Injection, I.P., B.P.
Protamine Zinc Insulin Injection, I.P.

II. ORAL ANTIDIABETIC AGENTS

1. CHLORPROPAMIDE

This is a derivative of urea. NH_2-CO-NH_2. To one nitrogen is attached p-chlorobenzenesulphonyl (Cl-C_6H_4-SO_2-) group. To the other nitrogen is attached a propyl (–$CH_2CH_2CH_3$) group. Therefore the systematic name for chlorpromide is *N-p-chlorobenzenesulphonyl-N′-propylurea.*

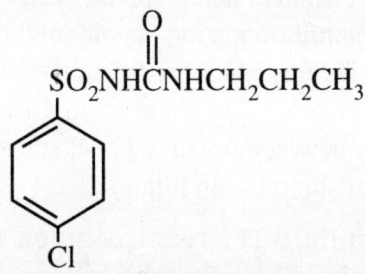

CHLORPROPAMIDE
(N-p-Chlorobenzenesulphonyl-N′-propylurea)

Physical Properties

Chlorpropamide is a white, odourless, crystalline powder. It is practically insoluble in water, freely soluble in chloroform and acetone, soluble in ethanol and slightly soluble in ether. It dissolves in solutions of alkali hydroxides. It melts between 126° and 130°C.

Chemical Properties

The compound can be disintegrated by heating with anhydrous sodium carbonate at dull red heat and the chlorine is now present as sodium chloride. It is extracted with water and detected by adding dilute nitric acid and silver nitrate solution. A white precipitate is produced.

Stability and Storage

Keep it in well-closed containers.

Uses

Oral hypoglycaemic. The oral antidiabetic agents induce a brisk release of insulin from the pancreas. Since chlorpropamide is long-acting, it can cause prolonged hypoglycaemia.

Official

Chlorpropamide, I.P., B.P.
Chlorpropamide Tablets, I.P., B.P.

Brand Names

Diabinese, Diabigon, Melitase, Adiaben etc.

2. TOLBUTAMIDE

In this compound, to one nitrogen is attached toluene-p-sulphonyl (tosyl) (CH_3-C_6H_5-SO_2-) group and to the other nitrogen a butyl (-$CH_2CH_2CH_2CH_3$) group. Therefore tolbutamide is *N-toluene-p-sulphonyl-N′-butylurea.*

Physical Properties

Tolbutamide is a white, odourless, crystalline powder. It melts between 126° and 130°C. It is practically insoluble in water, soluble in ethanol, acetone and chloroform and slightly soluble in ether.

Chemical Properties

Tolbutamide can be disintegrated by boiling with sulphuric acid. After cooling in ice, a crystalline precipitate of 4-toluene-sulphonamide is formed. This has a melting range between 135° and 140°.

Stability and Storage

Keep it in well-closed containers.

Uses

Oral hypoglycaemic. It is somewhat weaker and short-acting. However it does not cause any problem in those who easily develop hypoglycaemia.

Official

Tolbutamide, I.P., B.P.
Tolbutamide Tablets, I.P., B.P.

Brand Names

Rastinon, Artosin, Oralin, Glyconon, Diasulfon etc.

3. GLIBENCLAMIDE

Glibenclamide can also be considered as a sulphonylurea derivative. However the sulphonyl group attached to one of the nitrogens carries a rather complicated aromatic group while the other nitrogen has only a cyclohexyl group attached to it.

Physical Properties

Glibenclamide is a white or almost white, crystalline powder. It melts between 169° and 174°C. It is practically insoluble in water and ether and slightly soluble in ethanol and methanol. It dissolves in dilute solutions of alkali hydroxides.

Chemical Properties

If a little of glibenclamide is dissolved in concentrated sulphuric acid, the solution remains colourless but exhibits a blue fluorescence under ultraviolet light (365 nm). If a little chloral hydrate is added and allowed to dissolve, a deep yellow colour is produced. This changes to a brownish tinge after 20 minutes.

Stability and Storage

Keep in well-closed containers.

Uses

Oral Hypoglycaemic. It is a potent but slow-acting drug. It may be effective when other drugs fail.

Official

Glibenclamide, I.P., B.P.
Glibenclamide Tablets, I.P., B.P.

Brand Names

Daonil, Euglucon, Betanese, Micronase etc.

4. PHENFORMIN

This is a derivative of biguanide, the nitrogens being numbered as shown.

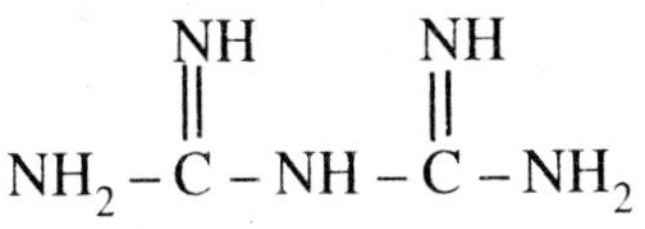

$$NH_2 - \overset{\overset{\displaystyle NH}{\|}}{C} - NH - \overset{\overset{\displaystyle NH}{\|}}{C} - NH_2$$

BIGUANIDE

A phenylethyl or phenethyl ($C_6H_5CH_2CH_2-$) group is attached to the first nitrogen to give phenformin. Phenformin hydrochloride is the salt clinically used.

$$
\text{C}_6\text{H}_5\text{—CH}_2\text{CH}_2\text{NHCNHCNH}_2.\text{HCl}
$$

with NH, NH groups above the C atoms.

PHENFORMIN HYDROCHLORIDE

Its systematic name is *1-(2-phenylethyl) biguanide hydrochloride.*

Physical Properties

Phenformin hydrochloride is a white or almost white, crystalline powder which is without odour. It melts between 175° and 179°C. It is freely soluble in water, soluble in ethanol and practically insoluble in chloroform and ether.

Chemical Properties

If, to an aqueous solution of phenformin hydrochloride, are added sodium hydroxide solution, 1-naphthol solution and dilute sodium hypochlorite solution with shaking, a red precipitate is produced. It darkens on standing. In another colour test, the aqueous solution of the substance may be mixed with a mixture of solutions of sodium nitroprusside, potassium ferri-cyanide and sodium hydroxide and allowed to stand for 20 minutes. A wine-red colour is slowly produced.

Stability and Storage

Keep in well-closed containers.

Uses

Oral hypoglycaemic. It is not very much used because of its tendency to cause lactic acidosis.

328

Official

Phenformin Hydrochloride, I.P.
Phenformin Hydrochloride Tablets, I.P.

Brand Names

DBI, DBI-TD, Diaphen, Diabis, Glucopostin etc.

5. METFORMIN

Metformin has an equally simple structure like phenformin in that only a dimethyl group, $-(CH_3)_2$, is attached to the first nitrogen of the biguanide. So metformin is *1,1-dimethylbiguanide*. It is clinically used as the hydrochloride.

Physical Properties

Metformin hydrochloride is a white or almost white, crystalline, hygroscopic powder. It melts between 222° and 226°C. It is freely soluble in water, slightly soluble in ethanol and practically insoluble in acetone, chloroform and ether.

Chemical Properties

It answers the same colour reactions as phenformin. However in the first reaction in which the aqueous solution of metformin hydrochloride is mixed with sodium hydroxide solution, 1-naphthol solution and dilute sodium hypochlorite solution with shaking, an orange-red colour, which darkens on standing, is produced unlike phenformin which gives a red precipitate. However in the other colour reaction useing sodium nitroprusside, potassium ferricyanide and sodium hydroxide, a wine-red colour only is produced by both the compounds. But whereas in the case of metformin the colour is produced within 3 minutes, in the case of phenformin it is produced more slowly.

Stability and Storage

Since it is hygroscopic, store it in tightly-closed containers.

Uses

Oral hypoglycaemic. It acts like phenformin but the incidence of lactic acidosis is less.

Official

Metformin Hydrochloride, I.P., B.P.
Metformin Hydrochloride Tablets, I.P.
(Metformin Tablets, B.P.)

Brand Names

Glyciphage, DMGG, Diabetosan, Fluamine etc.

Other oral hypoglacaemics are *acetohexamide, tolazamide, glipizide, gliclazide etc.*

CHAPTER - 28

LOCAL ANAESTHETICS

Local anaesthetics are drugs which produce localized insensitivity to pain which means that by using these drugs locally one is not aware of the pain. The transmission of impulses by the nerves is blocked by the local anesthetics. However the effect is reversible.

Local anaesthetics may be used in four different ways. Some of the local anaesthetics, which have good penetrating power, are applied on the surface, that is on the skin or mucous membrane. They block sensory nerve endings in these parts. Benzocaine, cocaine, amethocaine and lignocaine are good examples.

Some others are used as infiltration anaesthetics. Here the local anaesthetic is injected subcutaneously around the site of pain and paralyses the nerves there, thereby making the patient become insensitive to or unaware of the pain. This is very much used in dental extractions. Most hospitals treat scorpion sting only by injecting a local anaesthetic around the site of pain. Procaine and lignocaine are good examples. Usually adrenaline is added to give vasoconstriction which will keep the drug at the site for a longer time.

Nerve block anaesthesia is some times done by injecting a local anaesthetic around the nerve trunk or ganglia. By this it is possible to paralyse regions of the body.

In spinal anaesthesia, the local anaesthetic is injected into the subarachnoid space around the spinal cord. Adrenaline should not be added. Examples are amethocaine and cinchocaine.

CLASSIFICATION

I. The Esters

a) Simple Esters

Benzocaine

b) Amino Esters

Procaine

II. The Amides

Lignocaine

1. BENZOCAINE

Benzocaine is *ethyl p-aminobenzoate*. It is the ester of p-aminobenzoic acid NH_2-C_6H_4-COOH and ethyl alcohol.

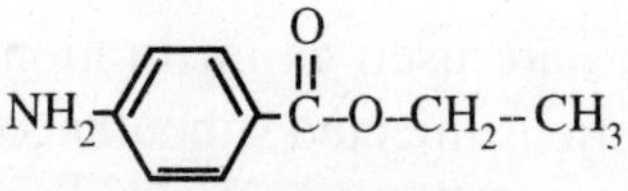

BENZOCAINE
(Ethyl p-aminobenzoate)

Physical Properties

Benzocaine consists of colourless crystals or occurs as a white, crystalline powder. It has no odour. It melts between 88° and 92°C. It is very slightly soluble in water and freely soluble in ethanol, chloroform and ether. It dissolves in dilute acids. When it is boiled with water, it is destroyed. It is also decomposed by alkali hydroxides. It is affected by light.

Chemical Properties

Since benzocaine contains an aromatic primary amino group, it can be diazotised by treatment with hydrochloric acid and sodium nitrite and coupled with 2-naphthol in alkaline solution to form a deep red azo dye. When benzocaine is dissolved in hydrochloric acid and iodine is added, a precipitate is produced. This distinguishes benzocaine from orthocaine. If potassium mercuri-iodide is added to the hydrochloric acid solution of benzocaine, no precipitate is produced. This distinguishes benzocaine from procaine.

Stability and Storage

Since benzocaine is affected by light, store it in well-closed, light-resistant containers.

Uses

Local anaesthetic. Benzocaine is used as dusting powder and ointment to relieve the pain in ulcers and wounds. It is used to relieve pain after dental surgery and internally in gastric ulcers. Benzocaine lozenges are used for sore throat and stomatitis (inflammation of the mouth).

Official

Benzocaine, I.P., B.P.

Brand Names

Proctoquinol, Anaesthesin, Orthesin, Parathesin.

2. PROCAINE

Procaine is also an ester of p-aminobenzoic acid. But the alcohol is an aminoalcohol. It is 2-diethylaminoethylalcohol. Therefore procaine is *2-diethylaminoethyl-p-aminobenzoate.*

$$\text{NH}_2\!\!-\!\!\bigcirc\!\!-\!\!\overset{\overset{\displaystyle O}{\|}}{C}\!-\!O\!-\!CH_2\!-\!CH_3N\!\!\underset{\text{Et}}{\overset{\text{Et}}{\diagup}}$$

PROCAINE

(2-Diethylaminoethyl-p-aminobenzoate)

Physical Properties

Procaine is used only as the hydrochloride. Procaine hydrochloride is a white, odourless, crystalline powder melting at 153° to 158°C. It is very soluble in water, soluble in ethanol, slightly soluble in chloroform and practically insoluble in ether. It is stable at pH 3.6 but is affected by light.

Chemical Properties

Like benzocaine, procaine also contains an aromatic primary amino group and so can be diazotised and coupled with 2-naphthol in alkaline solution to give a red azo dye like benzocaine. It decolourises acidified potassium permanganate immediately. When procaine is treated with fuming nitric acid, evaporated to dryness on a water bath, the residue dissolved in acetone and alcoholic potash is added, a brownish red colour is produced.

Stability and Storage

Since it is affected by light, store it in well-closed, light-resistant containers.

Uses

Local anaesthetic. It is widely used in dental surgery and for producing spinal anaesthesia. It is usually given with adrenaline in small operations like dental extractions and to relieve the pain in scorpion sting. After the introduction of lidocaine, its popularity is declining. It combines with benzyl penicillin to give a poorly soluble procaine penicillin.

334

Official

Procaine Hydrochloride, I.P., B.P.
Procaine Hydrochloride and Adrenaline
Bitartrate Injection, I.P.

Brand Names

Novocaine, Ethocaine, Syncaine, Jurocaine, Topocaine etc.

3. LIGNOCAINE (LIDOCAINE)

Lignocaine is an amide. It is formed by the combination of the carboxylic acid, N-diethylaminoacetic acid and the amino compound, 2 : 6-xylidine.

The alpha carbon atom of the acetic acid carries a diethylamino group in diethylaminoacetic acid. In 2 : 6 -xylidine, there are two methyl groups in the 2nd and 6th positions and a primary amino group in between them in the first position. Therefore lignocaine is *N-diethylaminoacetyl-2:6-xylidine.*

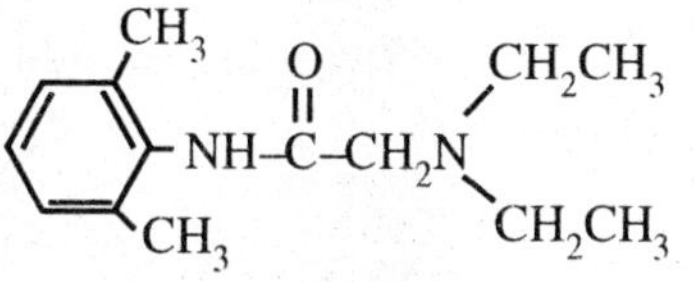

LIGNOCAINE
(N-diethylaminoacetyl 2 : 6-xylidine)

Physical Properties

Lignocaine is used as the hydrochloride. Lignocaine hydrochloride is a practically odourless, white, crystalline powder. It melts between 74° and 79°C. It is very soluble in water, freely soluble in ethanol and chloroform and practically insoluble in ether. It has slightly bitter, numbing taste.

335

Chemical Properties

When it is treated with fuming nitric acid, evaporated to dryness on a water bath, cooled, the residue dissolved in acetone and alcoholic potash is added, a green colour is produced (compare with procaine which gives a brownish red colour). An aqueous solution of lignocaine hydrochloride may be made alkaline with sodium hydroxide solution and filtered. The residue which is lignocaine base may be dissolved in alcohol and cobalt chloride solution is added. A bluish-green precipitate is produced. Since lignocaine is a base, it combines with picric acid to give lignocaine picrate which melts at about 229°C.

Stability and Storage

Since it is stable in air, store it in well-closed containers.

Uses

Local anaesthetic and antiarrhythmic. It is an excellent local anaesthetic which is useful for surface, nerve block, infiltration, spinal and intravenous regional block anaesthesia. At present it is the most popular local anaesthetic. It is also useful in treating cardiac arrhythmias. For this purpose it is injected intramuscularly.

Official

Lignocaine, B.P.
Lignocaine Hydrochloride, I.P., B.P.
Lignocaine Hydrochloride Gel, I.P.
(Lignocaine Gel, B.P.)
Lignocaine and Chlorhexidine Gel, B.P.
(Lignocaine Injection, B.P.)
Lignocaine Hydrochloride and Adrenaline Bitartrate
Injection, I.P.

(Lignocaine and Adrenaline Injection, B.P.)
Lignocaine Hydrochloride and Dextrose Injection, I.P.

Brand Names

Xylocaine, Gesicaine, Lidocain, Lidothesin etc.

Other local anaesthetics clinically used are *cocaine, tetracaine, bupivacaine, dibucaine, mepivacaine, benoxinate, cyclomethycaine, oxethazine etc.*

CHAPTER - 29

THYROID HORMONES AND ANTITHYROIDS

Thyroid gland secretes two iodine-containing hormones levothyroxine and liothyronine. For this purpose, it removes inorganic iodides from the blood. The thyroid hormones are responsible for the maintenance of basal metablic rate. Any deficiency leads to hypothyroidism marked by lowering of the basal metabolic rate and congenital deficiency leads to cretinism in which growth is stunted and mental development is retarded. Over-secretion of the hormones produces thyrotoxicosis or hyperthyroidism marked by increase in basal metabolic rate, cardiac acceleration, restlessness and anxiety.

Hypothyroidism is treated by administration of dried thyroid gland and thyroid hormones, whereas hyperthyroidisim is treated by synthetic antithyroids.

Structure of thyroxine and liothyronine

The basic compound is thyronine. Thyroxine contains 4 iodine atoms in the 3,5,3′ and 5′ positions. Thyronine is an aminoacid which is chemically p-4-hydroxyphenoxy phenylalanine. In liothyronine only three iodine atoms are present in the 3,5 and 3′ positions.

THYROXINE (X = I)

LIOTHYRONINE (X = H)

Antithyroid

Antithyroids are drugs which reduce the synthesis of the thyroid hormones by the thyroid gland. So they are useful in hyperthyroidism and also as a pre-operative treatment before the thyroid gland is removed surgically. They are administered orally.

CLASSIFICATION

1. Thiouracils
   a) Propylthiouracil
   b) Methylthiouracil

2. Imidazolines
   Methimazole

1. THYROXINE

Thyroxine, as already stated above, is $3,5,3',5'$ - *tetraiodothyronine*. It is synthesized and stored in the thyroid gland as part of a protein known as thyroglobulin. The secretion of thyroxine and the other hormone liothyronine is controlled by thyrotropin secreted by the anterior pituitary. Thyroxine is prepared either by extraction from the thyroid gland or by synthesis. It is official as thyroxine sodium.

Physical Properties

Thyroxine sodium consists of a fine, slightly coloured, crystalline powder or is an almost white or slightly brownish yellow powder. It turns slightly pink on exposure to light. It is very slightly soluble in water, slightly soluble in ethanol and practically insoluble in ether. It dissolves in aqueous solutions of alkali hydroxides.

Chemical Properties

If concentrated sulphuric acid is added to thyroxine sodium in a porcelain dish, violet vapours are evolved. If thyroxine sodium is disintegrated by heating with dilute sulphuric acid initially on a water bath and then by igniting at 600°C and dissolving the residue in water, the solution will answer tests for sodium.

Stability and Storage

Since it is affected by exposure to light, store it in tightly-closed, light-resistant containers.

Uses

Thyroid hormone. It is useful in thyroid deficiency states such as cretinism (congenital deficient thyroid secretion causing small stature, impaired mentality etc.), adult hypothyroidism, myxoedema (disease due to hypothyroidism marked by skin atrophy, swelling in the limbs and face and non-development of both mental and physical capacity), nontoxic goiter and papillary carcinoma (cancer) of the thyroid gland.

Official

Thyroxine Sodium, I.P., B.P.
Thyroxine Sodium Tablets, I.P.
(Thyroxine Tablets, B.P.)

Brand Names

Eltroxin, Roxin, Laevoxin, Synthroid sodium etc.

2. PROPYL THIOURACIL

Propylthiouracil is a synthetic compound which has a propyl group in the 6th position of thiouracil.

340

Physical Properties

Propylthiouracil consists of white or pale cream-coloured crystals or is a crystalline powder which is without odour. It is affected by light. It is very slightly soluble in water and ether and sparingly soluble in methanol and ethanol. It dissolves in aqueous solutions of alkali hydroxides. It melts between 217° and 221°C.

Chemical Properties

If bromine water is added to propylthiouracil, shaken for a few minutes, boiled until it is decolourised, allowed to cool, filtered and barium chloride solution is added, a white precipitate is produced.

Stability and Storage

Since it is affected by light, store it in well-closed, light-resistant containers.

Uses

Antithyroid. It depresses the production of the thyroid hormones and is used to control hyperthyroidism.

Official

Propylthiouracil, I.P., B.P.
Propylthiouracil Tablets, I.P., B.P.

Brand Names

Propasil, Procasil, Prothyran etc.

3. METHYLTHIOURACIL

In contrast to propylthiouracil, methylthiouracil carries a methyl group at the 6th position of thiouracil. It is not official in I.P. or B.P.

Properties

It is a white, crystalline powder with no odour. It melts at 326°-331°C with decomposition. It is affected by light. It is slightly soluble in cold water (more soluble in hot water), ether and chloroform. It is freely soluble in alkali hydroxide solutions and aqueous ammonia.

Stability and Storage

Since it is affected by light, store it in well-closed, light-resistant containers.

Uses

Antithyroid. It has the same uses as propylthiouracil.

Brand Names

Methicil, Muracil, Strumacil etc.

4. METHIMAZOLE

Methimazole is derived from imidazoline which is a partially saturated form of imidazole. Methylimidazole is *1-methylimidazole-2-thiol*. It is not official in I.P. or B.P.

Properties

Methimazole is a white to pale buff crystalline powder melting at 146° to 148°C. It has a faint, characteristic odour. It is freely soluble in water, soluble in alcohol, chloroform and ether and sparingly soluble in benzene and petroleum ether. It is affected by light.

Stability and Storage

Store it in well-closed, light-resistant containers.

Uses

Antithyroid. It is supposed to be more potent than propylthiouracil.

Brand Names

Mecazole, Tapazole, Strumazol etc.

Other antithyroids clinically used are *carbimazole, iodine, sodium and potassium iodides and radioactive iodine.*

CHAPTER - 30

STEROID HORMONES

Steroid hormones include the male sex hormones (androgens), female sex hormones (oestrogens and gestogens) and the adrenocortical hormones (corticosteroids).

The steroid nucleus is the basis of structure of all steroid hormones. It is made up of a fully saturated phenanthrene nucleus and a cyclopentane fused together (cyclopentanoperhydrophenanthrene) and has the structure and numbering given below:

STEROID NUCLEUS

Substitutes may be attached to any position in any of two possible orientations. If the substituent gets attached in such a way that it is oriented above the plane of the nucleus, it is said to beta-oriented. This is indicated by a continuous thick line. If, however, the substituent gets attached in such a way that it is oriented below the plane of nucleus, it is said to be alpha-oriented. This is indicated by a discontinuous broken line.

ANDROGENS

Androgens are male sex hormones. They are produced mainly in the testis and also in the adrenal cortex. The activity of androgens can be divided into two types: (1) *androgenic activity*, responsible for the development and maintenance of secondary sex characters, libido and virility in the male and (2) *anabolic activity*, responsible for the skeletal growth and protein synthesis (nitrogen retention). The natural hormone testosterone secreted by the testes has both types of activity and over the years research has been directed towards synthesizing compounds with only anabolic activity and little androgenic activity.

1. TESTOSTERONE

The basic hydrocarbon in the structure of androgens is 5-androstane which has two angular methyl groups 18 and 19

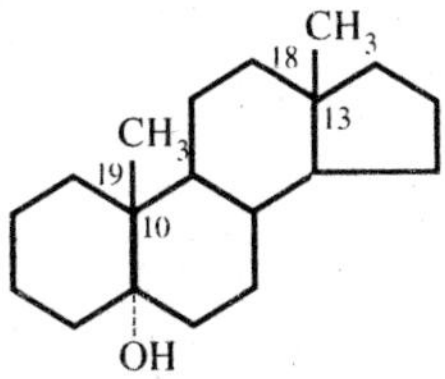

5α-ANDROSTANE

attached to carbon atoms nos 10 and 13. The hydrogen attached to the 5th position is alpha-oriented.

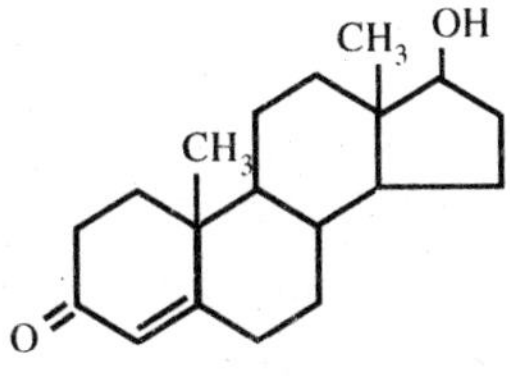

TESTOSTERONE

Chemically testosterone is *17β–hydroxy–4–dndrostene–3–one*; there is a hydroxyl group at the 17th position, a double bond between 4 and 5 positions and a keto group at the 3rd position. Testosterone may be administered either as such or as one of its esters such as propionate or phenylpropionate. Mostly they are administered as oily solutions by intramuscular injection. Testosterone may be administered in aqueous suspension by injection or as an implant. Methyltestosterone is a semisynthetic derivative of testosterone which can be given orally. It has an extra α-methyl group in the 17th position.

Properties

Testosterone is a white, almost odourless, crystalline powder melting at 155°C. It is practically insoluble in water, freely soluble in ethanol, soluble in chloroform, ether and vegetable oils and slightly soluble in ethyl oleate. It is affected by light. Esters of testosterone such as the acetate, cypionate (cyclopentanepropionate), decanoate, enanthate (heptanoate), isocaproate, undecanoate and phenylpropionate are all used in clinical medicine. Testosterone propionate is administered by injection and it is a sterile solution in ethyl oleate or suitable fixed oil or any mixture of these solvents.

Stability and Storage

It should be stored in a well-closed container and protected from light.

Uses

Androgen and anabolic steroid. It is used in cases of hypogonadism (defective development of the gonads, in this case the testicles). It is also used to treat postmenopausal breast carcinoma (cancer of the breast after menopause) and osteoporosis (fragility of bones).

Official

Testosterone, B.P.
Testosterone Implants, B.P.

Testosterone Decanoate, B.P.
Testosterone Enanthate, B.P.
Testosterone Isocaproate, B.P.
Testosterone Propionate, I.P., B.P.
Testosterone Propionate Injection, I.P., B.P.

Brand Names

Aquaviron, Testoviron, Parendren, Testanon, Testoviron depot, Sustanon etc.

2. NANDROLONE

Nandrolone is *19-nortestosterone* which means that it has almost the same structure as testosterone except for the fact that it has no angular methyl group corresponding to the 19th carbon atom. The removal of the methyl group has given it increased anabolic activity and reduced androgenic activity. It is used mainly in the form of its esters, the phenyl propionate and the decanoate. Other esters of nandrolone are cylohexylpropionate, benzoate, hemisuccinate and laurate.

Properties

Nandrolone decanoate is a white to creamy white, crystalline powder with a faint and characteristic odour. It is practically insoluble in water and freely soluble in ethanol, ether, chloroform, fixed oils and oily esters such as ethyl oleate. It melts at a very low temperature of 35°C and should be carefully stored. Nandrolone phenylpropionate melts at 97°C.

Stability and Storage

It should be stored under nitrogen at a temperature of 2° to 8°C and protected from light.

347

Uses

Anabolic steroid. It is mainly used for increasing body weight after acute illness etc.

Official

Nandrolone Decanoate, I.P., B.P.
Nandrolone Decanoate Injection, I.P., B.P.
Nandrolone Phenylpropionate, I.P., B.P.
Nandrolone Phenylpropionate Injection, B.P.

Brand Names

Durabolin, Decadurabolin, Laurabolin V, Decadurabol etc.

Other androgens and anabolic steroids in clinical use are *methyltestosterone, ethyloestrenol, methandienone, oxymetholone, oxandrolone, stanozolol, fluoxymesterone etc.*

OESTROGENS

Oestrogens are female sex hormones. They are required for the development and maintenance of secondary sex characters in the females. They are also required for maintaining the normal menstrual cycle and also for maintenance of pregnancy. They are also anabolic to some extent.

Oestrogens are formed in the ovary, placenta and adrenal cortex. They are commercially extracted from human or mare urine, or made synthetically. Oestradiol is the functioning oestrogenic hormone. Oestrone and oestriol are oxidation products of oestradiol. The parent hydrocarbon of oestrogens is 5α–oestrane.

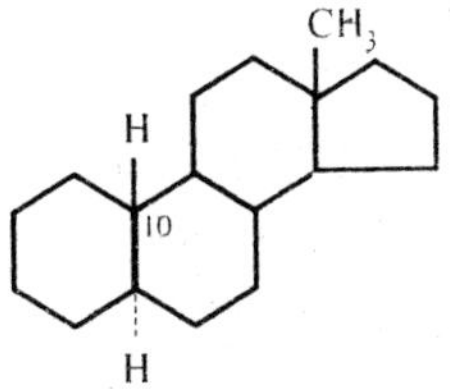

5α–OESTRANE

There is no CH_3 group corresponding to the 19th carbon atom and the hydrogen at the 5th position is alpha–oriented. The oestrogens are derivatives of 5α–oestrane.

OESTRADIOL

Oestradiol has the structure given below:

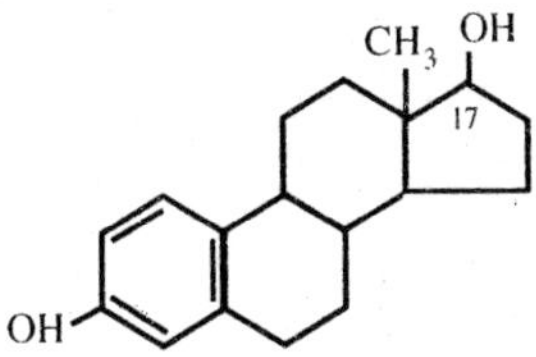

OESTRADIOL
[1,3,5(10)–Oestratriene–3β, 17β–diol]

The first ring is aromatic, there are two hydroxyl groups at positions 3 and 17. The hydroxyl group at position 3 is phenolic because of the benzenoid (aromatic) character of the ring. The hydroxyl group at position 17 is secondary alcoholic. Since there are three double bonds at positions. 1, 3, 5 (10), the systematic names is *1, 3, 5 (10)–oestratriene–3β, 17β-diol*. The third double bond at position 5 is between positions 5 and 10 and not between 5 and 6. Oesteradiol benzoate and oestradiol dipropionate are the two esters used clinically.

349

Physical Properties

Oestradiol benzoate occurs as colourless crystals or as a white, odourless, crystalline powder. It melts between 191° and 198°C. It is practically insoluble in water, slightly soluble in ethanol and fixed oils and sparingly soluble in acetone. Its solution in a suitable fixed oil is used as an injection. The injection should be sterilized by heating at 150°C for one hour. It is affected by light.

Chemical Properties

Oestradiol is slightly acidic since it contains a phenolic–OH group. With phenol sulphonic acid and sulphuric acid, oestradiol gives a magenta colour. In another reaction, oestradiol is treated with ammonium molybdate in sulphuric acid. A yellowish green colour is produced. It exhibits an intense green fluorescence when examined under ultraviolet light (365 nm). If concentrated sulphuric acid and water are added, the solution becomes pink and exhibits a yellowish fluorescence.

Stability and Storage

Store oestradiol benzoate in well-closed, light-resistant containers.

Uses

Oestrogen. It is used to treat deficiency states, menopausal syndromes and delayed onset of puberty in females. It is also used to control prostatic carcinoma (cancer of the prostate gland).

Official

Oestradiol Benzoate, I.P., B.P.
Oestradiol Benzoate Injection, I.P.
(Oestradiol Injection, B.P.)

Brand Names

Ovocyclin, Progynon depot, Gynergan, Gynoestril etc.

Ethinyl oestradiol is a derivative of oestradiol prepared by introducing an α–ethinyl (–C≡CH) group at the 17th position into oestradiol. It is orally active.

Mestranol is the 3–methyl ether of ethinyl oestradiol. Its structure is given below:

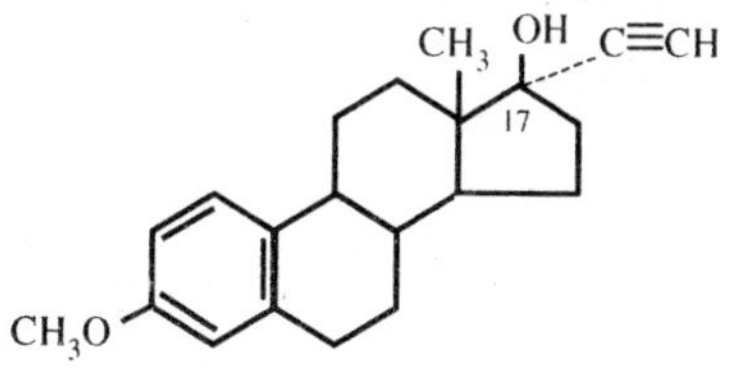

MESTRANOL

Mestranol is administered in oral contraceptive formulations along with a progestogen.

Stilboestrol is a synthetic non–steroidal compound which possesses oestrogenic properties. It has a comparatively simpler structure but its stereochemical representation shows a striking resemblance to the structure of oestradiol which is probably responsible for its action.

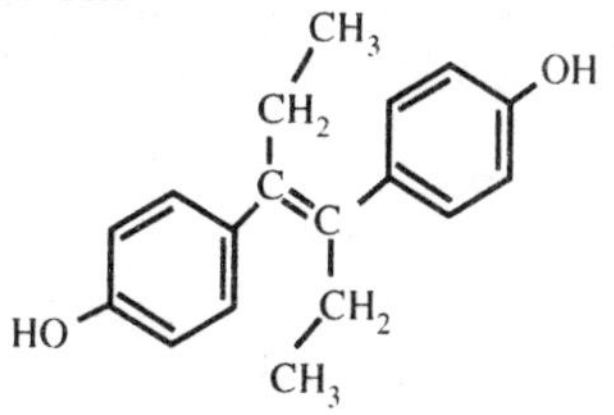

STILBOESTROL

It is a derivative of stilbene (1,2–diphenylethylene) and so it is called as stilboestrol.

351

Other synthetic oestrogens in clinical use are *dienoestrol, hexosterol, chlorotrianisene, benzestrol etc.*

PROGESTOGENS

Progesterone is a hormone secreted by the corpus luteum and the placenta. It is necessary for the preparation for and maintenance of pregnancy. It causes mild sodium retention and nitrogen catabolism. Whereas progesterone is given only by injection, other substances with similar activity but orally administered have also been synthesized. Progestogens in combination with oestrogens are useful as oral contraceptives. The basic hydrocarbon of the progestogens is 5α–pregnane which has 21 carbons including a two–carbon side chain attached to position 17.

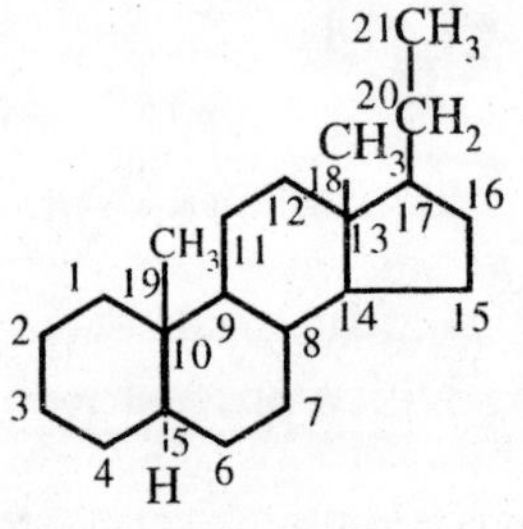

5α–PREGNANE

PROGESTERONE

Progesterone is a 5α–pregnane derivative which has a double bond between positions 4 and 5 and two keto groups at positions 3 and 20. Therefore its systematic name is *4–pregnene–3, 20–dione.*

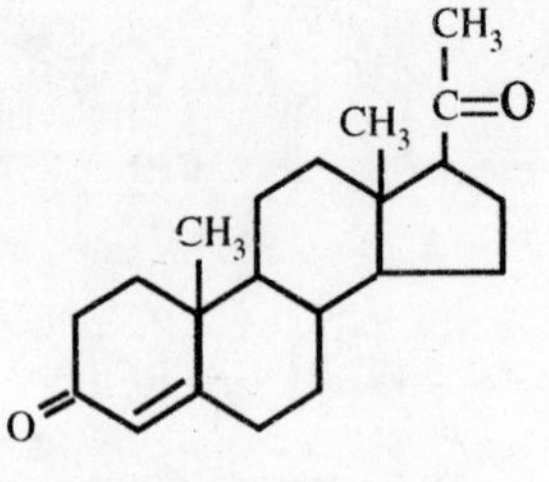

PROGESTERONE
(4–Pregnene–3, 20–dione)

352

Properties

Progesterone is a colourless or white or yellowish white, crystalline powder. It is dimorphous, that is, it exists in two crystalline forms, α–progesterone (prisms melting at 128°C) and β–projesterone (needles melting at 121°C). It is practically insoluble in water, very soluble in chloroform, freely soluble in absolute ethanol and sparingly soluble in acetone, ether and fixed oils. It is sensitive to alkalies and light.

It has the usual properties of ketones, forming a dioxime. It forms a bisdinitrophenylhydrazone on treatment with 2, 4–dinitrophenylhydrazine. This was the basis of its gravimetric assay method previously. It is administered by intramuscular injection as an oily solution.

Stability and Storage

It should be kept in a well-closed container and protected from light.

Uses

Progestogen. It is used to treat threatened or habitual abortion, dysfunctional uterine bleeding, endometriosis (the presence of membranous material of the kind lining the womb at other sites within the cavity of the pelvis), dysmenorrhoea (painful or difficult menstruation), premenstrual tension and endometrial carcinoma (cancer of the mucous membrane lining the uterus).

Official

Progesterone, B.P.
Progesterone Injection, B.P.

Brand Names

Progestin, Proluton, Lutocycline, Corlutin, Nolutron etc.

Many synthetic substitutes of progesterone are used clinically. Ethisterone is one such.

Ethisterone : In ethisterone the two carbon side chain at position 17 in progesterone is replaced by a hydroxyl group with beta orientation. In addition at the same position an ethinyl group with alpha orientation ($...C \equiv CH$) is present

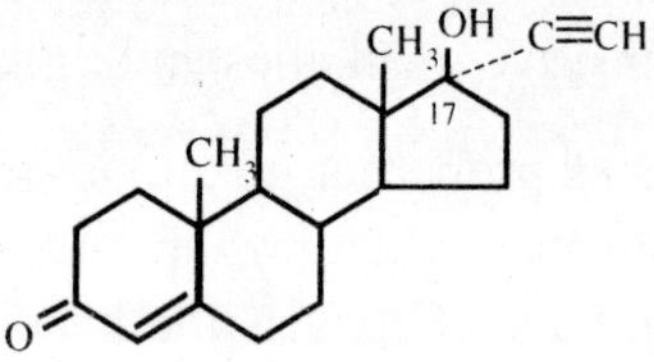

ETHISTERONE

Other progestogens used clinically are *hydroxy-progesterone caproate, medroxyprogesterone acetate, dydrogesterone, norethisterone, lynoestrenol, allylestrenol etc.*

ADRENOCORTICAL HORMONES

The adrenocortical hormones produced in the adrenal cortex are also known as corticosteroids. They assist in maintaining a constant internal environment and their release is under the control of the adrenocorticotrophic hormone (ACTH) of the anterior pituitary. They are specially important in controlling states of stress. They fall into two main groups according to their function although these overlap to some extent:

(1) Glucocorticoids [eg: cortisone] control the production of glycogen from protein and have various other effects. They also have antirheumatic, anti-inflammatory and antiallergic properties.

(2) Mineralocorticoids [eg: aldosterone] are concerned with electrolyte and water metabolism. They cause sodium and water retention and potassium excretion. They are used in Addison's disease. Deoxycortone is another important mineralocorticoid.

Structures and Structural Details

The basic hydrocarbon for the corticosteroids and also progestogens is 5α – pregnane.

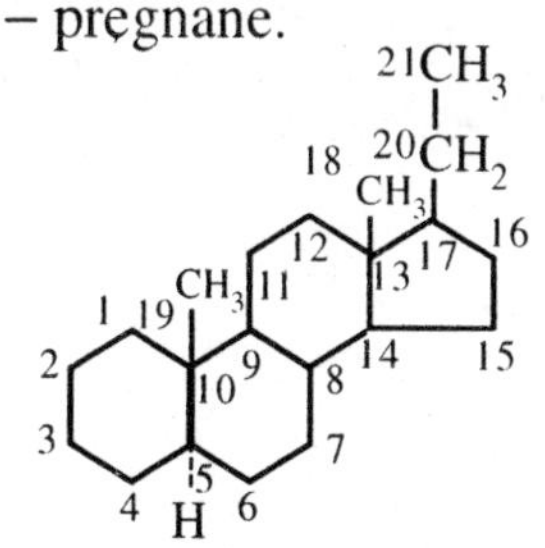

5α-PREGNANE

In the corticosteroids there is 20, 21–ketol function, that is, there is a keto group at the 20th carbon atom and a hydroxyl group at the 21st carbon. There is also a 3-keto group and a 4, 5 - double bond. Since these are all common features for all corticosteriods excepting aldosterone, another basic compound may be used for easy understanding of the structures of all corticosteroids. The basic compound referred to here which has all the features mentioned so far and also has a β-hydroxyl group at the 11th position is corticosterone. Its formula is given below:

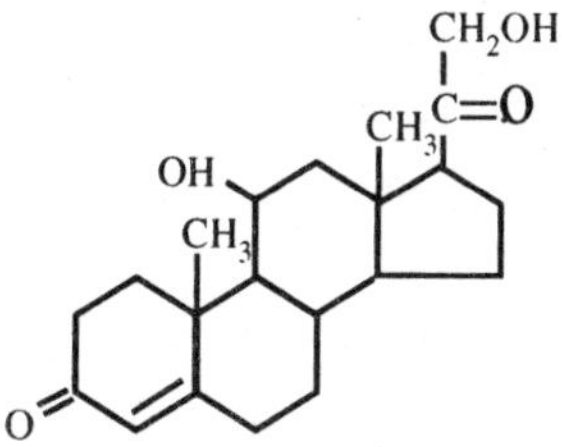

CORTICOSTERONE

355

1. HYDROCORTISONE

Hydrocortisone has the same structure as corticosterone and has a α–hydroxyl group in the 17th position extra. Therefore it is known as *17α–hydroxycorticosterone.*

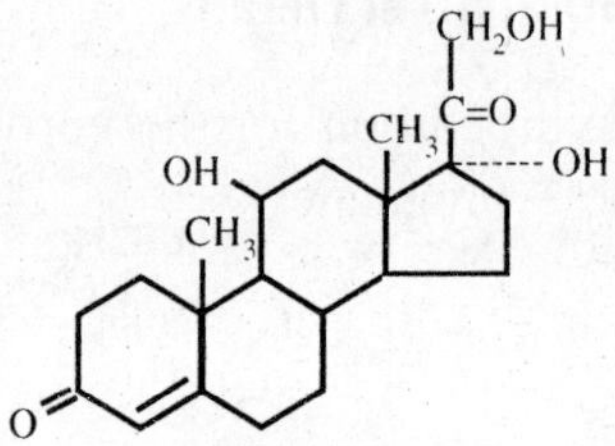

HYDROCORTISONE

Physical Properties

Hydrocortisone is a white to practically white, odourless, bitter, crystalline powder. It crystallises from ethanol in prisms melting at 217° to 220°C. It is practically insoluble in water, slightly soluble in chloroform, very slightly soluble in ether and sparingly soluble in 95% ethanol. The C_{21} sodium hydrogen succinate of hydrocortisone is soluble 1 in 3 water and so its solution in water is conveniently used as injection. The acetate, the C_{21} dihydrogen phosphate, the tertiary butylacetate and the hemisuccinate are also used. Hydrocortisone is affected by light.

Chemical Properties

If, to a solution of hydrocortisone in ethanol, concentrated sulphuric water is added, an intense yellow colour is produced. It also exhibits a green fluorescence. It is found to be particularly intense under ultraviolet light (365 nm). Even if the solution is diluted with water, the fluorescence at 365 nm does not disappear.

Stability and Storage

Store hydrocortisone in well-closed, light-resistant containers.

Uses

Adrenocortical steroid (glucocorticoid). It has antiinflammatory, antirheumatic and antiallergic uses. So it is useful in rheumatoid arthritis, oesteoarthritis and asthma. It is also used to treat collagen diseases, autoimmune diseases, severe allergic reactions, eye diseases, skin diseases, inflammatory intestinal diseases such as ulcerative colitis etc.

Official

Hydrocortisone, I.P. B.P.
Hydrocortisone Cream, B.P.
Hydrocortisone and Neomycin Cream, B.P.
Hydrocortisone Ointment, B.P.
Hydrocortisone and Clioquinol Ointment, B.P.
Hydrocortisone Acetate, I.P., B.P.
Hydrocortisone Acetate Cream, B.P.
Hydrocortisone Acetate and Clioquinol Cream, B.P.
Hydrocortisone Acetate and Neomycin Ear Drops, B.P.
Hydrocortisone Acetate and Neomycin Eye Drops, B.P.
Hydrocortisone Acetate Eye Ointment, I.P.
Hydrocortisone Acetate Injection, I.P., B.P.
Hydrocortisone Acetate Ointment, B.P.
Hydrocortisone Hydrogen Succinate, B.P.
(Hydrocortisone Hemisuccinate, I.P.)
Hydrocortisone Sodium Succinate Injection, I.P., B.P.

Brand Names

Lycortin-S, Efcorlin, Efcorlin soluble, Wycort etc.

357

2. CORTISONE

This has the same structures as hydrocortisone with the only difference that it has no hydroxyl group at the 11th position but an oxygen (keto group) only. Therefore it is known as *17α–hydroxy–11–dehydrocorticosterone*. Both cortisone and hydrocortisone are used as their acetates.

CORTISONE

Physical Properties

Cortisone acetate is a white or almost white, odourless, crystalline powder. It melts at 235° to 238°C. It is practically insoluble in water and cortisone acetate injection is a sterile suspension of the very fine powder of cortisone acetate in sodium chloride solution containing suitable dispersing agents. It is soluble in chloroform, sparingly soluble in acetone and slightly soluble in ethanol. It is affected by light.

Chemical Properties

When it is dissolved in concentrated sulphuric acid, a faint yellow colour is produced. When it is diluted with water, the yellow colour disappears and a clear solution is obtained. It reduces at room temperature ammoniacal silver nitrate.

Stability and Storage

Keep cortisone acetate in a well-closed container protected from light.

Uses

Adrenocortical steroid. It has the same uses as hydrocortisone.

Official

Cortisone Acetate, I.P., B.P.
Cortisone Acetate Injection, I.P.
Cortisone Acetate Tablets, I.P.
(Cortisone Tablets, B.P.)

Brand Names

Corlin, Incortin, Cortone, Cortistab, Cortelan etc.

3. PREDNISOLONE

In an effort to get increased glucocorticoid activity and reduced mineralocorticold activity some new substances were synthesized. Prednisolone is one such. In this the glucorticoid and antiinflammatory activity is increased 3 to 5 times but the mineralocorticoid activity is reduced. Prednisolone has the same structure as hydrocortisone but also has an extra double bond between positions 1 and 2. It can be called as *1–dehydrohydrocortisone*. Prednisolone is used as such and also as the acetate, pivalate and sodium phosphate.

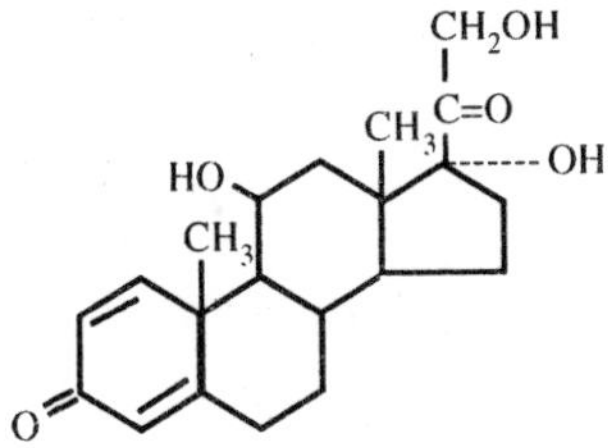

PREDNISOLONE
(1-Dehydrohydrocortisone)

359

Physical Properties

Prednisolone is a white or almost white, hygroscopic crystalline powder. It melts at about 230°C with decomposition. It is slightly soluble in water but soluble in methanol and ethanol, sparingly soluble in acetone and slightly soluble in chloroform. It is affected by light.

Chemical Properties

When prednisolone is dissolved in concentrated sulphuric acid, an intense red colour is produced. It has a reddish brown fluorescene in ultraviolet light (365 nm). When it is diluted with water, the colour fades and a yellow fluorescene is seen in ultraviolet light (365 nm).

Stability and Storage

Since it is hygroscopic and is also affected by light, store it in well-closed containers protected from light.

Uses

Adrenocortical steroid. Since it is 3 to 5 times more potent than hydrocortisone, it is used in lower doses. It is used to treat inflammatory, allergic, autoimmune diseases etc. and also in malignancies.

Official

Prednisolone, I.P., B.P.
Prednisolone Tablets, I.P., B.P.
Prednisolone Acetate, B.P.
Prednisolone Pivalate, B.P.
Prednisolone Sodium Phosphate, B.P.

Deltacortril, Hostacortin-H, Wysolone, Delta-cortef Nisolone etc.

4. BETAMETHASONE

This is another synthetic modification of hydrocortisone. It not only has the 1, 2-double bond as in prednisolone but also has a 9α-fluro and 16β–methyl groups. Therefore it can be called either as *9α–fluoro–16β–methylprednisolone* or as *1–dehydro–9α–fluoro–16β–methylhydrocortisone*. Betamethasone is used as such and also as sodium phosphate and valerate.

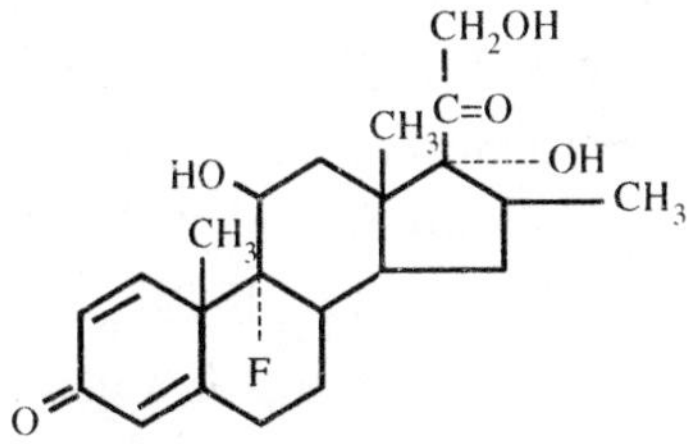

BETAMETHASONE
(1-Dehydro–9α–fluoro–16β–methylhydrocortisone)

In this steroid the glucocorticoid and antiinflammatory activity is increased but the mineralocorticoid activity is very much reduced.

Properties

Betamethasone is a white to creamy white odourless powder. It melts at about 242°C with decomposition. It is practically insoluble in water, very slightly soluble in chloroform and sparingly soluble in ethanol. It is affected by light.

Stability and Storage

Keep it in well-closed, light-resistant containers.

Uses

Adrenocortical steroid. It is a very potent glucocorticoid and is used in inflammatory and allergic conditions. It is also used topically in ointments and creams to treat certain skin conditions. The 16α-methyl epimer is known as dexamethasone and it is also useful in the same way.

Official

Betamethasone, I.P., B.P.
Betamethasone Tablets, I.P., B.P.
Betamethasone Sodium Phosphate, I.P. B.P.
Betamethasone Eye Drops, B.P.
Betamethasone Sodium Phosphate Injection, I.P.
(Betamethasone Injection, B.P.)
Betamethasone Sodium Phosphate Tablets, I.P., B.P.
Betamethasone Valerate, I.P., B.P.
Betamethasone Valerate Scalp Application, B.P.
Betamethasone Valerate Cream, B.P.
Betamethasone Valerate Lotion, B.P.
Betamethasone Valerate Ointment, I.P., B.P.

Brand Names

Betnesol, Betacortril, Betacorlan, Celestan, Visubeta etc.

Other corticosteroids in clinical use are *prednisone, methylprednisolone, fludrocortisone acetate, fluocinolone acetonide, beclomethasone dipropionate, fluocortolone, clobetasol propionate, triamcinolone and acetonide, paramethasone, desoxycorticosterone acetate (DOCA) etc.*

CHAPTER - 31

VITAMINS

Vitamins are essential nutrients which do not give energy but are required in small quantities for the maintenance of normal metabolism. They are relatively simple organic compounds. Since they are usually nitrogenous compounds and originally thought to be necessary for life, they were called as 'vitamines' which was later shortened to vitamins.

Deficiency of vitamins may give rise to several diseases such as beri-beri, scurvy, rickets etc. and they are rapidly relieved by the administration of the required vitamins. They were first designated by letters and figures but later on when we came to know more about their chemical structure, they were given appropriate chemical names also. Most vitamins act physiologically by being integral parts of coenzymes. Food is the most desirable and cheapest source of vitamins.

CLASSIFICATION

Vitamins can be broadly classified into two types depending on their solubility in fats and water.

(1) Fat-Soluble Vitamins
Vitamins A, D, E and K.

(2) Water-Soluble Vitamins
(a) Vitamin B Complex
1. Vitamin B_1 (Aneurine or Thiamine)
2. Vitamin B_2 (Riboflavine)
3. Vitamin B_6 (Pyridoxine)
4. Nicotinic acid (Niacin)
5. Folic acid (Pteroylglutamic acid)
6. Vitamin B_{12} (Cyanocobalalamin)

(b) Vitamin C or Ascorbic Acid.

FAT SOLUBLE VITAMINS

1. VITAMIN A

Vitamin A occurs in the form of A_1 (retinol) and A_2 of which Vitamin A_1 has the most widespread occurrence. It can also be formed in the body from a number of dietary precursors or provitamins which can be converted to the active vitamin A by the liver. The most important of these provitamins are alpha, beta and gamma-carotenes and cryptoxanthine. The carotenes are plentiful in carrots and green vegetables. Yellow corm contains cryptoxanthine. The most important dietary sources of preformed Vitamin A are dairy products such as milk and butter, liver and kidney.

Vitamin A deficiency causes night blindness in the early stages and finally xerophthalmia which is due to failure of the mucous and tear secretions which lubricate and moisten the eyes. The maintenance of epithelial tissues in proper condition and the resistance of the body to infection are dependant on vitamin A. Halibut liver oil, shark liver oil and cod liver oil are the most frequently used therapeutic sources of vitamin. It can be isolated from the fish liver oils or made synthetically.

Structure : Vitamin A_1 (retinol) is a complex organic primary alcohol.

VITAMIN A_1 (RETINOL)

Physical Properties

Pure vitamin A is a pale yellow, crystalline substance which melts at 62-64°C. It is optically inactive and isotropic.

As a fat-soluble vitamin, it is practically insoluble in water but soluble in oils, fats and organic solvents such as ether, chloroform and petroleum spirit. It is partially soluble in 96% alcohol. Vitamin A and its solutions are stable to heat but it is destroyed by oxidation by the oxygen of the air. Addition of antioxidants protects it. Exposure to light is quite destructive and ultraviolet light inactivates vitamin A. It occurs in nature usually in the form of its esters. The esters of vitamin A are more stable to oxidation. Solutions of vitamin A exhibit a characteristic green fluorescence.

Vitamin A is official in I.P. and B.P. in the form of solutions of its esters. In the I.P., Vitamin A Concentrate (oily form) [Synthetic Vitamin A Concentrate (oily form), B.P.] and Vitamin A Concentrate (water-miscible form) [Synthetic Vitamin A Concentrate (water-miscible form), B.P.] are official. In addition Vitamin A Ester Concentrate (Natural) is official in B.P.

Vitamin A Ester Concentrate (Natural) consists of a natural ester or a mixture of natural esters of vitamin A. It may also be a solution of the ester or mixture of esters of vitamin A in arachis oil or any other suitable vegetable oil. So this means that fish liver oils such as those of the halibut, cod etc. may be used in this form provided the vitamin A content conforms to the standards laid down. This may be ensured by diluting with a suitable vegetable oil, if necessary. It is permitted to contain a suitable antioxidant or antioxidants. This is a yellow oil which may contain some crystalline material. On warming it becomes a homogeneous yellow oil with a faint, characteristic odour.

Vitamin A Concentrate (oily form) consists of a solution of an ester or a mixture of esters of vitamin A which is prepared by synthesis. This may be diluted with a suitable vegetable oil, if necessary. It is permitted to contain antioxidants. It is a yellow to brownish-yellow oily liquid with a faint and characteristic odour.

Vitamin A Concentrate (powder form) consists of a single ester or a mixture of esters of vitamin A which is prepared by synthesis and dispersed in gelatin, acacia or any other suitable material. So this is a solid (powder) since vitamin A has been dispersed in a solid matrix such as gelatin or acacia. It is permitted to contain antioxidants. It is a yellow powder usually consisting of uniform size particles. If the matrix is any other material other than gelatin or acacia, it will be practically insoluble in water. If the matrix is gelatin it will swell in water. But if it is acacia, it will form an emulsion with water, since acacia is an emulsifying agent.

Vitamin A Concentrate (water-dispersible form) is a single ester or a mixture of esters of vitamin A prepared by synthesis. It contains, in addition to antimicrobial preservatives and antioxidants, suitable solubilisers also. It is a yellow liquid which may have different viscosity and opalescence at different periods. It has a charcteristic odour. If it is added to water, the insoluble esters of vitamin A are solubilised by the solubilisers giving what is almost a solution. If the solution is very much concentrated, it may become cloudy at low temperatures or it may become a gel at room temperature.

Chemical Properties

If vitamin A is dissolved in chloroform and antimony trichloride solution is added, a transient bright blue colour is produced immediately. If concentrated sulphuric acid is added to vitamin A, a violet colour is produced.

366

Stability and Storage

All the concentrates should be stored in a light-resistant, airtight container (since vitamin A is affected by light and oxygen) at a temperature between 8° and 15°C. Those concentrates which are liquids must also be stored in well-filled containers. Once the container is opened, the contents should be used quickly. If there is anything left unutilised, it should be stored and protected by providing an atmosphere of an inert gas such as nitrogen.

Uses

Antixerophthalmic vitamin. It is therapeutically used for relieving deficiency of vitamin A during pregnancy, childhood and lactation. It is also useful in skin diseases such as acne, psoriasis and icthyosis. It is used to treat night blindness and xerophthalmia (ulceration of the cornea due to vitamin A deficiency), for the maintenance of ephithelial tissue in proper condition and to tone up the body resistance to infection.

Official

Vitamin A Ester Concentrate (Natural), B.P.
Vitamin A Concentrate (Oily Form), I.P.
[Synthetic Vitamin A Concentrate (Oily Form), B.P.]
Vitamin A Concentrate (Powder Form), I.P.
[Synthetic Vitamin A Concentrate (Powder Form), B.P.]
Vitamin A Concentrate (Water-dispersible Form), I.P.
[Synthetic Vitamin A Concentrate (Water-dispersible Form), B.P.]
Vitamin A and D Capsules, I.P.
Concentrated Vitamins A and D Solution, I.P.

367

Brand Names

Aquasal, Arovit, Carofral, Axerophthol, Afaxin etc.

2. VITAMIN D

This term is applied to a group of closely related fat-soluble substance which are necessary for the proper calcification of bones. Deficiency causes the disease rickets. It occurs in butter, cream and milk. Fish liver oils such as the cod liver oil are the richest sources. It is also produced by the irradiation of ergosterol or 7-dehydrocholesterol present on the human skin which is irradiated when one is exposed to direct sunlight as in tropical countries.

The different vitamins D are given below:

a) Vitamin D₂ (calciferol or ergocalciferol)
obtained by the irradiation of ergosterol from yeast.

b) Vitamin D₃ (cholecalciferol)
obtained by the irradiation of 7-dehydrocholesterol or by isolation and extraction from fish liver oils.

Structures : These are derivatives of sterols.

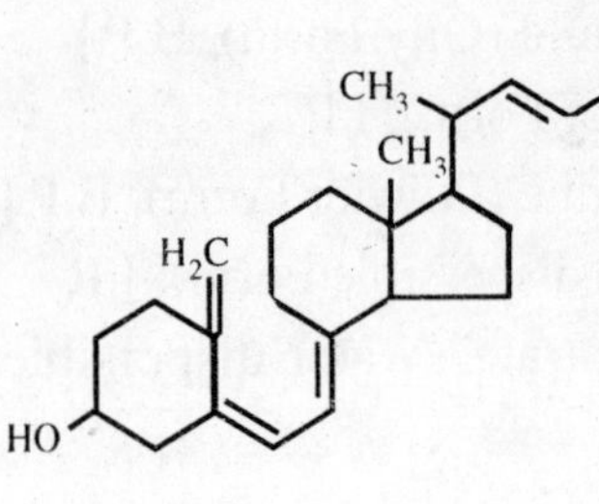

ERGOCALCIFEROL 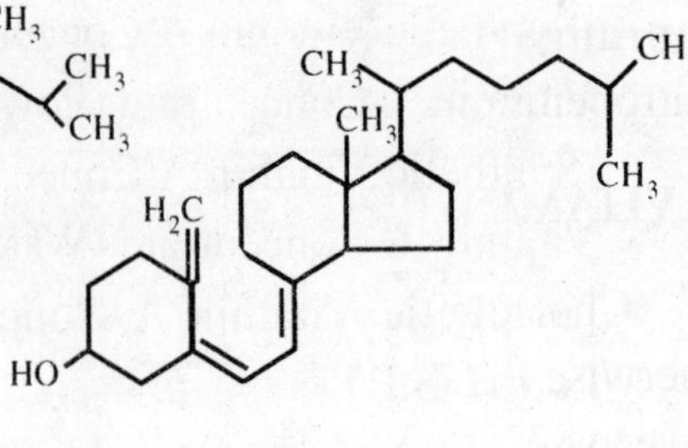   CHOLECALCIFEROL

(c) Dihydrotachysterol : Tachysterol is an intermediate in the conversion of ergosterol to ergocalciferol and when one of the three double bonds in tachysterol is hydrogenated, dihydrotachysterol is obtained. It has slight antirachitic actioity.

DIHYDROTACHYSTEROL

A) VITAMIN D₂ (ERGOCALCIFEROL OR CALCIFEROL)

Vitamin D_2 is official in the B.P. as ergocalciferol.

Properties

Ergocalciferol consists of white or almost white crystals or is a white or slightly yellowish crystalline powder. It is affected by air, heat and light. It is practically insoluble in water, freely soluble in chloroform, ether and ethanol and soluble in fixed oils. Since solutions in volatile solvents are unstable, they should be used immediately after preparation. It melts between 112° and 117°C. With antimony trichloride in chloroform it produces an orange-yellow colour. It forms an ester with 3:5 dihitrobenzoyl chloride.

(B) VITAMIN D₃ (CHOLECALCIFEROL)

Cholecaliferol consists of white or almost white crystals. Otherwise it has the same properties as ergocalciferol. It melts between 82° and 87°C. It is official in the B.P. as Cholecalciferol Concentrate (Oily Form) which is a solution of cholecalciferol

369

in a suitable vegetable oil, Cholecalciferol Concentrate (Powder Form) which is prepared by dispersing an oily solution of cholecalciferol in a suitable matrix of gelatin and other suitable carbohydrates and Cholecalciferol Concentrate (Water-dispersible Form) which is a solution of cholecalciferol in a suitable vegetable oil containing suitable solublisers. All these forms contain suitable antioxidants. Like califerol it gives an orange-yellow colour with antimony trichloride in chloroform and also forms a 3 : 5-dinitrobenzoic ester.

(C) DIHYDROTACHYSTEROL

It consists of colourless crystals or occurs as a white crystalline powder. It has no odour. It is practically insoluble in water, very soluble in chloroform, freely soluble in ether, soluble in ethanol and sparingly soluble in arachis oil.

It gives a red colour with antimony trichloride in chloroform solution.

Stability and Storage

All forms of vitamin D should be kept under nitrogen in an airtight container which is protected from light and stored at a temperature between 2° and 8°C. If any container is opened, its contents should be used immediately.

Uses

Antirachitic vitamin. It is useful in the prophylactic treatment of obstructive jaundice, steatorrhoea (passage of pale, bulky, offensive stools with a high fat content and which tend to float on water) etc. and treatment of metabolic rickets, postmenopaused osteoporosis (fragility of bones due to reabsorption of calcium after menopause in women) and hypoparathyroidism (diminished function of parathyroid glands).

Official

Ergocalciferol, B.P.
Calciferol Capsules, I.P.
Calciferol Injection, I.P., B.P.
Calciferol Oral Solution, I.P., B.P.
Calciferol Tablets, I.P., B.P.
Cholecalciferol, I.P., B.P.
Cholecalciferol Concentrate (Oily Form), B.P.
Cholecalciferol Concentrate (Powder Form), B.P.
Cholecalciferol Concentrate (Water-dispersible Form), B.P.
Cod-liver Oil, B.P.
Halibut-liver Oil, B.P.
Halibut-liver Oil Capsules, B.P.
Vitamins A and D Capsules, I.P.
Concentrated Vitamins A and D Solution, I.P.
Concentrated Vitamin D Solution, I.P.
Dihydrotachysterol, B.P.

Brand Names

Vitamin D$_2$: Calciferol, Ergocalciferol, Ostelin, Decaps, Deltalin, Mulsiferol etc.

Vitamin D$_3$: Oleovitamin D$_3$, Cholecalciferol, Vigontal, Deparal etc.

Dihydrotachysterol : AT 10, Parterol, Tachyrol, Antitanil etc. **Cod-liver Oil**: Seven Seas cod-liver oil.

3. VITAMIN E

This is a fat-soluble substance present in the oil from the embryo of the wheat seed and in other seed oils of plants. It is also present in green leaves such as those of lettuce. Its absence from the diet of rats causes sterility. Its role in human nutrition has not been clearly established.

There are four compounds of vitamin E group known as tocopherols (alpha, beta, gamma and delta). They·are derivatives of 2, 3-benzpyran and are used as antioxidants. Of these alphatocopherol is the most important.

ALPHATOCOPHEROL *(5, 7, 8-trimethyltocol)*

Properties

Alphatocopherol is a clear, colourless or yellowish-brown, viscous oil. It melts at 2°-4°C and boils at 200-220°C. It is odourless. It is practically insoluble in water and freely·soluble in absolute alcohol, acetone, chloroform, ether and fixed oils. It is stable to heat provided oxygen is excluded. It is stable to visible light but not to ultraviolet light. It is particularly susceptible to oxidation. It is slowly oxidized by oxygen of the air and quickly by silver and ferric salts. It is official as alphatocopherol and as the acetate.

Stability and Storage

It should be kept in an airtight container under an inert gas and protected from light.

Uses

Vitamin. It is used in the prevention and treatment of vitamine E deficiencies. It acts in the body as an antioxidant preserving unsaturated lipids in cell membranes, certain coenzymes etc. from damage by peroxides formed by free radicals. It is reported to be of value in delaying ageing.

Official

Alpha Tocopherol, B.P.
Alpha Tocopheryl Acetate, B.P.
(Tocopheryl Acetate, I.P.)
Alpha Tocopheryl Acetate Concentrate (Powder Form),
B.P.

Brand Names

Evion, Covitol, Syntopherol, Etavit etc.

4. VITAMIN K

This term is applied to a group of napthoquinone derivatives which are used for prothrombin synthesis in the liver and are therefore necessary for the normal coagulation of blood. Vitamin K_1 (phytomenadione) is synthesized by plants and Vitamin K_2 by bacteria inhabiting the intestine. Vitamin K_1 occurs in fresh green vegetables, fruits and egg-yolk. Synthetic substitutes of vitamin K are menadione (menaphthone) and acetomenadione (acetomenaphthone).

Chemically, vitamin K_1 is a derivative of 1, 4 naptho-quinone. It contains a methyl group in the second position and

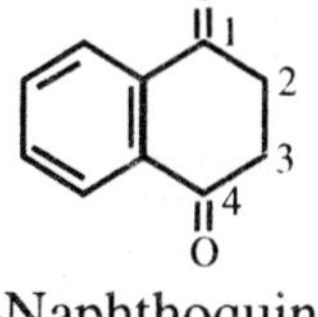

(1, 4-Naphthoquinone)

a phytyl group in the third position:

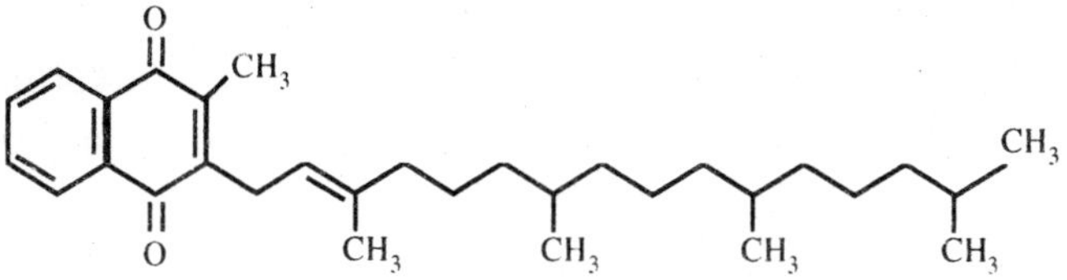

VITAMIN K_1 (PHYTOMENADIONE)
(2-Methyl-3-phytyl-1, 4-naphthoquinone)

373

Physical Properties

Phytomenadione (Vitamin K_1) is a clear, deep yellow oil with almost no odour. It is practically insoluble in water, sparingly soluble in ethanol and freely soluble in chloroform, ether and fixed oils. It decomposes on exposure to light. It is stable to air and moisture. It is destroyed by reducing agents and in alkali hydroxide solutions. It is not affected by acids. It exhibits a characteristic fluorescence when exposed to the light from an argon lamp.

Chemical Properties

When phytomenadione is treated with methanol and solution of potassium hydroxide in methanol, a green colour is produced. If it is heated gently, the colour becomes purple and when it is allowed to stand for some time, it becomes reddish brown.

Stability and Storage

Since it is affected by light, it should be kept in a well-closed container protected from light.

Uses

Prothrombogenic vitamin. It is used to correct deficiency of vitamin K either due to dietary deficiency (which is very rare) or due to prolonged antibacterial therapy or due to obstructive jaundice or due to liver disease. It is also used to treat the heamorrhagic disease of the new born and to block the effect of overdose of anticoagulants.

Official

Phytomenadione, B.P.
Phytomenadione Injection, B.P.
Phytemenadione Tablets, B.P.

Brand Names

Vitamin K, Phytomenadione, Mephyton, Mono-kay, Konakion etc.

5. MENADIONE

See the Chapter on **"Coagulants and Anticoagulants"**

Menadione sodium bisulphite is a water-soluble derivative used as injection. Similarly menadiol sodium phosphate is a water-soluble derivative used in a similar way. Menadiol is prepared by reducing menadione to the diol.

6. ACETOMENAPHTHONE (ACETOMENADIONE)

If 2-methyl-1, 4-naphthoquinone is reduced, the resulting compound is 2-methyl 1,4-naphthoquinol.

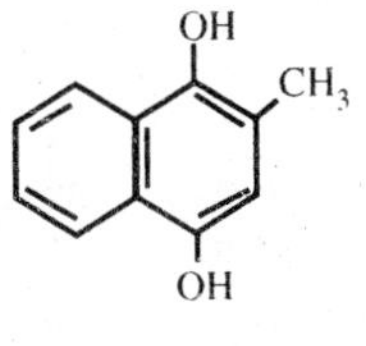

2-methyl-1, 4-naphthoquinol

If the hydroxyl groups at both the 1 and 4 positions are acetylated, acetomenaphthone is got.

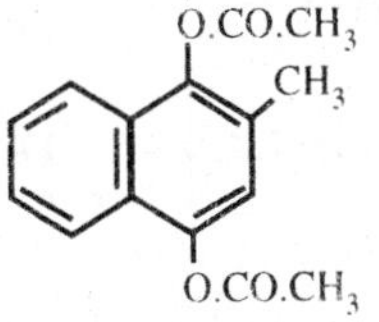

Acetomenaphthone
(1, 4-Diacetoxy-2-methylnaphthalene)

Physical Properties

Acetomenaphthone is a white, crystalline powder having no odour or an odour reminding that of acetic acid. It has a bitter taste. It is practically insoluble in water, slightly soluble in cold ethanol and freely soluble in boiling ethanol.

Chemical Properties

It responds to the test for acetyl groups. In this test the acetomenaphthone is hydrolysed by phosphoric acid and the vapour allowed to react with a drop of lanthanum nitrate solution. When the drop is mixed with one drop of ammonia, a blue colour appears at the junction of the two drops after one or two minutes.

Stability and Storage

Since it may be affected by atmospheric moisture, store it in well-closed containers.

Uses

Prothrombogenic vitamin (synthetic substitute of vitamin K). It has the same uses as phytomenadione.

Official

Acetomenaphthone, I.P.'85
Acetomenaphthone Tablets, I.P.'85

Brand Names

Acetomenadione, Kapilin etc.

WATER SOLUBLE VITAMINS

1. THIAMINE (VITAMIN B_1 OR ANEURINE)

Deficiency of this vitamin in humans leads to beri-beri, the corresponding condition in other animals especially birds is polyneuritis. The richest sources are rice polishings, yeast, eggs, liver and pork. Green leafy vegetables come next, while milk, fish and meat also contain small quantities of it. Thiamine is concerned with carbohydrate metabolism in the body.

Structure : This vitamin is a compound of basic character. In the molecule there is a pyrimidine ring linked by a methylene group to a thiazole ring. The nitrogen of the thiazole ring is cationic and a chloride ion is associated with it. The weakly basic $-NH_2$ group in the pyrimidine ring also forms a hydrochloride.

$$CH_3 \quad N \quad N \quad CH_2 \quad N^+ \quad CH_3 \quad .Cl^-.HCl \quad NH_2 \quad S \quad CH_2CH_2OH$$

THIAMINE HYDROCHLORIDE

Physical Properties

Thiamine hydrochloride is a white or almost white, crystalline powder or it consists of colourless crystals with a slight and characteristic odour. It absorbs water from the atmosphere forming a hydrate. It is freely soluble in water, slightly soluble in ethanol and practically insoluble in ether and chloroform. The commercial sample contains about 4% of water which can be removed by drying at 100°C. It is fairly stable to heat but temperatures above 100°C are quite injurious. It is destroyed by alkalies and substances with an alkaline reaction. Aqueous solutions are acidic and are stable at a pH of 3.5 to 5. Alkaline pH is quite injurious. The decomposition of thiamine in aqueous solution is catalysed by certain metals.

Chemical Properties

It combines with diazonium salts to form coloured azo dyes. It is precipitated by Mayer's reagent, picric acid, iodine, mercuric chloride, tamins etc. It is oxidized in alkaline solution

377

to a fluoroscent substance known as thiochrome by potassium ferricyanide. Thiochrome can be extracted by adding n-butanol and the solution exhibits an intense light blue fluorescence especially when exposed to ultraviolet light (365 nm).

Stability and Storage

For the reasons stated under "Physical Properties" it should be stored in tightly-closed, light-resistant, non-metallic containers.

Uses

B complex vitamin. In the body it is converted to thiamine pyrophosphate which serves as a coenzyme in carbohydrate metabolism. It is used to treat beriberi. It is also used to treat certain neurological and cardiovascular disorders.

Official

Thiamine Hydrochloride, I.P., B.P.
Thiamine Hydrochloride Injection, I.P., (Thiamine Injection, B.P.)
Thiamine Hydrochloride Tablets, I.P. (Thiamine Tablets, B.P.)
Vitamin B and C Injection, B.P.
Thiamine Mononitrate, I.P.
(Thiamine Nitrate, B.P.)

Brand Names

Berin, Beneuron, Betabion, Betaxin, Thiadoxine etc.

2. RIBOFLAVINE (VITAMIN B$_2$)

Riboflavine deficiency in man is characterised by inflammation and scalines of the lips. The growth of the young is retarded and in adults premature ageing is caused. These symptoms respond rapidly when riboflavine is administered. It is present in eggs, milk, green leafy vegetables and meat. Liver and yeast contain higher amounts.

It has the following structure:

It is a derivative of the complex heterocyclic isoalloxazine system. There are two methyl groups at the 6 and 7 positions and a D–ribityl group derived from the sugar D–ribose at the 9th position. Therefore chemically it *is 9–1′–ribityl–6, 7–dimethyl isoalloxazine.*

$CH_2(CHOH)_3CH_2OH$

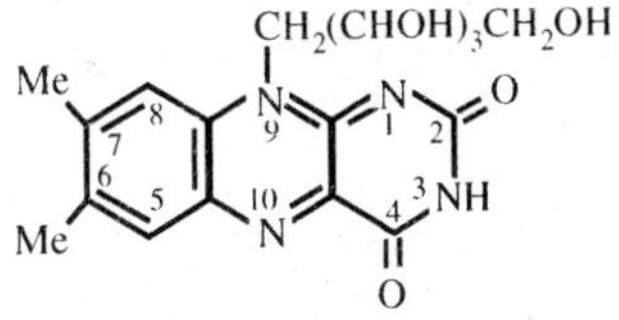

RIBOFLAVINE
(9–1′–ribityl–6, 7–dimethylisoalloxazine)

Physical Properties

RibolaVine is a yellow to orange yellow, crystalline powder with a slight odour and a bitter taste. It melts at 278°C to 282°C with decomposition. It is very slightly soluble in water and practically insoluble in ether, ethanol and chloroform. It is more easily soluble in saline solution. It deteriorates rapidly in alkaline solution and the decomposition is more when it is exposed to light. It gives an intense yellowish green fluorescence when dissolved in water and the fluorescence is maximum when the solution is neutral. It disappears on the addition of mineral acids or alkalies. It is fairly stable to heat and mineral acids and oxidising agents. However, as already stated, it deteriorates rapidly in alkaline solution.

Chemical Properties

It is reduced to a colourless leuco compound and in the presence of air the colour reappears. When it is exposed to sun light or ultraviolet light in alkaline solution, it decomposes forming a yellow compound known as lumiflavin which is insoluble in water but soluble in chloroform and gives the same yellowish green fluorescence like riboflavine. When riboflavine is exposed to light in dilute methyl alcoholic solution, it forms a different compound known as lumichrome. Lumichrome exhibits an intense sky blue fluorescence.

Stability and Storage

Keep it in tightly-closed containers protected from light.

Uses

B Complex Vitamin : It is used to treat ariboflavinosis (group of symptoms caused by deficiency of riboflavine).

Official

Riboflavine, I.P., B.P.
Riboflavine Tablets, I.P.
Riboflavine Sodium Phosphate, I.P., B.P.
Vitamin B and C Injection, B.P.

Brand Names

Lipabol, Riboflavin, Lactoflavine, Beflavine etc.

3. PYRIDOXINE (VITAMIN B₆)

In nature it occurs as a mixture of three related pyridine derivatives, pyridoxine, pyridoxal and pyridoxamine. In the body all three forms are converted into pyridoxal phosphate. Dietary sources include yeast, rice bran, wheat germ, molasses and liver.

PYRIDOXAL   PYRIDOXINE   PYRIDOXAMINE

Chemically pyridoxine is *3–hydroxy– 4, 5-di(hydroxymethyl)– 2–methylpyridine*.

It is official as the hydrochloride.

Physical Properties

Pyridoxine hydrochloride is a white or almost white, crystalline powder with no odour. It is freely soluble in water, slightly soluble in ethanol and practically insoluble in ether and chloroform. It melts at about 205°C with decomposition. It is affected by light.

Chemical Properties

It is easily oxidized by oxidising agents such as hydrogen peroxide. It gives a deep reddish brown colour with aqueous ferric chloride.

Stability and Storage

Since it is affected by light, store it in well-closed, light-resistant containers.

Uses

B Complex vitamin. It is necessary for normal growth and is involved in protein, aminoacid and carbohydrate metabolism. Deficiency symptoms are oedema, hair loss and convulsions. It is also used to treat sideroblastic anaemia, neuropathy due to poisoning by isoniazid, morning sickness, muscular weakness, acne (condition particularly occurring among adolescents, resulting from hormonally induced hyperactivity of the sebaceous glands and characterized by black heads and pustules occurring commonly on the face, neck, and chest), radiation sickness, nausea and vomiting in pregnancy and suppression of lactation in women. It is converted to pyridoxal phosphate in the body.

Official

Pyridoxine Hydrochloride, I.P., B.P.
Pyridoxine Hydrochloride Tablets, I.P. (Pyridoxine Tablets, B.P.)
Vitamins B and C Injection, B.P.

Brand Names

Compoviton 6, Hexobion, Hexabetalin, Becilan etc.

4. NICOTINIC ACID (NIACIN) AND NICOTINAMIDE

Nicotinic acid functions in the body as the amide. Deficiency of nicotinic acid produces black tongue in dogs and pellagra in man. Therefore nicotinic acid is also known as pellagra preventive factor (pp factor). Dietary sources are yeast, wheat germ, green leafy vegetables, legumes, liver, kidney, milk and fish. The amide is a constituent of coenzymes diphosphopyridine nucleotide (DPN) and triphosphopyridine nucleotide (TPN) which are concerned with hydrogen transport in several biological oxidation-reduction systems.

Structures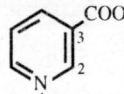

NICOTINIC ACID   NICOTINAMIDE
(Pyridine–β–carboxylic acid) (Pyridine–β–carboxamide)

Physical Properties

Nicotinic acid is a creamy-white or white powder melting between 234° and 240°C. It sublimes without decomposition. It is soluble in boiling water and boiling ethanol, sparingly soluble in cold water, very slightly soluble in chloroform and practically insoluble in ether. Since it is an acid, it dissolves in dilute solutions of alkali hydroxides and carbonates. It is affected by light.

Nicotinamide occurs as colourless crystals or as a white, crystalline powder with a faint and characteristic odour. It melts between 128° and 131°C. It is freely soluble in water and ethanol and slightly soluble in chloroform and ether.

Chemical Properties

When nicotinic acid is heated with soda lime, it is decarboxylated and pyridine is produced. When it is dissolved in water, neutralised with dilute sodium hydroxide solution and copper sulphate solution is added, a blue precipitate is slowly produced. A solution of nicotinic acid gives with cyanogen bromide and aniline a golden yellow colour.

When nicotinamide is heated with dilute sodium hydroxide solution, ammonia is evolved. With cyanogen bromide and aniline, it gives a golden yellow colour like nicotinic acid.

Stability and Storage

Keep nicotinic acid in well-closed, light-resistant containers and nicotinamide in well-closed containers.

Uses

B Complex vitamin and vasodilator. The acid only is the vasodilator and not the amide. It is used to treat pellagra. Pellagra is characterised by dermatitis, diarrhoea and dementia (hallucinations in the brain).

Official

Nicotinic Acid, I.P., B.P.
Nicotinic Acid Tablets, I.P., B.P.
Nicotinamide, I.P., B.P.
Nicotinamide Tablets, I.P., B.P.
Vitamins B and C Injection, B.P.

383

Brand Names

For nicotinic acid – Nicacid, Niconacid, Akotin, Daskil etc.

For nicotinamide : Nicofort, Benicol, Aminicotin etc.

5. FOLIC ACID (PTEROYLGLUTAMIC ACID)

Folic acid occurs in yeast, green vegetables, liver and many other foods. It is also prepared by synthesis. It is necessary for cell division and for normal production of red blood cells. It is also concerned with synthesis from one-carbon units in metabolic processes. Deficiency produces diarrhoea, glossitis, loss of weight and appearance of immature red blood cells in the blood known as megaloblasts.

Structure : It is a pteridine derivative. It is made up of pteridine, p–aminobenzoic acid and L–glutamic acid. There may be several glutamic acid residues present depending on the source.

| pteridine | p-aminobenzoic acid | L-glutamic acid |

Physical Properties

Folic acid crystallises from water as orange yellow needles or occurs as a yellowish or orange, crystalline powder. It is almost odourless. It has no definite melting point but darkens and chars and decomposes above 250°C. It is practically insoluble in water and in most organic solvents but is more soluble in ether, acetone, benzene and chloroform. By virtue of

384

its amphoteric character, it dissolves in dilute acids and in alkaline solutions. It is decomposed readily in the dry state or in dilute solutions by sun light or ultraviolet light. It is destroyed more readily by cooking compared to other water soluble vitamins. Its sodium salt is more soluble in water and is used in injections.

Folic acid occurs in nature in combination with a chain of glutamic acid residues such as pteroyltriglutamic acid and pteroylheptaglutamic acid.

Chemical Properties

Pteroylglutamic acid can be reduced by zinc amalgam to p-aminobenzoylglutamic acid. Since the latter contains a primary aromatic amino group, it can be diazotised with sodium nitrite and dilute hydrochloric acid and coupled in acid solution with N-(1-naphthyl) ethylenediamine hydrochloride to give an orange red azo dye. In fact this is the assay method prescribed for folic acid in the I.P. and the B.P.

Stability and Storage

As it is affected by light and also is easily oxidised, it must be kept in tightly closed, light-resistant containers.

Uses

B complex vitamin (heamotopoietic). It is used in the treatment of certain megaloblastic anaemias, macrocytic anaemia and pernicious anaemia. It is reduced in the body to tetrahydrofolate which functions as the coenzyme for the synthesis of DNA.

Official

Folic Acid, I.P., B.P.
Folic Acid Tablets, I.P., B.P.

Brand Names

Folvite, Vitamin M, Folacin, Foliamin etc.

6. CYANOCOBALAMIN (VITAMIN B$_{12}$)

Vitamin B$_{12}$ is necessary for normal growth, normal production of red blood cells and for the proper maintenance of epithelium.

It is made by culturing of various Streptomyces bacteria. It occurs in kidney, liver, eggs, muscle tissue and milk. Daily requirement is 1 microgram. Deficiency causes pernicious anaemia. Usually it is the failure to absorb vitamin B$_{12}$ from the gastrointestinal tract due to lack of intrinsic factor which causes pernicious anaemia. Therefore the condition is immediately relieved by injection of vitamin B$_{12}$ or by giving vitamin B$_{12}$ and the intrinsic factor orally.

Structure : Cyanocobalamin has a very complex structure. Structurally it is related to porphyrin and contains a cobalt atom and a cyanide group. The cyanide may be replaced by hydroxyl or nitro group in other naturally produced compounds which are also active.

Physical Properties

Cyanocobalamin is a dark red, crystalline powder which is very hygroscopic. When exposed to air, it absorbs about 12% of moisture. It is very sensitive to cyanide and light. Aqueous solutions stored in the dark at pH 6 to 7 are stable.

It is rapidly inactivated by acids and alkalies. Hydroxocobalamin is less stable than cyanocobalamin. It is sparingly soluble in water and ethanol and practically insoluble in chloroform, ether and acetone.

Chemical Properties

When cyanocobalamin is mixed with potassium sulphate and 0.5 M sulphuric acid, heated to redness, allowed to cool and water, saturated solution of ammonium thiocyanate and benzyl alcohol added and shaken, a blue colour is formed and it is extracted into the benzyl alcohol layer.

Stability and Storage .

Cyanocobalamin is very hygroscopic and is also affected by light. So it should be kept in an airtight container and protected from light.

Uses

B complex vitamin (haematopoietic). It acts as a coenzyme in the synthesis of proteins, nucleic acids and lipids. It is used in the treatment of pernicious anaemia and subacute combined degeneration of the spinal cord and neuritis. Hydroxocobalamin is better retained in the body. In the absence of intrinsic factor, cyanocobalamin may be given by i.m. or s.c. injection only. It should not be given intravenously.

Official

Cyanocobalamin, I.P., B.P.
Cyanocobalamin Injection, I.P., B.P.
Cyanocobalamin Tablets, B.P.

Brand Names

Macrabin, Redisol, Calomide, Cobaltamin-S etc.

Hydroxocobalamin : Macrabin-H, Redisol-H.

7. ASCORBIC ACID (VITAMIN C)

The lack of this vitamin causes a well-known disease called scurvy and hence the name ascorbic acid. The early symptoms of the diseases are weakness in the joints and spongy gums. When the disease is more advanced, subcutaneous haemorrhage, loose teeth, fragility of bones and often oedema result.

It is the most abundant of the vitamins. The most abundant sources are fresh vegetables and citrus fruits like lemon and orange.

It is a strong reducing agent and probably helps to maintain oxidation-reduction systems in enzymatic processes. It is required for the development of cartilage, bone and teeth. It is also required for the maturing of red blood cells and for the healing of wounds. It may be extracted from the juices of citrus fruits or capsicum annuum or prepared synthetically.

Structure : Ascorbic acid has the following structure:

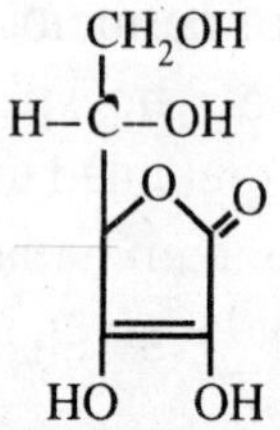

$$CH_2OH$$
$$H-\overset{|}{C}-OH$$

ASCORBIC ACID

It has a furanose structure and has acid properties because of the α–ketonediol group.

Physical Properties

Ascorbic acid occurs in the form of colourless crystals or as a white to very pale yellow, crystalline powder. It is odourless and melts at 190°–192°C. It has a pleasant, sharp, acidic taste. When it is adequately protected from oxidation it can be crystallised from water, alcohol and acetone. It is freely soluble in water, sparingly soluble in ethanol and insoluble in chloroform, ether and benzene. Even though it may be stable in the dry state, in solution it darkens rapidly on exposure to air due to oxidation. This oxidation is catalysed by light, alkalies and certain metals such as iron, copper and manganese. An 1% solution has a pH of 2.7 which indicates the intensely acidic nature of ascorbic acid. It combines with metals to form salts.

388

Chemical Properties

Ascorbic acid gives an intense violet colour with ferric chloride solution. It is easily precipitated by lead acetate. The most characteristic property of ascorbic acid is its strong reducing action. It reduces iodine, potassium permanganate, ammoniacal silver nitrate etc. It decolourises 2, 6-dichloro-phenolindophenol (a dye). In these reactions, ascorbic acid is oxidised to dehydroascorbic acid. Ascorbic acid answers many colour reactions. For example when a solution of ascorbic acid is treated with freshly prepared solution of sodium nitroprusside and sodium hydroxide solution and hydrochloric acid is added drop by drop and stirred, the yellow colour of the solution becomes blue. In another colour reaction when to a solution of ascorbic acid, sodium bicarbonate and ferrous sulphate are added, shaken and allowed to stand, a deep violet colour is produced. When dilute sulphuric acid is added, the colour is discharged or disappears.

Stability and Storage

See the Physical Properties again. It can be understood that ascorbic acid is the least stable of all vitamins. So it must be stored in tightly closed, light-resistant containers avoiding contact with metals.

Uses

Antiscorbutic vitamin and antioxidant.

Ascorbic acid is found to be necessary for the synthesis of collagen and is very important for maintenance of intercellular connective tissue. It is used in the prevention and treatment of scurvy and to enhance healing of wounds. The severity of common cold may be reduced by treatment with ascorbic acid.

Official

Ascorbic Acid, I.P., B.P.
Ascorbic Acid Injection, I.P., B.P.
Ascorbic Acid Tablets, I.P., B.P.
Vitamins B and C Injection, B.P.

Brand Names

Celin, Redoxon, Cecon, Ascorvit, Cevitan etc.

CHAPTER - 32

ANTINEOPLASTIC AGENTS
(ANTICANCER DRUGS)

Cancer is a disease in which there is abnormal growth of some cells in the body producing tumours. It is believed to be caused by viruses, exposure to x-rays, uv rays and ionizing radiation, heavy smoking and continuous irritation to any body tissue due to any reason including tobacco chewing, snuff taking etc. Antineoplastic agents are drugs used to treat cancer.

The treatment of cancer is now limited to exposure to ionizing radiation, surgery and using chemotherapeutic agents. The drugs increase survival time and provide relief from pain. They are able to do this by suppressing the growth of the tumour. They are also able to provide cure or prolonged remission (remission is a lessening in the severity of symptoms or their temporary disappearance during the course of an illness) in certain leukemias, lymphomas and sarcomas. They are also now used along with surgery, radiotherapy and immunotherapy for treating certain solid tumours and also metastasis (transfer or spreading of a disease from one organ to another, especially cancer). Drugs are also used to destroy any residual cancer cells remaining after surgery or radiotherapy.

CLASSIFICATION

1. Alkylating agents

  a) Nitrogen mustards
    1. Cyclophosphamide
    2. Chlorambucil

  b) Alkyl sulfonate
    Busulphan

2. Antimetabolites
a) Purine antagonist
1. Mercaptopurine
2. Azathoprine
b) Pyrimidine antagonist
5-Fluorouracil
c) Folate antagonist
Methotrexate

3. Antibiotics
1. Actinomycins
2. Daunorubicin
3. Mytomycin

4. Miscellaneous
Cisplatin

1. CYCLOPHOSPHAMIDE

Cyclophosphamide is a nitrogen mustard. It is a derivative of a cyclic oxazophosphorine which means that it is a six membered ring with oxygen, nitrogen and phosphorus in the ring.

Physical Properties

Cyclophosphamide is a white or almost white, crystalline powder. It melts at 49.5°C to 53°C. It is soluble in water, freely soluble in ethanol and slightly soluble in ether. It is thermoliabile and should be stored at a temperature at or below 30°C.

Chemical Properties

Cyclophosphamide contains chlorine in the side chain since a dichloroethylamino group is present attached to the nuclear phosphorus atom. When it is dissolved in water, it is *slowly* hydrolysed to the ethyleneimmonium ion and liberates chloride ions.

So when cyclophosphamide is dissolved in water and silver nitrate solution added, there is no precipitate. But if the solution is boiled, hydrolysis is hastened and chloride ions are liberated. So a white precipitate is produced. It is insoluble in nitric acid but dissolves in dilute ammonia solution and can be reprecipitated by adding dilute nitric acid.

Cyclophosphamide can also be disintegrated by dissolving it in a mixture of concentrated nitric and sulphuric acids and heating. The phosphorus atom is oxidised to phosphate which can be detected by adding ammonium molybdate solution. A bright yellow precipitate is slowly produced.

Stability and Storage

As already stated, it is thermolabile. So long exposure to temperatures above 30°C should be avoided. Therefore store it in a well-closed container in a cold place.

Uses

Anticancer drug (cytotoxic). By itself it is inactive and is converted into active metabolites in the liver which are responsible for the antitumour action. It has good immunosuppressant activity as well. It is used in the treatment of many malignant diseases such as leukemia, Hodgkin's disease, Burkitt's lymphoma, myeloma, cancer of the breast etc.

Official

Cyclophosphamide, I.P., B.P.
Cyclophosphamide Injection, I.P., B.P.
Cyclophosphamide Tablets, I.P., B.P.

Brand Names

Endoxan, Cycloxan, Sandoxan, Procytox etc.

2. CHLORAMBUCIL

Chlorambucil is a substituted butyric acid with a simpler structure than that of cyclophosphamide.

Physical Properties

Chlorambucil is a white, crystalline or granular powder melting at 64°C to 67°C. It is practically insoluble in water, freely soluble in acetone, chloroform and ethanol. It is affected by light.

Chemical Properties

As in the case of cyclophosphamide, chlorambucil contains a bisdichloroethylamino group and will undergo slow hydrolysis when it is put into water. The hydrolysis is hastened when the suspension is boiled and chloride ions are liberated and they give the white precipitate with silver nitrate.

Thus when a solution of chlorambucil in water is poured into water and nitric acid and silver nitrate solution are added, no opalescence is produced immediately. But if it is heated on a water bath, an opalescence develops.

Stability and Storage

Since it is affected by light, it should be kept in a well-closed container and protected from light.

Uses

Anticancer agent (cytotoxic). It is also a nitrogen mustard and is a very slow alkylating agent. It is used in the treatment of chronic lymphoid leukemia, Hodgkin's disease and some solid tumours.

Official

Chlorombucil, I.P., B.P.
Chlorambucil Tablets, I.P., B.P.

Brand Names

Leukeran, Amboclorin, CB 1348.

3. BUSULPHAN

Busulphan has a much simpler structure than cyclophosphamide and chlorambucil. It is an alkyl sulfonate and is *tetramethylene di(methane sulfonate)*.

$$CH_3\text{-}SO_2\text{-}O(CH_2)_4O\text{-}SO_2\text{-}CH_3$$

BUSULPHAN

Physical Properties

Busulphan is a white or almost white, crystalline powder melting at about 116°C. It is very slightly soluble in water, ethanol and ether and freely soluble in acetone and chloroform. It is affected by light.

Chemical Properties

The compound can be disintegrated by fusing with solid potassium nitrate and potassium hydroxide. The sulphur is oxidised to sulphate which can be detected by dissolving the residue in water and adding dilute hydrochloric acid and barium chloride. A white precipitate is produced.

Stability and Storage

Since it is affected by light, store in tightly-closed, light-resistant containers.

Uses

Anticancer agent (cytotoxic). It is the drug of choice in chronic myeloid leukemia.

Official

Busulphan, I.P., B.P.
Busulphan Tablets, I.P., B.P.

Brand Names

Myleran, Misulban, Myelosan, Meilucin etc.

4. MERCAPTOPURINE

Mercaptopurine has a simple structure. It has a mercapto or thiol group (-SH) in the sixth position of the purine nucleus. So it is *6-mercaptopurine*.

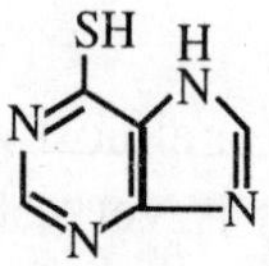

MERCAPTOPURINE

Physical Properties

Mercaptopurine is a yellow, odourless, crystalline powder, melting at 313°C to 314°C. It is practically insoluble in water, ether and acetone and slightly soluble in ethanol. It dissolves in solutions of alkali hydroxides. It is affected by light.

Chemical Properties

A white precipitate is produced when an ethanolic solution of mercaptopurine is heated and mixed with a solution of mercuric acetate in ethanol. A yellow precipitate is produced when the ethanolic solution of mercaptopurine is heated and mixed with a solution of lead acetate in ethanol.

Stability and Storage

Since it is affected by light, store it in well-closed containers protected from light.

Uses

Anticancer agent (cytotoxic). It acts as an antimetabolite for adenine in the synthesis of nucleotides. It interferes with the synthesis of nucleic acids. It is used in the treatment of acute childhood leukemia, some solid tumours and same auto-immune disorders.

Official

Mercaptopurine, I.P., B.P.
Mercaptopurine Tablets, B.P.

Brand Names

Leukerin, Mercaleukin, 6-MP, Purinethiol.

5. AZATHIOPRINE

Azathioprine is a derivative of mercaptopurine and contains a substituted imidazole ring attached to the thiol group in the 6th position. This imidiazole ring has a nitro group in the 4th position.

Physical Properties

Azathioprine is a pale yellow powder. It is practically insoluble in water, ethanol and chloroform. It is sparingly soluble in dilute mineral acids but dissolves in dilute solutions of alkali hydroxides. It forms azathioprine sodium with sodium hydroxide and azathioprine sodium is also used clinically as an injection. This solution has a pH of 9.8 to 10.

It is also affected by light.

Chemical Properties

A weak aqueous solution of the substance may be prepared by heating with a large quantity of water and filtering. The nitro group in the imidazole may be reduced to the amino group by treating the filtrate with hydrochloric acid and zinc powder. The solution becomes yellow. It is filtered, cooled in ice and treated with sodium nitrite solution, sulphamic acid and 2-napthol solution. A pale pink precipitate is produced.

Stability and Storage

Since it is affected by light, it should be kept in a well-closed container and protected from light.

Uses

Anticancer agent and immunosuppressant. It is primarily used as an immunosuppressant in organ transplantation. It is also used in rheumatoid arthritis, lupus erythematosus etc.

Official

Azathioprine, B.P.
Azathioprine Tablets, B.P.

Brand Names

Imuran, Transimune, Imurel, Azanin etc.

6. FLUOROURACIL

Fluorouracil is a pyrimidine derivative with a fluorine atom in the 5th position. It is actually *2,4-dioxo-5-fluorotetrahydropyrimidine.*

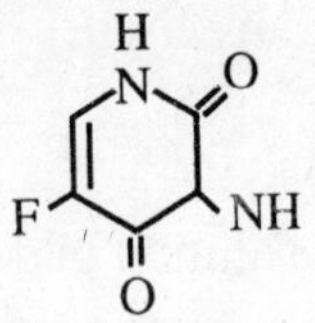

5-FLUOROURACIL

Physical Properties

Fluorouracil is a white or almost white, crystalline powder without odour and melting at 282°C to 283°C with decomposition. It is sparingly soluble in water, slightly soluble in ethanol and practically insoluble in chloroform and ether. It is affected by light.

Chemical Properties

If bromine water is added to an aqueous solution of fluorouracil, the colour of the bromine is discharged.

Stability and Storage

Since it is affected by light, store it in tightly-closed, light-resistant containers.

Uses

Anticancer agent (cytotoxic). It interferes with DNA synthesis and is used in the treatment of certain solid tumours such as breast cancer, colon cancer, cancer of the urinary bladder, liver cancer etc. It can be also be topically applied in cutaneous basal cell carcinoma.

Official

Fluorouracil, I.P., B.P.
Fluorouracil Cream, B.P.
Fluorouracil Injection, I.P., B.P.

Brand Names

Fluracil, FFU, Five Fluro, Adrucil, Timazin etc.

7. METHOTREXATE

Methotrexate has a structure similar to that of folic acid and so acts as a folate antagonist.

Properties

Methotrexate is a yellow to orange-brown, crystalline powder melting at 185° to 204°C with decomposition. It is practically insoluble in water, ethanol and ether. It is soluble in dilute solutions of mineral acids and in dilute solutions of alkali hydroxides and carbonates. It is affected by light.

Stability and Storage

Since it is affected by light, store it in well-closed containers protected from light.

Uses

Anticancer agent (cytotoxic). As already stated, it is a folate antogonist. It mainly inhibits DNA synthesis but also affects RNA and protein synthesis. It is used in choriocarcinoma, in acute leukemias, in psoriasias and as an immunosuppressant.

Official

Methotrexate, I.P., B.P.
Methotrexate Injection, I.P., B.P.
Methotrexate Tablets, I.P., B.P.

Brand Names

Neotrexate, Biotrexate, Emtexate, Aminopterin etc.

8. CISPLATIN

Cisplatin is a coordination complex of platinum.

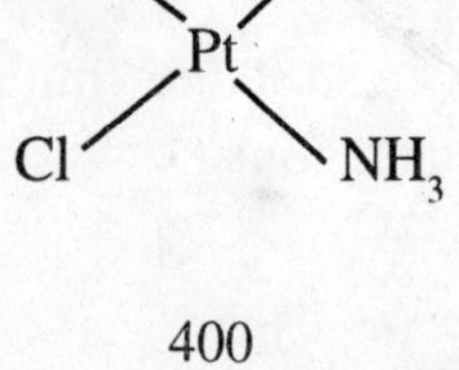

Properties

Cisplatin is a yellow powder or consists of orange-yellow crystals. It melts at 270°C with decomposition. It is slightly soluble in water, sparingly soluble in dimethylformamide and practically insoluble in ethanol. In aqueous solution it is changed to the *trans* form. It is affected by light.

Stability and Storage

Since it is affected by light, keep it in tightly-closed, light-resistant containers.

Uses

Anticancer agent (cytotoxic). It interferes with DNA synthesis and is very effective in ovarian and testicular carcinoma. It is an emetic and should be given by injection.

Official

Cisplatin, I.P., B.P.
Cisplatin Injection, I.P.

Brand Names

Cisplatin, Aquaplat, Cisplatyl, Neoplatin etc.

9. ACTINOMYCINS

These are antibiotics obtained from the growth products of certain species of Streptomyces such as *Streptomyces antibioticus*. They have potent antitumour and cytotoxic activity. The most important of the actinomycins are dactinomycin (actinomycin D) and daunorubicin.

Dactinomycin is obtained from *Streptomyces parvullus* and is a mixture of several substances. It is a bright red, crystalline powder which is hygroscopic. It melts at 241°C to 243°C with decomposition. It is soluble in water, freely soluble in ethanol and very slightly soluble in ether. It is affected by light, especially dilute solutions of the substance are very sensitive. It should be kept in air-tight containers protected from light at a temperature below 40°C. It is used as a potent anticancer agent especially in the treatment of Wilm's tumour and certain myosarcomas.

Daunorubicin (rubidomycin) is obtained from *Streptomyces peucetius*. It is a blue-violet, crystalline powder, soluble in water and ethanol. It is used as an anticancer agent in the treatment of acute leukemia. However it is very toxic to the heart.

10. MITOMYCIN C

Mitomycin C is a blue-violet, crystalline powder obtained from *Streptomyces caespisosus*. It is soluble in water and ethanol but is unstable in the presence of acids and alkalis. It is used in resistant cancers of stomach, colon, cervix, rectum, bladder etc.

Other naticancer agents in clinical use are *mechlorethamine (mustine hydrochloride), ifosfamide, melphalan, thiotepa, carmustine, lomustine, semustine, decarbazine, 6-thioguanine, ftorafur, cytarabine, vincristine, vinblastine, etoposide, doxorubicin, mitoxantrone, bleomycins, mithramycin, hydroxyurea, procarbazine, L-asparaginase, carboplatin etc.*

CHAPTER - 33

DIAGNOSTIC AGENTS

Diagnostic agents are substances which are used to find out whether an organ in the body functions normally or abnormally thereby helping us to know the underlying disease or pathological condition. Thus diagnostic agents help the physicians to arrive at the correct diagnosis of the disease(s). They are also useful in detecting any abnormality in any tissue or organ. They should be completely inert and should not have any pharmacological or physiological actions of their own.

CLASSIFICATION

I. Radioopaque substances
   a) Iopanoic acid
   b) Propyliodone

II. Drugs used to Test Organ Function
   a) Sulphobromophthalein sodium
   b) Indigotin disulphonate sodium (Indigo Carmine)
   c) Evans blue
   d) Congo red
   e) Fluorescein sodium

I. RADIOOPAQUE SUBSTANCES

These are also known as x-ray contrast media because they are able to absorb x-rays and cast a shadow on the x-ray film. So they are opaque to x-rays and are used to map out various organs such as the gastrointestinal tract, gall bladder, kidney etc.

1. IOPANOIC ACID

This is a simple butyric acid derivative and is actually 2–(3–amino–2, 4, 6–triiodobenzyl) butyric acid.

Physical Properties

It is a white or yellowish white powder. It is practically insoluble in water and soluble in absolute ethanol, ether and methanol. It is soluble in dilute solutions of alkali hydroxides. It melts at about 155°C with decomposition and is affected by light.

Chemical Properties

The compound can be disintegrated by heating in a small porcelain dish over a flame and the iodine escapes as a violet vapour.

Stability and Storage

Since it is affected by light, store it in a well-closed container protected from light.

Uses

Diagnostic agent. Radiopaque substance (used in cholecystography, that is, radiographic examination of the gall bladder and bile duct). It is given by mouth along with a light fat-free meal about 10-14 hours before the x-ray examination.

Official

Iopanoic Acid, B.P.
Iopanoic Acid Tablets, B.P.

Brand Names

Colepar, Teletrast, Iodopanoic acid etc.

2. PROPYLIODONE

Propyliodone is an ester of a substituted acetic acid. Actually it is the propyl ester of *1,4–dihydro–3, 5–diiodo–4–pyridone–1–acetic acid.*

Physical Properties

Propyliodone is a white or almost white, crystalline powder without odour. It melts at 187°C to 190°C. It is practically insoluble in water, slightly soluble in ethanol and chloroform and very slightly soluble in ether. It is affected by light.

Chemical Properties

Hydrolysis of propyliodone by boiling with sodium hydroxide and subsequent acidification give the basic acid, that is 1, 4–dihydro–3, 5–diiodo–4–pyridone–N–acetic acid. Since it is sparingly soluble, it is isolated by filtration. The melting point of the dry substance is about 245°C. When propyliodone is heated with sulphuric acid, it is disintegrated and violet vapours of iodine are evolved.

Stability and Storage

Since it is affected by light, store in a well-closed container protected from light.

Uses

Diagnostic agent. Radio-opaque substance used in bronchography (examination of the bronchial tract using radioopaque substance). It is also used in the investigation of fistulae (a fistula is a pathological communication between two epithelial surfaces or cavities, eg: rectovaginal fistula) and sinuses (a sinus is a passage leading from an abscess or some internal part to an external opening).

Official

Propyliodone, B.P.
Propyliodone Suspension, B.P.
Propyliodone Oily Suspension, B.P.

Brand Names

Dionosil, Propiodone.

II. DRUGS USED TO TEST ORGAN FUNCTION

Organs like the kidney, liver etc. may not function properly at times and this can be ascertained by the use of specific compounds.

3. SULPHOBROMOPHTHALEIN SODIUM

This is a phthalein derivative which is a dye used to test liver function.

Physical Properties

It is a hygroscopic, white, crystalline powder. It is soluble in water and practically insoluble in ethanol and acetone.

Chemical Properties

The compound can be disintegrated by mixing with sodium carbonate and igniting until thoroughly charred. The bromine atoms present in the compound are converted into sodium bromide which can be extracted by using hot water. The filtrate gives the reactions of bromides.

Stability and Storage

Since it is hygroscropic, store in tightly-closed containers.

Uses

Diagnostic agent. It is used to test liver function. The rate at which the dye is removed from the blood is found out and it is a measure of the hepatic function.

Official

Sulphobromophthalein Sodium, I.P.
Sulphobromophthalein Sodium Injection, I.P.

Brand Names

BSP, SBP, Bromthalein, Sulphobrompthal sodium etc.

4. INDIGOTINDISULPHONATE SODIUM (INDIGO CARMINE)

Indigo carmine is a dye. It is the sodium salt of a disulphonic acid obtained from the indigo plant, *Indigofera tinctoria Linn*. It can also be synthesised.

Physical Properties

It consists of a purplish-blue powder or blue granules with a coppery lustre. It is odourless and has a saline taste. It is soluble in water, slightly soluble in ethanol and practically insoluble in most other organic solvents. Its solution in water or ethanol has a purplish-blue or blue colour which is due to the chromophoric group, O=C-C=C-C=O, present in it. It is precipitated from aqueous solution by sodium chloride. It is affected by light. The official product is required to be pyrogen-free.

Chemical Properties

The blue colour of indigo carmine is discharged by oxidizing agents. Thus when nitric acid or bromine solution is added to the deep blue solution of indigo carmine, the colour is discharged. The colour is also discharged when alkaline reducing agents are added. Thus if sodium hydroxide solution and zinc powder are added to an aqueous solution of the dye, the colour is discharged. However, if sodium hydroxide solution alone is added, a yellow or olive-brown colour is produced.

Stability and Storage

Since it is affected by light and also by oxygen of the air, store it in tightly-closed containers protected from light.

Uses

Diagnostic agent. It is used for testing renal function. It appears in the urine within minutes of its administration and is excreted in the urine at a steady rate. It is also used as a reagent for nitrates and chlorates and to locate urethral orifices. It is also used as a food colour.

Official

Indigo Carmine, I.P.'66

Brand Names

Soluble indigo blue, Acid Blue 74. Food Blue I, Blue X etc.

5. EVANS BLUE

Evans blue is an azo dye and is also a disodium bisnaphthalene disulphate. It is obtained by synthesis.

Physical Properties

Evans blue is a blue or bluish-green or brown powder. It is odourless and is hygroscopic. It is very soluble in water, slightly soluble in ethanol and practically insoluble in ether and chloroform.

Chemical Properties

It is precipitated from aqueous solution by neutral salt solutions such as sodium chloride. In aqueous solution its colour is discharged by strong oxidizing and reducing agents. The compound can be disintegrated by ignition and an aqueous extract of the residue gives the reactions of sodium salts.

Stability and Storage

Since it is hygroscopic, store it in tightly-closed containers.

Uses

Diagnostic agent (blood volume estimation). It is used for the determination of blood or plasma volume. On being injected intravenously, it combines with the plasma proteins firmly and the binding is proportional to its concentration. It is estimated colorimetrically.

Official

Evans Blue, I.P.'66.

Brand Names

Azovan Blue, T-1824, C.I. Direct Blue - 53 etc.

6. CONGO RED

Congo red is also an azo dye and disodium binaphthalene disulphonate like Evans blue but it has a comparatively simpler structure.

Properties

Congo red is a reddish-brown powder soluble in water and ethanol. It is very slightly soluble in acetone and practically insoluble in ether.

Stability and Storage

Store in a well-closed container.

Uses

Diagnostic agent. It is used as a stain in the diagnosis of the disease amyloidosis (infiltration of the liver, kidneys, spleen and other tissues with amyloid, a starch-like substance). It is also used as an indicator in the laboratory and as a colouring agent in culture media.

Brand Names

C.I. 22120, C.I. Direct Red 28.

7. FLUORESCEIN SODIUM

Fluorescein is an important dye of the phthalein group to which also belong phenolphthalein, sulphobromophthalein, eosin etc.

Physical Properties

Fluorescein itself is a dark red powder which dissolves freely in aqueous sodium hydroxide forming fluorescein sodium. Fluorescein sodium is an orange-red powder with almost no odour and is hygroscopic. It is freely soluble in water and ethanol. The aqueous solution is strongly fluorescent and exhibits a yellowish green fluorescence. The fluorescence disappears when the solution is made acidic and reappears when it is made alkaline. It is affected by light.

Chemical Properties

If a filter paper is soaked in fluorescein sodium solution and dried, it becomes yellow. When this paper is exposed to bromine vapour and then to ammonia, the yellow colour of the paper becomes deep pink. This is because first tetrabromofluorescein or eosin is formed and this gives the deep pink colour on exposure to ammonia.

Stability and Storage

Since it is hygroscopic, store it in tightly-closed containers protected from light.

Uses

Diagnostic agent (dye used for detection of abrasions of the cornea). A sterile strip over the cornea and corneal ulcers, if any, will become visible because they will be stained green. It is also used as an auxiliary solution for the filling of hard contact lenses. It is used intravenously for the determination of circulation time.

Official

Fluorescein Sodium, I.P., B.P.
Fluorescein Sodium Eye Drops, I.P., B.P.
Fluorescein Injection, B.P.

Brand Names

Soluble fluorescein, Resorcinol phthalein sodium, Uranine yellow, Acid yellow, C.I.No.45350 etc.

Other diagnostic agents in clinical use are *diatrizoic acid, sodium diatrizoate, iothalamic acid, iodipamide, ipodate calcium, ipodate sodium, iodophthalein, iophendylate, aminohippuric acid, phenolsulphonphthalein, indocyanine green, histamine acid phosphate, inulin, pentagastrin, xylose etc.*

PREPARATION OF SIMPLE ORGANIC COMPOUNDS

Simple organic compounds may be prepared in the laboratory involving one-step synthesis only. They may be prepared by resorting to various reactions such as hydrolysis, oxidation, reduction, nitration, sulphonation etc., using suitable reagents and suitable starting materials. The product may be purified by recrystallisation from a suitable solvent if it is a solid and by fractional distillation usually if it is a liquid. Normal routine glassware & equipment such as the round bottomed flask, condenser, Buchner funnel etc. may be used in the preparations.

Given below are the preparations of three simple organic compounds.

1. PREPARATION OF SALICYLIC ACID FROM METHYL SALICYLATE (HYDROLYSIS)

Aim : To prepare as much of salicylic acid as possible from the given quantity of methyl salicylate.

Principle : Methyl salicylate is made to react with sodium hydroxide solution at water bath temperature for one hour. Methyl salicylate is hydrolysed by sodium hydroxide to give sodium salicylate. Subsequent addition of enough quantity of hydrochloric acid hydrolyses the sodium salicylate to liberate salicylic acid which is insoluble in water.

OH COOCH₃ ... OH COONa ... OH COOH reaction scheme

$$\underset{\text{Methyl salicylate}}{\text{OH, COOCH}_3} \xrightarrow{\text{NaOH}} \underset{\text{Sodium salicylate}}{\text{OH, COONa}} \xrightarrow{\text{HCl}} \underset{\text{Salicyclic acid}}{\text{OH, COOH}}$$

Methyl salicylate	Sodium salicylate	Salicyclic acid

Procedure

Methyl salicylate	-	3 ml
20% sodium hydroxide solution	-	20 ml
Concentrated hydrochloric acid	-	quantity sufficient

Take the methyl salicylate in a clean round bottomed flask, add the sodium hydroxide solution and heat on a water bath for at least one hour under a reflux or air condenser. Then transfer the contents to a beaker and acidify with concentrated hydrochloric acid. Filter the precipitated salicylic acid using a Buchner funnel. Recrystallise a part of the crude substance from hot water. Dry the crude preparation between folds of filter paper and weigh. Dry the recrystallised salicylic acid in the same way.

Yield : .... g.

Melting point : Between 158°C and 161°C (See Chapter 35).

2. PREPARATION OF PICRIC ACID FROM PHENOL (NITRATION)

Aim : To prepare as much of picric acid as possible from the given sample of phenol.

413

Principle : Phenol gives phenolsulphonic acid on sulphonation with concentrated sulphuric acid. This phenolsulphonic acid, on nitration with a mixture of concentrated sulphuric acid and concentrated nitric acid. is converted into trinitrophenol or picric acid.

| Phenol | Phenol sulphonic acid | Picric acid |

Procedure

Phenol	-	3 ml
Conc. sulphuric acid	-	4 ml
Conc. nitric acid	-	12 ml

Take conc. sulphuric acid in a round bottomed flask and add phenol to it slowly. Dissolve by warming on a water bath. Cool at the water tap after 15 minutes.

Take the conc. nitric acid in a round bottomed flask and add the phenol sulphonic acid solution to it (preferably from a dropping funnel) slowly with constant shaking. Cool at the tap from time to time so that the temperature may not exceed 50°C. Heat the flask in a boiling water both for two hours. Then cool and add a drop of the reaction mixture to cold water in a test tube. If a yellow precipitate is separating, the reaction may be deemed to be complete. Otherwise continue to heat and test periodically.

After the reaction is complete, remove the flask from the water bath and cool. Add cold water. Filter the precipitate of picric acid using a Buchner funnel. Wash and dry. Recrystallise a part of the precipitate from hot water containing a small quantity of hydrochloric acid.

Yield : .... g.

Melting point : About 122°C (See Chapter 35).

3. PREPARATION OF ASPIRIN FROM SALICYLIC ACID (ACETYLATION)

Aim : To prepare as much of aspirin as possible from the given quantity of salicylic acid.

Principle : Salicylic acid may be acetylated at the phenolic –OH group by using acetic anhydride. A small quantity of conc. sulphuric acid acts as a catalyst.

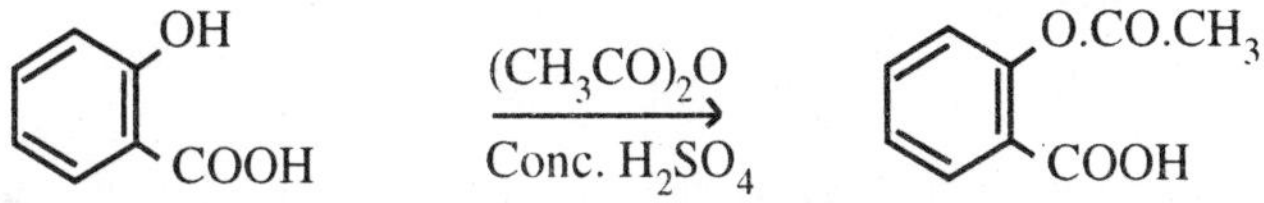

Salicylic acid   Aspirin
                        (Acetyl salicylic acid)

Procedure

| Salicylic acid | - | 5 g |
| Acetic anhydride | - | 7 ml |

Take the salicylic acid in a 100 ml conical flask and add the acetic anhydride. Then add a few drops of conc. sulphuric acid and mix thoroughly. Heat on a water bath for 30 minutes. Cool and add 75 ml of water. Filter the precipitated aspirin by using a Buchner funnel. Dry well and recrystallise a portion of it from hot toluene or warm alcohol.

Yield : .... g.

Melting point : About 142°C (See Chapter 35).

415

CHAPTER - 35

SYSTEMATIC QUALITATIVE ;ANALYSIS OF ORGANIC COMPOUNDS AND ORGANIC DRUGS

Systematic qualitative organic analysis enables us to find out the chemical nature of the organic compounds. The information obtained through qualitative analysis in a systematic manner can be as follows:-

1. Whether the organic compound is aliphatic or aromatic.
2. Whether it is saturated or unsaturated
3. What other elements are present apart from carbon, hydrogen and oxygen?
4. What is the nature of the functional groups present?

Again it is stressed that by this analysis it will be possible to ascertain only the chemical nature of the organic compound and not its identity. Specific identification tests and determination of melting point or boiling point will have to be done to establish the identity of the organic compound or organic drug conclusively. These identification tests are given in standard references such as the I.P. etc. Preparation of derivatives of the organic compounds will also help in establishing the identity.

The procedure for systematic qualitative analysis of organic compounds is given on the next page.

SYSTEMATIC PROCEDURE FOR QUALITATIVE ORGANIC ANALYSIS

EXPERIMENT	OBSERVATION	INFERENCE
1. Physical appearance and colour	a) Dark brown liquid	May be an amine or phenol
	b) Yellow solid or liquid	May be an aromatic nitro compound
	c) Colourless solid d) Colourless liquid	May be a hydrocarbon, aldehyde, ketone, ester etc.
2. Odour	a) Pleasant fruity odour	May be an ester
	b) Fishy odour	May be an amine
	c) Carbolic odour	May be a phenol
	d) Pungent odour	May be an aliphatic or aromatic halogen compound.
	e) Spirituous odour	May be a lower alcohol
	f) Camphor - like or kerosene - like odour	May be an aromatic hydro-carbon·

EXPERIMENT	OBSERVATION	INFERENCE
	g) Bitter almond odour	May be an aromatic aldehyde (benzaldehyde) or an aromatic nitro compound (nitrobenzene).
3. Solubility characteristics a) Take about 0.1 g of solid (0.5 ml of liquid) each in four separate test tubes and add 3 ml each of a) cold and hot water, b) 5% hydrochloric acid and c) 5% sodium hydroxide. Shake well and observe whether the substance is soluble.	a) Soluble in cold water	May be a sugar or lower aliphatic alcohol or polyhydric alcohol or aldehyde or ketone or amine etc.
	b) Soluble in hot water	May be an aromatic acid or phenolic acid etc.
	c) Soluble in acid	May be an organic base such as an amine.
	d) Soluble in alkali	May be a carboxylic acid or phenol
	e) Insoluble	May be an aromatic hydrocarbon or aromatic amine or a higher alcohol or a ketone or aldehyde or phenol or an ester.

EXPERIMENT	OBSERVATION	INFERENCE
4. Test for acidic or basic nature Dissolve 0.1g of the compound in 2 ml of water and place one drop of the solution on blue and red litmus each.	Blue litmus changes to red.	May be a carboxylic acid or phenol.
	Red litmus changes to blue.	May be a basic compound eg:amine.
5. Test for aromatic or aliphatic nature.		
a) Take a small quantity of the given organic compound on a clean nickel spatula and ignite (heat strongly).	a) Sooty flame	May be an aromatic compound.
	b) No sooty flame	May be an aliphatic compound.
b) Add 1 ml of conc. HNO_3 and 1 ml of conc. H_2SO_4 to a small quantity of the substance. Heat well and cool. Pour into a beaker of water.	a) Yellow solid separates or a yellow oil or solution is obtained.	May be an aromatic compound.
	b) No yellow colour is seen.	May be an aliphatic compound.

EXPERIMENT	OBSERVATION	INFERENCE
6. Test for saturation or unsaturation a) Add 2 or 3 drops of saturated bromine water to the substance and shake well.	a) The colour of bromine is discharged.	May be a saturated compound.
	b) The colour of bromine is not discharged.	May be a saturated compound.
	c) Bromine water is decolourised with formation of white precipitate.	May be an aromatic amine or phenol.
b) Add 1 ml of water and 2 drops of Baeyer's reagent (alkaline potassium permanganate) to a small quantity of the substance.	a) Pink colour is discharged.	May be an unsaturated compound.
	b) Pink colour is not discharged.	May be a saturated compound.

7. DETECTION OF ELEMENTS

Sodium Fusion Extract Tests or Lassaigne's Tests

Take a small piece of sodium metal (already dried between the folds of a filter paper) in an ignition tube and add a small quantity of the powdered organic compound. Heat gently at first and then strongly till the lower end of the tube becomes red hot. Plunge the ignition tube immediately into a China dish containing about 15 to 20 ml of water. The bottom of the tube is broken into small pieces. Grind the pieces with a pestle, boil, cool and filter. The clear filtrate is the sodium fusion extract. It is divided into several parts. In this test the organic compound is disintegrated by fusion with sodium metal and the elements present such as nitrogen, sulphur and halogens converted into water soluble sodium salts such as sodium cyamide, sodium sulphide and sodium halide (that is, chloride, bromide, and iodide as the case may be).

EXPERIMENT	OBSERVATION	INFERENCE
a) Test for nitrogen To 1 ml of the sodium fusion extract add 1 ml of ferrous sulphate solution. Add about 1 ml of dilute sulphuric acid.	A blue or green precipitate or solution is formed.	Indicates the presence of *nitrogen* in the organic compound.
b) Test for Sulphur To 1 ml of the sodium fusion extract add 3 drops of *freshly prepared* sodium nitroprusside solution.	A deep violet or purple colour is formed.	Presence of *sulphur.*
To another portion of the extract add 4 drops of lead acetate solution	A black precipitate is produced.	Confirms presence of *sulphur.*

EXPERIMENT	OBSERVATION	INFERENCE
c) Test for Chlorine To another portion of the extract add dilute nitric acid to acidify and silver nitrate solution (1 ml).	A curdy white precipitate is formed. It dissolves on adding excess of aqueous ammonia.	Presence of *chlorine.*
d) Test for Bromine and Iodine d) Acidify another portion of the extract with dil H_2SO_4 and add 1 ml of carbon tetrachloride and 1 ml of chlorine water. Shake well.	The carbon tetrachloride layer becomes orange-coloured. The carbon tetrachloride layer becomes violet-coloured.	Presence of *bromine.* Presence of *iodine.*
8. Test with conc. H_2SO_4. Add about 1 ml of conc. H_2SO_4 to a small quantity of the compound. Shake.	The substance is charred.	May be a carbohydrate.
9. Test with Tollen's reagent. Add 1 ml of Tollen's reagent. (ammoniacal silver nitrate) to a small quantity of the compound and heat over a water bath for 10 to 15 minutes.	A bright silver mirror is formed.	May be a reducing sugar or an aldehyde.

EXPERIMENT	OBSERVATION	INFERENCE
10. Test with Fehling's Reagent Add 1 ml of the Fehling's reagent to a small quantity of the compound and heat on a water bath for 15 minutes.	A reddish brown precipitate is produced.	May be a reducing sugar or an aldehyde.
11. Test with neutral FeCl₃ solution Add 1 ml of neutral ferric chloride solution to a small quantity of the compound.	Violet, blue or green colour is formed.	May be a phenol or a phenolic compound.

12. TESTS FOR FUNCTIONAL GROUPS

A) FOR CARBOXYLIC ACIDS

(i) Add a small quantity of the substance to sodium bicarbonate solution	Effervescence is seen.	May be a carboxylic acid.
(ii) Ester Test To a small quantity of the substance, add 1 ml of alcohol and 2 to 3 drops of conc. H_2SO_4. Heat over a water bath for 10 to 15 minutes and pour into dilute sodium carbonate solution.	Fruity odour is observed.	-do-

EXPERIMENT	OBSERVATION	INFERENCE
(iii) Phenolphthalein Test To a small quantity of the test add 1 ml of phenol and 1 ml of conc.H_2SO_4 Heat, cool and pour into dilute sodium hydroxide solution.	A pink colour is seen.	May be a dicarboxylic acid.
(iv) Fluorescein Test To a small quantity of the substance add double the quantity of resorcinol and 10 drops of conc. H_2SO_4. Heat, cool and pour into dilute sodium hydroxide solution.	A greenish yellow fluorescence is seen.	-do-
(B) FOR PHENOLS **(i) Liebermann's reaction** To a small volume of the substance add a little sodium nitrite and warm gently and cool. Add 0.5 ml of conc.H_2SO_4.	A deep blue colour is produced.	

EXPERIMENT	OBSERVATION	INFERENCE
Pour into water and then add sodium hydroxide solution.	The solution first turns red and then becomes blue.	May be a phenol.

(C) FOR CARBOHYDRATES

(i) Molisch's Test

EXPERIMENT	OBSERVATION	INFERENCE
To a solution of a small quantity of the substance add 1 ml of an alcoholic solution of β-naphthol. Add conc.H_2SO_4 carefully through the side of the test tube.	A violet or purple ring is formed at the junction of the two liquids.	May be a carbohydrate.
(ii) Repeat Tests 9 and 10 given above.	Answered.	May be a carbohydrate which is a reducing sugar.
	Not answered.	May be a carbohydrate which is non-reducing.

(iii) Barfoed's Test

EXPERIMENT	OBSERVATION	INFERENCE
To a small quantity of the substance add 1 ml of water and 5 ml of Barfoed's reagent. Heat on a boiling water bath for 10 to 15 minutes.	A red precipitate is immediately formed.	May be a reducing monosachloride.

EXPERIMENT	OBSERVATION	INFERENCE
	No red colour is formed. The rate of reduction is slow.	May be a reducing disaccharide.
(D) FOR ESTERS (i) To about 2 ml of the given liquid (esters are usually liquids) add 2 ml of sodium hydroxide solution. Heat for one minute and cool. Acidify with conc.HCl.	A white precipitate is formed.	May be an ester.
(ii) To 1 ml of the sample add 1 ml of hydroxylamine hydrochloride solution and also add alcoholic KOH till it is made alkaline. Heat for a minute, cool and acidify with dil. HCl. Add 1 ml of $FeCl_3$ solution.	A violet colour is produced.	-do-
(E) FOR ALDEHYDES (i) To 1 ml of the Schiff's reagent add 1 ml of the given liquid.	A purple colour is produced.	May be an aldehyde.

EXPERIMENT	OBSERVATION	INFERENCE
(ii) To 1 ml of the given liquid add 1 ml of ethyl alcohol and 10 drops of saturated sodium bisulphite solution and shake well.	A white crystalline precipitate is produced.	May be an aldehyde. (Both aldehydes and ketones produce crystalline sodium bisulphite compounds.)
(iii) Borsche's Test To 1 ml of the given liquid add 1 ml of ethyl alcohol and 5 drops of Borsche's reagent and warm.	An orange yellow precipitate is produced.	-do- (Both aldehydes and ketones give precipitates with Borsche's reagent).
(iv) Test with Baeyer's reagent To 1 ml of the given liquid add 1 ml of Baeyer's reagent (alkaline potassium permanganete) and shake for a few minutes.	Pink colour is discharged. A brown precipitate is formed.	May be an aldehyde
(v) Test with Tollen's Reagent To 1 ml of the given liquid add 1 ml of Tollen's reagent and heat on a water bath for 15 minutes.	A black precipitate or a silver mirror is formed.	-do-

EXPERIMENT	OBSERVATION	INFERENCE
(vi) Test with Fehling's reagent To 1 ml of the given liquid add 1 ml of Fehling's reagent and heat on a water bath for 15 minutes.	A reddish brown precipitate is formed.	-do- (Benzaldehyde does not reduce Fehling's solution)
(F) FOR KETONES (i) To 1 ml of the given liquid add 1 ml of saturated sodium bisulphite solution and shake well.	A white, crystalline precipitate is produced.	May be a ketone. (Both aldehydes and ketones produce crystalline sodium bisulphite compound).
(ii) Borsche's Test To 1 ml of the given liquid add 1 ml of Borsche's reagent and 2 drops of conc. HCl. Warm for 15 minutes and cool.	A pale yellow precipitate is produced.	May be a ketone. (Both aldehydes and ketones give precipitates with Borsche's reagent).
(iii) To 1 ml of the given liquid add 1 ml of sodium nitroprusside solution and 1 ml of sodium hydroxide solution and mix well.	An orange colour is produced.	

EXPERIMENT	OBSERVATION	INFERENCE
Add a little dilute acetic acid.	The colour becomes purple.	May be a ketone.
(iv) Iodoform Reaction To 1 ml of the given liquid add 1 ml of sodium hydroxide solution and 1 ml of iodine solution and warm on a water bath for 15 minutes.	A yellow precipitate with a typical smell is produced.	-do- (This reaction is given only by methyl ketones).
(v) Test with Schiff's reagent.	No pink or purple colour is produced.	May be a ketone (not an aldehyde)
(vi) Test with Tollen's reagent.	Not answered.	-do-
(vii) Test with Fehling's solution	Not answered.	-do-
(G) FOR PRIMARY AMINES		
(i) Test the given liquid with red litmus paper	Red litmus turns blue.	May be a basic compound like a primary amine.
(ii) Acetylation To 1 ml of the given liquid add 1 ml of acetic anhydride and heat. Pour into 10 ml of water.	A white, crystalline precipitate is produced.	May be a primary amine.

429

EXPERIMENT	OBSERVATION	INFERENCE
(iii) Benzoylation To 1 ml of the given liquid add 1 ml of sodium hydroxide solution and 1 ml of benzoyl chloride. Cork the test tube and shake well.	A white precipitate is produced.	May be a primary amine.
(iv) Dye Test Dissolve the given liquid in dil. HCl, add 1 ml of sodium nitrite solution and cool in ice. Add 1 ml of β-naphthol in sodium hydroxide solution.	An orange red to scarlet red azo dye is produced.	-do-
(v) Carbylamine Test To a few drops of the given liquid add 2 drops of chloroform and 2 ml of alcoholic potash. Mix well. Add conc. HCl and pour into the sink.	A very disagreable odour is produced.	-do- *(carbylamine is poisonous and should not be inhaled).*

(H) FOR NITRO COMPOUNDS

(i) To 2 ml of the given liquid add 2 ml of conc. HCl and a little zinc dust, heat strongly,	A red dye is produced.	May be a nitro compound.

430

EXPERIMENT	OBSERVATION	INFERENCE
cool and filter. To the filtrate add 1 ml of sodium nitrite solution and cool in ice. Add 1 ml of β-naphthol in sodium hydroxide solution.		
(ii) Mulliken and Barker Test To 2 ml of the given liquid add a little zinc dust and 1 ml of ammonium chloride solution, cool and filter. Divide the filtrate into two portions.		
To one portion add Tollen's reagent and warm on a water bath.	A black precipitate of silver is produced.	May be a nitro compound.
To the other portion add Fehling's solution and heat on a water bath for 15 minutes.	A reddish brown precipitate is produced.	-do-

(I) FOR AMIDES AND DIAMIDES

(i) To a little of the substance add 1 ml of sodium hydroxide solution and heat.	Ammonia is evolved (Test with moistened red litmus paper).	May be an amide or a diamide.

431

EXPERIMENT	OBSERVATION	INFERENCE
(ii) Biuret Test Heat a little of the substance strongly in a test tube and dissolve the white sublimate in distilled water. Add 1 ml of dilute solution of $CuSO_4$ and 1 ml of sodium hydroxide solution.	A violet to pink colour is produced.	May be a diamide
(iii) Dissolve a little of the substance in water and add 1 to 2 ml of conc.HNO_3.	A white, crystalline precipitate is produced.	-do-
(iv) Prepare a saturated solution of the substance in water and filter. Add to the filtrate 1 ml of saturated solution of oxalic acid.	-do-	-do-

PREPARATION OF DERIVATIVES

It is necessary to prepare suitable derivatives of the organic compounds so that the determination of the melting points of the derivatives will serve to further identify the organic compound specifically. The derivative prepared should be dry, solid and stable and should be able to melt sharply at a particular temperature. In the absence of any derivative being prepared, a

432

characteristic colour reaction should be sufficient to identify the compound.

The preparation of derivatives is a means of identification of the functional groups in the organic compounds and is detailed below:-

a) Derivative for Carboxylic Acids

The derivatives for carboxylic acids are usually esters prepared from suitable alcohols. However these esters are invariably liquids and will not serve the purpose. So the following ester which is a solid is prepared:-

Add enough sodium hydroxide solution to about 0.5 g of the acid so that it is fully dissolved. Now add an equal volume of S-benzylisothiouranium chloride reagent. A white precipitate is produced. Filter and dry well.

b) Derivatives for Phenols

Derivatives for phenols can be prepared either by benzoylating the phenol or preparing the tribromoderivative.

1. Add a slight excess of sodium hydroxide solution to about 0.5 g of the phenol. Add 2 ml of benzoyl chloride and shake vigorously. Pour it into water, filter the precipitate and dry well.

2. To 0.5 g of the phenol add 5 ml of water to dissolve. Add bromine water till the yellow colour of the bromine persists. Filter the precipitate and dry well.

c) Derivatives for Carbohydrates

Monosaccharides and other sugars which contain the carbonyl group in their open chain form combine with phenylhydrazine to form osazones which are coloured crystalline derivatives of the carbohydrates.

To 0.5 g of the carbohydrate add 0.5 g of phenylhydrazine hydrochloride. Add about 5 ml of water and 0.5 g of sodium acetate. Heat on a water bath for 30 minutes and cool. A yellow, crystalline precipitate is produced. Filter and dry well.

d) Derivatives for Aromatic Esters

Aromatic esters can be hydrolysed and the corresponding aromatic acid which is a solid is isolated.

Add to the given ester 3 ml of sodium hydroxide solution and heat for at least 10 to 12 minutes. Cool and acidify with conc.HCl. A precipitate is produced. Filter and dry well (See the preparation of Salicylic Acid-Chapter 34).

e) Derivatives for Aldehydes and Ketones (Carbonyl Compounds)

The carbonyl compounds produce dinitrophenyl-hydrozones on reaction with Borsche's reagent.

Dissolve 1 g of the given compound in enough ethyl alcohol and add 4 ml of Borsche's reagent. Heat on a water bath for 15 minutes and cool. Pour into water. A yellowish orange precipitate is formed. Filter and dry well.

f) Derivatives for Primary Amines

Derivatives for primary amines can be prepared by acetylating the primary amine and isolating the acetylated amine. Alternatively since the primary amine is basic, it can be reacted with picric acid to give the corresponding picrate.

1. Take 0.5 g of the given organic compound and dissolve in enough glacial acetic acid. Add 3 ml of acetic anhydride and heat on a water bath for at least 30 minutes. Pour into cold water surrounded by ice. A white precipitate is produced Filter and dry well.

2. Add enough ethyl alcohol to dissolve about 0.5 g of the given compound. Add 3 ml of an alcoholic solution of picric acid and shake well. A yellow precipitate is produced. Filter and dry well.

g) Derivatives for Nitro Compounds

First the nitro compound is reduced to the corresponding primary amine by zinc and acid. The primary amine is then acetylated or benzoylated and the acetylated or benzoylated primary amine is isolated.

To about 0.5 g of the given organic compound add an equal quantity of zinc dust and 2 ml of conc.HCl, heat strongly and filter. Make the filtrate slightly alkaline by adding sodium hydroxide solution. Add 5 ml of benzoyl chloride and shake well. A precipitate is produced. Filter and dry well.

h) Derivatives for Diamides

The diamide given for analysis is usually urea which gives precipitates with nitric acid (urea nitrate) and oxalic acid (urea oxalate).

1. Add enough water to dissolve about 0.5 g of the given organic compound and add 5 ml of conc.HNO$_3$. A white, crystalline precipitate is produced. Filter and dry well.

2. Prepare urea solution in the same way as given under (1) and add 5 ml of saturated solution of oxalic acid in water. A white, crystalline precipitate is produced. Filter and dry well.

435

DETERMINATION OF MELTING POINT

Melting point determination is one of the methods of determining not only the identity of an organic compound but also its state of purity. A pure compound melts sharply at a particular temperature but an impure compound melts below its melting point and also not at a particular temperature but over a range. Thus the purity of an organic compound can be easily found out by determining the temperature at which it melts and also the sharpness of the melting point. Further an organic compound can be identified by preparing a suitable derivative as outlined above and the derivative itself is identified by the determination of its melting point.

The procedure for determination of the melting point of any organic (or inorganic) compound is given below:-

The substance is taken in fine powder form. A capillary tube is sealed at one end by means of heat sealing and the powder is put into the open end of the tube little by little and tapping gently till a compact column of the powder about 3-4 mm long is at the bottom of the tube (sealed end). The filled capillary tube is attached to the lower end of a thermometer by wetting it with the bath liquid which is concentrated sulphuric acid. The capillary tube will be sticking to the thermometer due to the effect of the surface tension of the liquid. The thermometer carrying the capillary tube may be fixed into a bored cork which is fixed to an iron stand. The thermometer is lowered into the bath liquid kept in a beaker so that the bulb of the thermometer is immersed in the liquid and also taking care to see that the open end of the capillary tube is above the surface of the bath liquid. See figure on page 436.

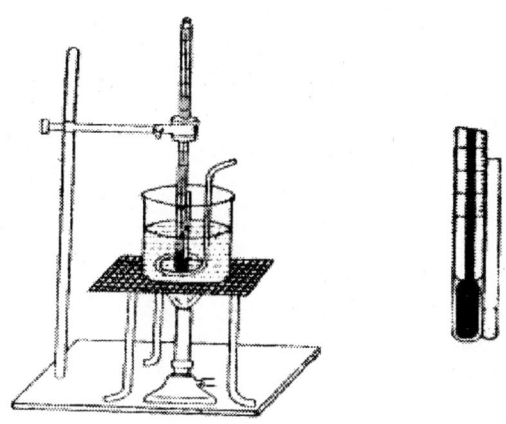

Determination of Melting Point

Keep the beaker over a wire guaze and start heating gently with a bunsen burner. Continue heating, at the same time observing the powder in the capillary tube. Note the temperature at which the powder melts. Remove the burner and allow the bath liquid to cool below the melting point. Again heat and observe the temperature at which the powder melts. Like this three readings should be taken and the mean of the three readings is the melting point of the substance.

DETERMINATION OF BOILING POINT

Determination of boiling point not only serves to identify the compound but also its purity as in the case of melting point for solids. If the liquid is available in large quantity, its boiling point may be determined by resorting to distillation. The constant temperature at which the liquid boils and distils over is found out. If the liquid is available in small quantity only, then the following method may be used to find out the boiling point:-

An ignition tube is filled to less than half with the given liquid and attached to the bottom end of a thermometer by means of a rubber band or thread. A capillary tube, sealed at one end, is put into the liquid in the ignition tube (immersing the open end into the liquid). The thermometer is clamped to an iron stand and immersed into the bath liquid (sulphuric acid). The thermometer bulb is immersed in the bath liquid but the rubber band should be above the surface of the liquid. The closed end of the capillary tube also should be above the surface of the liquid in the ignition tube. See figure given below:-

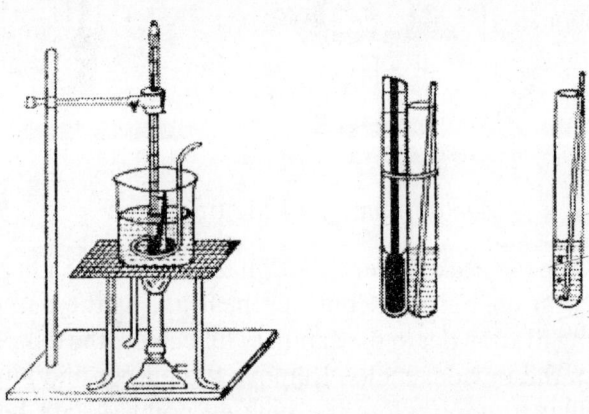

Determination of Boiling Point

Heat the bath liquid gently at first and stir it well. As the heating is continued, observe the liquid in the ignition tube continuously. When a stream of bubbles escapes from the bottom of the capillary tube, remove the burner and stir the bath liquid. Note the temperature at which the evolution of the bubbles stops. Heat the bath liquid and repeat the process. Take the mean of three readings to give the boiling point of the liquid.

CHAPTER - 36

TESTS FOR IDENTIFICATION OF SELECTED GROUPS OF DRUGS

Pharmacy students should be able to perform some identification tests in case of doubt as to the identity of any drug. For this purpose the tests for identification given in the individual monographs in the pharmacopoeia should prove to be useful. Given below are not only official tests but also non-official tests, where relevant, so that the identity of the drugs may be well established and confirmed. Drugs belonging to particular groups such as sulphonamides and barbiturates may be tested by some general tests sometimes with slight variations for the individual compounds. Only chemical tests are given here and the other tests such as the spectrophotometric and thin layer chromatographic tests are omitted, since they are not relevant here. Compounds official in both the current and earlier I.P.s are discussed.

SULPHONAMIDES

Sulphonamides are derived from sulphanilamide which has the formula given below:-

$$H_2N-\!\!\!\left\langle\!\!\!\bigcirc\!\!\!\right\rangle-\!SO_2NH_2$$

The nitrogen of the sulphonamido group is named as N^1. The nitrogen of the para amino group is named N^4. Mostly sulphonamides are derived by the substitution of the sulphonamido group. Examples are sulphacetamide, sulphaguanidine, sulphadiazine, sulphadimethoxine, sulpha-dimidine, sulphadoxine, sulphafurazole, sulphamethoxazole, sulphaphenazole etc.

However there are also other sulphonamides which are made by the substitution of both the sulphonamido and the para amino groups. Examples are succinysulphathiazole and phthalysulphathiazole.

Since sulphonamides contain both nitrogen and sulphur they answer the tests for elements for these two elements.

Some of the sulphonamides such as sulphanilamide decompose on strong heating in a dry test tube and produce a mass of residue which may vary from yellow to dark violet in colour.

The N^4 substituted sulphonamides have a free primary aromatic amino group (first group above). Therefore they can be diazotised by treating with sodium nitrite and dilute hydrochloric acid and coupled with β-napthol containing sodium acetate to give an orange-red azo dye precipitate. The N^1 and N^4 substituted sulphonamides (second group above) cannot give this reaction since the primary aromatic amino group is not free but substituted. They will give this reaction only after acid hydrolysis to release the primary aromatic amino group.

Many of the sulphonamides on treatment with sodium hydroxide and copper sulphate solutions give different colours. For example sulphadimethoxine gives a yellow precipitate. Sulphadiazine gives an olive-green precipitate which soon becomes purple-grey on standing.

The sulphonamides dissolve on addition of alkali forming the alkali salts. However they are precipitated by the addition of acids. Salts such as sulphacetamide sodium precipitate the basic compounds when acids are added to their aqueous solutions. Individual sulphonamides can also be tested by certain special tests.

IDENTIFICATION OF SULPHONAMIDES

1. SULPHANILAMIDE

EXPERIMENT	OBSERVATION
1. Tests for Elements. **Preparation of Sodium Fusion Extract** Take a small piece of sodium metal (already dried between the folds of a filter paper) in an ignition tube and add a small quantity of the powdered organic compound. Heat gently at first and then strongly till the lower end of the tube becomes red hot. Plunge the ignition tube immediately into a china dish containing about 15 to 20 ml of water. The bottom of the tube is broken into small pieces. Boil the contents of the china dish and filter. The filtrate is the sodium fusion extract.	
Test for Nitrogen To 1 ml of the sodium fusion extract add 1 ml. of ferrous sulphate solution and boil for one minute. Add about 1 ml of dilute sulphuric acid. Shake well.	A green or deep blue or greenish blue colour is formed indicating the presence of nitrogen.
Test for Sulphur To 1 ml of the sodium fusion extract add 3 drops of freshly prepared sodium nitroprusside solution.	A deep violet colour is formed indicating the presence of sulphur.

EXPERIMENT	OBSERVATION
2. Action on Heating Heat about 0.1 g. of the substance in a dry test tube until it melts.	A dark violet residue is left.
3. Dye Test To about 0.1 g. of the substance add 2 ml of dilute hydrochloric acid and 2 ml of sodium nitrite solution. Cool in ice and pour the mixture into 2 ml of β–napthol solution containing 1 g of sodium acetate.	An orange-red precipitate (dye) is produced.

2. SULPHADIAZINE

EXPERIMENT	OBSERVATION
1. Tests for Elements (Refer Sulphanilamide).	Tests for nitrogen and sulphur answered.
2. Action on Heating Heat about 50 mg in a dry test tube until it melts.	A reddish brown residue is produced.
3. Dye Test	Answered. An orange red dye is formed.

EXPERIMENT	OBSERVATION
4. Copper Sulphate Test Dissolve about 10 mg. of the substance in a mixture of 10 ml of water and 2 ml 0.1 N sodium hydroxide solution and add 0.5 ml of copper sulphate solution.	An olive-green precipitate is produced. It becomes purple-grey on standing.

BARBITURATES

Barbiturates are hypnotics and sedatives used as sodium salts. When an acid is added to the solution of a sodium salt of a barbiturate, the sodium part of the salt is neutralised and a precipitate of the free barbiturate is released. Barbiturates contain nitrogen and answer the test for nitrogen in the tests for elements. Thiobarbiturates answer the test for sulphur also.

Many barbiturates give a colour or a coloured precipitate when treated with copper sulphate solution in pyridine and sodium hydroxide in the cold. For example barbitone gives a reddish violet colour. Individual barbiturates can also be identified by some special tests.

IDENTIFICATION OF BARBITURATES

1. BARBITONE SODIUM

EXPERIMENT	OBSERVATION
1. Dissolve 0.2 g in 5 ml. of water. Add 1 ml of dilute hydrochloric acid.	A white precipitate is produced.
2. Tests for elements (Refer sulphanilamide)	Test for nitrogen is answered.

EXPERIMENT	OBSERVATION
3. Dissolve 0.1 g of barbitone sodium in a mixture of 5 ml. of sodium hydroxide and 2 ml of 10% w/v of pyridine. Add 8 ml of pyridine and 1 ml of copper sulphate solution and set aside for 10 minutes.	A reddish violet precipitate is produced.
4. Boil 0.2 g of the substance with 5 ml of sodium hydroxide solution.	Ammonia is evolved (identified by its smell).
5. Dissolve 0.2 g of the substance in 5 ml of distilled water and add 0.5 ml of potassium antimony tartrate solution.	A white crystalline precipitate is formed (presence of sodium).
6. Dissolve 0.2 g of the sample in 5 ml of distilled water and add 0.5 ml of zinc uranyl acetate solution.	-do- (If the sample is only barbitone and not barbitone sodium, these two tests (5 and 6) will not be answered.)

2. PHENOBARBITONE SODIUM

EXPERIMENT	OBSERVATION
1. Dissolve 0.2 g of the substance in 5 ml of water. Add 1 ml of dilute hydrochloric acid.	A white precipitate is produced.

EXPERIMENT	OBSERVATION
2. Tests for Elements.	Test for nitrogen is answered.
3. Boil 0.2 g of the sample with 5 ml. of sodium hydroxide solution.	Ammonia is evolved.
4. Copper sulphate test (refer barbitone sodium)	A lilac precipitate is produced.
5. Dissolve about 0.1 g of the sample in 2 ml of concentrated sulphuric acid. Add one or two crystals of sodium nitrite.	A golden yellow colour is produced.
6. Dissolve about 20 mg of the sample in 5 ml of alcohol. Add one drop of cobalt chloride solution and one drop of dilute ammonia solution.	A violet colour is produced.
7. Potassium antimony tartrate test (Refer barbitone sodium)	Answered (presence of sodium).
8. Zinc uranyl acetate test.	-do-

CARBOHYDRATES

Carbohydrates were dealt with in some detail in the previous chapter. The three important sugars are dextrose (glucose), sucrose and lactose. They answer all the general tests for carbohydrates such as charring on heating, charring on addition of concentrated sulphuric acid and Molisch's test.

445

Dextrose and lactose are reducing sugars and reduce Fehling's solution and Tollen's reagent. They also form osazones. Sucrose, being a non-reducing sugar, does not answer these tests. However after it is hydrolysed to invert sugar (a mixture of dextrose and fructose) by boiling with dilute sulphuric acid, it answers all the reduction tests and also forms the osazone.

IDENTIFICATION OF CARBOHYDRATES

1. DEXTROSE

EXPERIMENT	OBSERVATION
A. General Tests for Carbo-hydrates.	
1. Heat a little of the substance strongly in a clean, dry test tube.	Charring takes place. A black residue is left
2. To a little of the substance add 1 ml of concentrated sulphuric acid. Warm gently.	The solution turns black.
3. Molisch's test Dissolve about 0.1 to 0.2 g of the substance in 2 ml of water. Add 3 drops of alcoholic solution of α-naphthol (1%). Add through the sides of the test tube about 2 ml of concentrated sulphuric acid so that the acid forms a heavy layer at the bottom.	A deep violet ring or colouration is produced.

EXPERIMENT	OBSERVATION
B.Special Tests for Dextrose	
1. Reduction Tests	
a) Reduction of Barfoed's Reagent	
Prepare a dilute solution of the substance in water. Add 2 ml of this solution to 1 ml of Barfoed's reagent and heat on a boiling water bath.	The blue solution turns red within one or two minutes. This test indicates that the same is a reducing mono-saccharide.
b) Reduction of Fehling's Solution	
To about 0.2 g of the substance add 2 ml of a mixture of Fehling's solution I and II (or A and B) in equal parts. Heat to boiling.	A brick red colour or precipitate is formed.
c) Reduction of Tollen's Reagent	
Dissolve about 0.3 g of the substance in 3 ml of water. Add 2 ml of Tollen's ragent (ammoniacal silver nitrate) and heat on a boiling water bath for five minutes.	A silver mirror is formed.
2. Osazone Test	
Dissolve 0.3 g of the substance in 5 ml of water. Add 0.4 g of phenylhydrazine hydrochloride and 0.7 g of crystalline sodium acetate or 2 ml of glacial acetic acid. Heat on a water bath for about 10 minutes and cool.	A yellow precipitate separates out.

EXPERIMENT	OBSERVATION
Examine a little of the precipitate under a microscope.	Bundles of needles of glucosazone are seen.

2. LACTOSE

EXPERIMENT	OBSERVATION
A. General tests for Carbo-hydrates (Refer dextrose).	
1. Action of heat.	Charring.
2. Action of conc. sulphuric acid.	Black solution.
3. Molisch's test.	Deep violet colouration or ring.
B. Special Tests for Lactose **1. Reduction Tests** (Refer dextrose)	
(a) Reduction of Barfoed's reagent.	The blue solution does not turn red. This indicates that lactose is a disaccharide.
(b) Reduction of Fehling's solution.	A brick red colour or a brick red precipitate is formed.
(c) Reduction of Tollen's reagent.	A silver mirror or a black solution is formed.

EXPERIMENT	OBSERVATION
2. Osazone Test (Refer dextrose).	A yellow precipitate is formed.
Examine under microscope.	Clusters of crystals are seen.
C. Confirmatory Tests	
(a) Heat 5 ml of a 5% solution of the substance in water with 5 ml of strong ammonia solution in a water bath at 80°C for ten minutes.	A red colour develops.
(b) To about 0.1 g of the substance add 1 ml of lead acetate solution. Boil for one minute. Add dilute ammonia drop by drop till a distinct precipitate is obtained and boil again.	The precipitate becomes deep cream in colour.

3. SUCROSE

EXPERIMENT	OBSERVATION
A. General Tests for carbo-hydrates	
(a) Action of Heat	Charring.
(b) Action of conc. sulphuric acid.	Black solution.
(c) Molisch's test	Deep violet colouration or ring.

EXPERIMENT	OBSERVATION
B. Special Tests for Sucrose	
1. Reduction Tests	
(a) Reduction of Barfoed's reagent.	Not answered. Sucrose is a disaccharide.
(b) Reduction of Fehling's solution.	Not answered. Sucrose is a non-reducing sugar.
(c) Reduction of Tollen's reagent.	-do-
2. Osazone Test	
3. Dissolve 1 g of the substance in 5 ml of water and add 2 ml of dilute sulphuric acid. Heat to boiling and cool. Divide the solution into four parts and do the above three reduction tests using three parts.	All the reduction tests are now answered.
4. Do the osazone test on the fourth part of the solution obtained in (3).	Yellow precipitate.
Examine a little of the precipitate under a microscope.	Sheaves of fine needles are seen.

ALKALOIDS

The following alkaloids can be identified easily because they answer the general tests mostly and also answer some special tests. In the tests for elements, alkaloids answer for nitrogen and also any other element like sulphur, if present.

IDENTIFICATION OF ALKALOIDS

1. ATROPINE SULPHATE

EXPERIMENT	OBSERVATION
A. General Tests for Alkaloids	
(1) Mayer's Regent	
To about 10 mg of the substance add 1 ml of dilute hydrochloric acid and shake well. Add 0.5 ml of Mayer's reagent.	A yellowish white precipitate is produced.
(2) Dragendorff's or Kraut's Reagent	
To about 10 mg of the substance add 1 ml of dilute hydrochloric acid and shake well. Add 0.5 ml of Dragendorff's reagent.	An orange red precipitate is produced.
(3) Wagner's Reagent	
To about 10 mg of the substance add 1 ml of dilute hydrochloric acid and shake well. Add 0.5 ml of Wagner's reagent.	A brown precipitate is produced.
(4) Hager's Reagent	
To about 10 mg of the substance add 1 ml of dilute hydrochloric acid and shake well. Add 0.5 ml of Hager's reagent.	A brown precipitate is produced.

EXPERIMENT	OBSERVATION
B. Special Tests for Atropine Sulphate **(1) Vitali's Test** To about 10 mg of the substance in a china dish add 2 drops of concentrated nitric acid and evaporate to dryness on a water bath. Add to the residue one drop of solution of potassium hydroxide in acetone.	An intense violet colour is produced.
(2) Test for Sulphate To about 10 mg of the substance add 1 ml of dilute hydrochloric acid. Add 0.5 ml of barium chloride test solution.	A white precipitate is produced.

2. QUININE SULPHATE

EXPERIMENT	OBSERVATION
A. General Tests for Alkaloids **(Refer atropine sulphate)** (1) Mayer's reagent. (2) Dragendorff's reagent (3) Wagner's reagent (4) Hager's reagent	All answered.

EXPERIMENT	OBSERVATION
B. Special Tests for Quinine Sulphate	
(1) Fluorescence Test To about 0.1 ml of a 0.5% solution of the substance add an equal volume of dilute sulphuric acid.	A strong light blue fluorescence is produced.
(2) Thalleioquin Test To 5 ml of a 0.1% solution of the substance add 2 or 3 drops of bromine solution and 1 ml of dilute ammonia solution.	An emerald green colour or precipitate is produced.
(3) Test for Sulphate (Refer atropine sulphate)	A white precipitate is produced.

3. CAFFEINE

EXPERIMENT	OBSERVATION
A. General Tests for Alkaloids (1) Mayer's reagent	Not answered. No precipitate is formed.
(2) Dragendorff's reagent	
(3) Wagner's reagent	All answered.
(4) Hager's reagent	

EXPERIMENT	OBSERVATION
B. Special Tests for Caffeine **1. Murexide Reaction** To 10 mg. of the substance in a china dish add 1 ml. of concentrated hydrochloric acid and 3 or 4 drops of concentrated nitric acid. Evaporate to dryness on a water bath. Add to the reddish brown residue one drop of ammonia.	A deep purple colour is produced.
2. Reaction with Tannic Acid To 1 ml. of a saturated aqueous solution of caffeine add a few drops of tannic acid.	A white precipitate is produced (caffeine tannate).
Add excess of tannic acid solution.	The precipitate dissolves and a clear solution is produced.
3. Reaction with Iodine. (Refer reaction with Wagner's reagent) To 5 ml of a saturated aqueous solution of caffeine add 2 ml of N/10 iodine.	No precipitate is produced.
Add 1 ml. of dilute hydrochloric acid.	A brown precipitate is produced.
Add enough sodium hydroxide solution to neutralise.	The precipitate dissolves and clear solution is produced.

PHENOTHIAZINES

Phenothiazines are tricyclic heterocyclic compounds with nitrogen and sulphur in the central ring. So they will answer tests for elements, that is, nitrogen and sulphur and any special tests. Those which are hydrochlorides will also answer the test for chlorine in the tests for elements.

PROMETHAZINE HYDROCHLORIDE

EXPERIMENT	OBSERVATION
1. Tests for Elements (Refer sulphanilamide) A. Test for nitrogen B. Test for sulphur	Answered.
C. Test for halogens To 1 ml. of the sodium fusion extract, add 1 ml of dilute nitric acid and 1 ml of silver nitrate solution.	A curdy white precipitate is produced.
2. Dissolve 0.1 g. of the substance and add 1 ml of nitric acid drop by drop.	Initially a precipitate is produced. It dissolves quickly to give a red solution. The solution then slowly becomes orange and finally yellow.
Heat the solution to boiling.	It becomes orange once again and an orange-red precipitate is produced.

ANTIBIOTICS

PENICILLINS

The penicillins, in addition to answering the tests for elements, also answer certain colour tests in which distinctive colours are obtained.

1. PHENOXYMETHYLPENICILLIN POTASSIUM

EXPERIMENT	OBSERVATION
1. Tests for Elements (Refer sulphanilamide). a. Test for nitrogen b. Test for sulphur	Answered.
2. Test for Potassium Dissolve about 50 mg of the substance in water and add 1 ml. of dilute acetic acid and 1 ml. of a freshly prepared 10% w/v solution of sodium cobaltinitrite.	A yellow or orange precipitate is formed immediately.
3. Special test Take 2 mg of the substance and add 2 mg of chromotropic acid sodium salt and 2 ml of concentrated sulphuric acid. Immerse in an oil bath at 150°C. Shake and examine every 30 seconds.	The solution is colourless at first but becomes pale pink and then purple. It then becomes bluish violet and finally dark blue.
4. Special Test Place a little of the substance in a test tube and moisten it with enough water. Add 2 ml of a mixture of formaldehyde solution and concentrated sulphuric acid.	The solution becomes reddish brown in colour.

EXPERIMENT	OBSERVATION
Immerse the test tube in a water bath at 100°C for one minute.	The solution becomes dark reddish brown.

2. AMPICiLLIN SODIUM

EXPERIMENT	OBSERVATION
1. Test for Elements a. Test for nitrogen ⎫ b. Test for sulphur ⎭	Answered.
2. Test for Sodium To the solution of the substance add a little dilute acetic acid to make it acidic. Then add a large excess of magnessium uranyl acetate solution.	A yellow, crystalline precipitate is produced.
3. Special Test Carry out the test no.3 given under phenoxymethylpenicillin potassium.	The solution is colourless at first, then becomes purple and deep purple. It then becomes violet. Finally the substance is charred.
4. Special Test Carry out the test no.4 given under phenoxymethylpenicillin potassium.	The solution is almost colourless on adding the formaldehyde-sulphuric acid mixture but becomes dark yellow when it is heated at 100°C for one minute.

3. CLOXACILLIN SODIUM

EXPERIMENT	OBSERVATION
1. Tests for Elements (Refer sulphanilamide) a) Test for nitrogen ⎫ b) Test for sulphur ⎬ c) Test for chlorine ⎭ (Refer promethazine hydro-chloride).	Answered
2. Test for Sodium Carry out the test no.2 given under ampicillin sodium.	Answered
3. Special Test Carry out the test no.3 given under phenoxymethylpenicillin potassium	The solution is colourless at first and becomes pale yellow, greenish yellow, green, greenish purple and finally purple.
4. Special Test Carry out the test no.4 given under phenoxymethylpenicillin potassium.	The solution becomes slightly greenish yellow on adding the formal-dehyde-sulphuric acid mixture but becomes yellow on heating at 100°C for one minute.

The other antibiotics such as the streptomycins and the tetracyclines also give colour reactions by which they can be easily identified.

1. STREPTOMYCIN SULPHATE

EXPERIMENT	OBSERVATION
1. Tests for Elements (Refer sulphanilamide) a) Test for nitrogen b) Test for sulphur	Answered
2. Test for Sulphate To a little of the substance dissolved in water, add 1 ml of dilute hydrochloric acid and barium chloride solution.	A white precipitate is produced.
3. Special Tests a) Dissolve about 10 mg of the substance in 5 ml of water and add 1 ml. of dilute sodium hydroxide solution. Heat in a water bath and add a slight excess of dilute hydrochloric acid and two drops of a 10% solution of ferric chloride.	A violet colour is produced. (By alkaline hydrolysis, maltol is produced from streptomycin and it gives the violet colour with the ferric chloride solution).
b) Dissolve about 10 mg of the substance in 5 ml of water and add 1 ml of dilute 1-naphthol solution and 2 ml of dilute sodium hypochlorite solution.	A red colour is produced.

2. OXYTETRACYCLINE HYDROCHLORIDE

EXPERIMENT	OBSERVATION
1. Test for Elements (Refer sulphanilamide) **a) Test for Nitrogen** **b) Test for Chlorine** (Refer promethazine hydrochloride).	Answered.
2. Special Tests a) To a little of the substance, add 2 ml of concentrated sulphuric acid.	A red colour is produced.
Add the solution to a little water.	The colour now becomes yellow.
b) Dissolve a small quantity of the substance in about 5 ml of dilute sodium carbonate solution. Add 2 ml of diazotised sulphanilic acid solution.	An orange-red to brownish-red colour is produced.
3. Test for Chloride To a small quantity of the substance dissolved in water, add 1 ml. of dilute nitric acid and 1 ml of silver nitrate solution.	A curdy white precipitate is produced.